DISCOVERING PRECISION HEALTH: PREDICT, PREVENT, AND CURE TO ADVANCE HEALTH AND WELL-BEING

DISCOVERING PRECISION HEALTH
Predict, Prevent, and Cure to Advance Health and Well-Being

LLOYD MINOR, MD
Dean, Stanford University School of Medicine

MATTHEW REES

WILEY Blackwell

Registered Office(s)
John Wiley & Sons, Inc., 111 River Street, Hoboken, NJ 07030, USA
John Wiley & Sons Ltd, The Atrium, Southern Gate, Chichester, West Sussex, PO19 8SQ, UK

Editorial Office
9600 Garsington Road, Oxford, OX4 2DQ, UK

For details of our global editorial offices, customer services, and more information about Wiley products visit us at www.wiley.com.

Wiley also publishes its books in a variety of electronic formats and by print-on-demand. Some content that appears in standard print versions of this book may not be available in other formats.

Library of Congress Cataloging-in-Publication Data
Names: Minor, Lloyd, author. | Rees, Matthew, 1968– author.
Title: Discovering precision health : predict, prevent, and cure to advance
   health and well-being / Lloyd Minor, Matthew Rees.
Description: Hoboken, NJ : Wiley-Blackwell, 2020. | Includes
   bibliographical references and index.
Identifiers: LCCN 2019049521 (print) | LCCN 2019049522 (ebook) | ISBN
   9781119672692 (hardback) | ISBN 9781119672685 (adobe pdf) | ISBN
   9781119672746 (epub)
Subjects: MESH: Delivery of Health Care | Healthcare Disparities | Health
   Services Accessibility | Socioeconomic Factors | Precision Medicine |
   United States
Classification: LCC RA418 (print) | LCC RA418 (ebook) | NLM W 84 AA1 |
   DDC 362.1–dc23
LC record available at https://lccn.loc.gov/2019049521
LC ebook record available at https://lccn.loc.gov/2019049522

Cover Design: David Armario Design
Cover Image: © kentoh/Shutterstock

Set in 10/12pt TimesLTStd-Roman by SPi Global, Pondicherry, India

Printed in the United States of America

10 9 8 7 6 5 4 3 2 1

This book is dedicated to my colleagues at Stanford whose creativity, insight, and dedication are advancing the biomedical revolution in Precision Health, and to the people we serve through tailored care and cutting-edge research.

TABLE OF CONTENTS

ABOUT THE AUTHORS

Lloyd Minor, MD, is a scientist, surgeon, and academic leader. He is the Carl and Elizabeth Naumann Dean of the Stanford University School of Medicine, a position he has held since December 2012. He is also a professor of otolaryngology–head and neck surgery and a professor of bioengineering and of neurobiology, by courtesy, at Stanford University.

As dean, Dr. Minor plays an integral role in setting strategy for the clinical, research, and teaching missions of Stanford Medicine, an academic medical center that includes the Stanford University School of Medicine, Stanford Health Care, and Stanford Children's Health and Lucile Packard Children's Hospital Stanford. Dr. Minor led the first integrated strategic planning process for Stanford Medicine. With his leadership, Stanford Medicine has established a strategic vision to lead the biomedical revolution in Precision Health (predict, prevent, and cure—*precisely*), a fundamental shift to more proactive and personalized health care that empowers people to lead healthy lives.

Before coming to Stanford, Dr. Minor was provost and senior vice president for academic affairs of Johns Hopkins University. Prior to his appointment as provost in 2009, Dr. Minor served as the Andelot Professor and director (chair) of the Department of Otolaryngology–Head and Neck Surgery in the Johns Hopkins University School of Medicine and otolaryngologist-in-chief of the Johns Hopkins Hospital.

With more than 140 published articles and chapters, Dr. Minor is an expert in balance and inner ear disorders. In the medical community, he is perhaps best known for his discovery of superior canal dehiscence syndrome, a debilitating disorder characterized by sound- or pressure-induced dizziness. He subsequently developed a surgical procedure that corrects the problem and alleviates symptoms.

In 2012, Dr. Minor was elected to the National Academy of Medicine.

Matthew Rees is the founder of Geonomica, an editorial consulting firm that works with clients on speeches, books, articles, white papers, and other written materials. He is the co-author, with former IBM CEO Samuel J. Palmisano, of *Re-Think: A Path to the Future*, a book about the globally integrated enterprise and the emergence of the global economy.

Mr. Rees is also a senior fellow at Dartmouth's Tuck School of Business. He was the founder of *FT Newsmine*, a weekly email brief he produced in partnership with the *Financial Times* from 2009 to 2017.

Mr. Rees's government experience includes serving as a speechwriter for President George W. Bush; the national security adviser, Condoleezza Rice; and the U.S. trade representative, Robert Zoellick. He also served as a speechwriter and senior adviser for the chairman of the Securities and Exchange Commission, William Donaldson.

During a 10-year career in journalism, Mr. Rees wrote for many of America's most respected publications. He was employed in Washington for the *Weekly Standard*, the *Economist*, and the *New Republic*, and in New York and Brussels for the *Wall Street Journal*. Mr. Rees's writing has also appeared in the *New York Times*, the *Washington Post*, the *International Economy*, *Reader's Digest*, and *Finance & Development* (a publication of the International Monetary Fund). He is a frequent contributor of book reviews to the *Wall Street Journal*. A native of Lafayette, California, Mr. Rees is a graduate of Wesleyan University.

ACKNOWLEDGMENTS

The idea for a book describing Stanford Medicine's vision for Precision Health was suggested to me in 2016 during discussions with faculty and staff who were working on plans for the initiatives that have become a part of this vision. Bob Harrington, chair of the Department of Medicine, and Priya Singh, chief strategy officer and senior associate dean for Stanford Medicine, were leaders of this planning process. It has been heartening to see the engagement of our communities in the planning, communication, and execution of the strategy for Precision Health. Those who encouraged me to write the book were correct that the process of writing would help us to shape ideas and plans for the future. The book is also a reflection of a dictum, first emphasized to me by Jay Goldberg (my scientific mentor at the University of Chicago), that concepts only become meaningful and incisive when they are written, revised, and refined.

I have the honor of working every day with wonderful colleagues at Stanford. Their work is a constant source of inspiration for me and for so many others. The patients who entrust their care to us provide a grounding and focus to our scientific and educational pursuits. Our partnership with them is a privilege never to be taken for granted.

Although this book turned into a larger and lengthier project than initially envisioned, I want to express my regret that I could not describe all of the people, projects, and activities that are having a transformative impact. The same can be said for my description of companies focused on digital health, where there are also many more than I can cover here.

I want to thank Harry Clark for introducing me to Matt Rees. Matt's keen insights and his assistance with the interviews and writing enabled this book to be completed. Jessica Best, director of strategic initiatives and communications, is an exceptionally talented writer and gave us valuable feedback on the manuscript. Sandy Yujuico, chief of staff in the Dean's Office, arranged and coordinated the interviews and helped us keep the project on track. Esmond Harmsworth, our literary agent, provided valuable assistance during every step of the process.

Finally, and most importantly, I want to express my appreciation to my family. Lisa Keamy, my wife, has been my partner, companion, and adviser for these past 32 years. Her love and support energize and motivate me every day. Our children, Emily and Sam, amaze and inspire us as we watch their journey through life. Phoebe and Watson, our canine companions, make even the most challenging days seem a lot better.

Lloyd Minor
Stanford, California 2019

Working on this book has been the most intellectually stimulating project of my professional life. It has been a privilege to collaborate with Lloyd Minor and help explain his inspiring vision for a new approach to health and well-being. I am particularly grateful to Lloyd for enabling me to interview so many distinguished members of the faculty at Stanford's School of Medicine, as well as a remarkable collection of entrepreneurs and investors. Harry Clark is a valued friend who introduced me to the School of Medicine's leadership—making this one more in a long line of fascinating projects he has referred to me. I want to thank my wife, Nina, and my daughter, Sophia, for their everyday love and support, and for accommodating my sometimes-chaotic schedule. My parents, Don Rees and Marilyn Rees, both Stanford graduates, laid the foundation that has enabled me to have a rewarding career and a fulfilling life.

Matthew Rees
McLean, Virginia 2019

THE POWER OF PRECISION HEALTH

Imagine yourself in the not-too-distant future. Routine genomic screening tests, available at the time of birth, have shown that you have genetic variants that place you at high risk for pancreatic cancer in your adult years. Because of this propensity, you have elected to participate in a regular program of non-invasive screening tests that are designed to provide early detection of any tumor development in your pancreas. Every six months you take a pill that will cause a pancreatic tumor (if one exists) to shed a novel synthetic biomarker that can be detected in the urine.

Several days after you take one of the early cancer detection pills, your home's "smart toilet" automatically detects the synthetic biomarker in your urine. A device that is part of the smart toilet sends an alert to you on your smart phone, and to your primary care physician, who has your consent to receive information about these screening tests. To ensure the signal from the smart toilet is not a false positive, the signal is monitored in your urine over several days.

You follow the physician's recommendation to undergo imaging studies with molecular tracers that will identify the location of the tumor and ensure the toilet device was correct. A pancreatic tumor is detected that measures 1 cubic millimeter and there is no evidence that it has spread to other sites. You are given targeted therapies, which activate your immune system and destroy the tumor while it is still at an early stage of development. You continue the plan of close surveillance and monitoring with an early cancer detection pill every six months.

As I will describe in the pages that follow, all the components of this scenario are within our grasp today. We are in the midst of a revolution in science and technology related to the mechanisms of disease and, of equal importance, to the determinants of health and well-being. The impact of these advances and their broad dissemination are going to have a profound effect on our ability not just to treat diseases but to prevent them from developing in the first place. And in those instances when diseases cannot be prevented, they will be diagnosed much earlier and therefore treated much more effectively.

Discovering Precision Health: Predict, Prevent, and Cure to Advance Health and Well-Being,
First Edition. Lloyd Minor and Matthew Rees.
© 2020 John Wiley & Sons Ltd. Published 2020 by John Wiley & Sons Ltd.

The example above illustrates just how transformative the results of this revolution are going to be. With pancreatic cancer today, there are no good tools for early detection, which means it is typically diagnosed much later in the course of tumor progression. In 80–95 percent of diagnoses, the cancerous tumor is locally advanced or metastatic [1]. As a result, 74 percent of all people with pancreatic cancer die within one year of diagnosis [2]. In 2017, this cancer resulted in the deaths of more than 43,000 people in the United States [3].

This vignette is emblematic of what the future of medicine should look like—and what I think it *will* look like—soon. Because for the first time in history, the world is starting to see the possibility of a new kind of medicine and health care. Instead of a race to cure disease after the fact, we can win the race before it even begins by preventing disease before it strikes—and curing it decisively if it does.

This approach is what we in Stanford Medicine have labeled "Precision Health" because it helps individuals thrive based on all factors specific to them, from their genetics to their lifestyle choices to their environment. It is based on the powerful idea that health care should promote health and wellness as much as it defeats disease.

Simply stated, the goals of Precision Health are to predict, prevent, and cure, *precisely*. And in that order, because more accurate prediction of propensity for disease will lead to more specific approaches for prevention. Even in cases where disease cannot be prevented altogether, diagnosing diseases much earlier in their course will mean that our ability to achieve cures will be greater than now. All too often today we identify diseases much too late to have the type of treatment outcome all of us would like to achieve.

THE PRECISION HEALTH PAST—AND PRESENT

The principles underpinning Precision Health reach back many years. The authors of a paper presented at a meeting of the American Public Health Association in 1873 wrote that "the custom of society must be changed so that the physician is employed to prevent rather than to cure diseases" [4]. Twenty years later, William Osler—often thought of as the originator of modern medicine—helped to found the medical school at Johns Hopkins University. And he was clear about the need for patient-centered medicine. "The good physician," said Osler, "treats the disease; the great physician treats the patient who has the disease." As a staunch advocate of prevention, Osler was well ahead of his time. He believed in both the power of scientific evidence and the power of bedside medicine. Precision Health is Osler's heir—the modern incarnation of his dual focus on rigorous science and the enduring physician-patient bond.

A focus on prevention was also at the heart of groundbreaking research that began in 1948. That year marked the launch of the Framingham Heart Study, which was an in-depth exploration of cardiovascular disease. At the time, the disease affected one of every three men in the United States, and it was twice as common as cancer [5]. Yet its cause was unknown. To better understand cardiovascular disease, an arm of the National Institutes of Health recruited more than 5,200 volunteers, between the ages of 30 and 59, in the Massachusetts town of Framingham to participate in a study. Each of the volunteers would be examined every two years, for a period of 20 years.

It became the most comprehensive such study ever undertaken and it continues today, with its third generation of participants. The discoveries it has brought forth have greatly expanded our understanding of the causes of cardiovascular disease and how to prevent it, through diet, exercise, and avoiding tobacco. Data from the study is the foundation of several risk prediction calculators for heart conditions, along with diabetes, fatty liver disease, and hypertension [6].

The knowledge unlocked by the Framingham Heart Study is a reminder of why researchers need to continue exploring the causes of different diseases—and to focus on preventing those diseases. Looking into the future, Project Baseline, a contemporary sequel to the Framingham study, holds the promise of dramatically increasing our understanding of health and disease by analyzing an enormously greater number of parameters. Like the Framingham study, Project Baseline, which I describe in more detail in the conclusion, is a longitudinal cohort study. One of its goals is tracking these parameters, and the health of the study volunteers, for a period of years.

KEY PRINCIPLES OF PRECISION HEALTH

There are many different dimensions of Precision Health, which I will elaborate on in this chapter and throughout the book. But some of the key features include the following:

Predictive and Preventive

Precision Health draws on the enablers of precision medicine—genomics, big data science, and regenerative medicine—but applies them in a predictive and proactive way. While precision medicine implies that individuals who get sick are treated precisely, Precision Health is focused on a holistic approach to keeping people healthy through targeted interventions and stopping disease before it starts. It seeks to understand the features of disease that explain why some people get sick when others do not, and which treatments, tests, and lifestyle changes will help prevent disease in each individual. When it isn't possible to altogether prevent a disease, Precision Health seeks to improve diagnostics such that diseases are detected much earlier and treated more effectively.

Personalized and Precise

With Precision Health, all forms of health and medical care are tailored to individual variations. That means doctors are able to provide every therapy based on what's known about a patient: their genetics, their metabolomics, all their

-omics, their imaging, everything about them. As my colleague Thomas Robinson says, Precision Health is about identifying the right interventions, for the right person, at the right place, at the right time, in the right sequence. And information technology is deployed so that health professionals can confidently tell their patients, "You are going to benefit most from doing the following."

Patient-Centered

Health care today is often a complex and confusing journey, characterized by fragmentation and care on a disease-by-disease basis. Precision Health makes providers own the complexity of care for their patients, providing care that is seamless, coordinated around their needs, and based on the best science.

Participatory

Precision Health is focused on empowering individuals to monitor their own health. It breaks with the long-standing practice of people interacting with the medical system sporadically (the annual "check-up")—or when driven by illness or disease. Patients and their families get involved in the care delivery experience through practices such as continuous monitoring (as in the example provided in the scenario above). A rough parallel comes from the way in which financial institutions use algorithms to monitor their customers' spending. If there's suspicious activity, customers may be contacted and asked to confirm certain transactions. We are getting to a point where technologies can do the same monitoring of our bodies, and immediately alert us—or our health care team—if something is amiss.

Preeminent

The United States performs poorly on some broad measures of health compared to other developed nations. Precision Health delivers value by focusing on ways to both improve outcomes and cut costs. These two goals can be achieved in tandem. Precision Health seeks to lower costs through early detection, prevention, accurate risk assessment, and efficiencies in care delivery.

Precision Health applies to people of all ages, and it's an attempt to understand all the different trajectories of life. But the health care of children, coupled with maternal and fetal health, are given special emphasis, since they are at the beginning of life's trajectory. Mothers have an extraordinary influence on the future life of their children—and that influence begins even before they become pregnant. New technologies and new approaches are being used to look at pregnancy in entirely new ways. Everything we learn becomes part of large data sets to create a comprehensive picture of pregnancy. We can then extract information for the purpose of predicting—and preventing—certain outcomes.

"High Touch" and "High Tech"

In the "high touch" environment we want to develop, physicians will return to some of the wisdom of figures like William Osler. Doctors need to recognize the intimate bonds with their patients when performing hands-on examinations and listen to their concerns with empathy. This is part of a time-honored ritual and enables health professionals to gain critical information that differs from what they learn through lab tests and radiological scans. This kind of rich, nuanced data—what is important to patients, what they fear, how their symptoms manifest and how they feel—must also factor into a truly holistic approach to health care. As my Stanford colleague Abraham Verghese has written, "True clinical judgment is more than addressing the avalanche of blood work, imaging and lab tests; it is about using human skills to understand where the patient is in the trajectory of a life and the disease, what the nature of the patient's family and social circumstances is and how much they want done" [7].

Precision Health can—and should—strengthen the doctor-patient relationship, and it should allow each of us to be more participatory in decisions as well as activities that have an impact on our health and wellbeing. As Stanford's Sanjiv "Sam" Gambhir points out, Precision Health

> creates an opportunity for the entire health care team, including physicians, to utilize more detailed and comprehensive health data sets to be better informed about their patients' individualized health. In turn, it allows physicians to more accurately address their patient's health risk profile and tailor monitoring methods and early intervention to that individual. This type of approach will empower doctors to be more focused and directed in how they treat patients [8].

For patients, says Gambhir,

> increased health monitoring allows them to more proactively engage in their own health—in some cases in real time—and see how it relates to their lifestyle and other health factors. Rather than simply follow a standard appointment schedule, patients would only visit their physician when needed, but they could still have contact with their health care team through a secure health portal [9].

The emphasis on "high touch" is complemented by a focus on "high tech." Technology has spawned new fields like genomics, nanoscience, regenerative medicine, and biomedical data science. It is enabling health care professionals to piece together a high-resolution picture of human health at the population level. Euan Ashley, a professor of cardiology at Stanford, explains, "The fundamental concept of precision health is the idea of defining disease better in order to target it more precisely. And how do we define disease better? We do it with new technology. If you look at the history of medicine, we've always defined disease according to the state-of-the-art tools of the time." He points out that in decades past, a cardiologist sought to diagnose heart disease by listening to the sounds coming through the stethoscope. "But when someone invented the electrocardiogram, we started to define heart disease according to the electrical signals from the heart" [10].

The ultimate objective of Precision Health is not just to glimpse the finer details of health and disease—it's to consistently track and actively apply the findings to detect disease earlier, if not prevent it altogether [11].

THE TIME IS RIGHT FOR PRECISION HEALTH

The three fundamental components of Precision Health (predict, prevent, and cure) share many of the same enablers. Specifically, they are all being driven by ongoing advances in science and technology. The ability to achieve precision is based on progress in our understanding of biological processes and the application of this knowledge to specific challenges and opportunities in human health.

These expansions of understanding are driving a scientific revolution. If the 19th century was all about chemistry and the 20th century about physics, the 21st century will be about biology. There is enormous excitement about the present and future being about biology, given its evolution into a quantitative discipline after being transformed by chemistry and physics.

With biomedical knowledge having grown exponentially over the past two decades, we have new insights into how life works. Astonishing advances are offering up possibilities that were unimaginable just a few years ago. New tools that will allow us not only to heal disease, but to predict and prevent it, are finally within our reach. New technologies are accelerating medical discoveries and help to tailor care to each individual's unique situation. We live in a time of remarkable progress in medicine.

The biomedical sciences are undergoing unprecedented changes as the pace of discovery accelerates. We can now build on fundamental research taking place in genomics, proteomics, metabolomics, data science, regenerative medicine, artificial intelligence, nanoscience, biotechnology, and engineering to deliver Precision Health that is predictive and preventive.

Fundamental, discovery-based research will be of central importance to all future advances in predicting, preventing, and curing disease. There has never been a more exciting time for investigator-initiated research aimed at understanding the way living systems work at the cellular and molecular level—because the more we learn, the more we also recognize how much we don't know. In the chapters that follow, I will describe some of these transformative discoveries and share the stories of remarkable scientists who have done and are doing this work.

In addition to the prodigious pace at which discovery-based research is advancing, our ability to translate these discoveries into direct benefits for human health is accelerating at an ever-increasing pace. The time from "bench to bedside"—shorthand for the time it takes between when therapies are being researched and when they are being used—is being accelerated in many areas. Further, direct observations and studies of health and disease are now being taken back to the laboratory to drive discovery-based research in ways that were unimaginable just a decade ago. In the chapters that follow, I will provide an overview of the processes of translational medicine by sharing examples of areas of transformative impact that we are already seeing.

Advances in digital technology are also fueling the success and impact of Precision Health. It is a curious fact that up until very recently, consumer technology has had relatively little impact on the way health care is delivered or the way each of us obtains information about our health. This is in sharp contrast to every other aspect of the economy where technology has radically transformed our lives. From the way we order goods and services to the way we conduct financial transactions, many day-to-day activities today are radically different than they were just a decade ago. Yet all too frequently today we still transmit medical records by fax machines and compact discs. Information about our health remains trapped within electronic medical records and health care delivery systems in ways that make it challenging to access and even more difficult to analyze. This landscape needs to change. In the chapters that follow, I will explore some of the exciting enablers in digital health at the level of both consumer-facing devices and technologies and artificial intelligence applied to large biomedical and health-related data sets.

But there is more to the Precision Health revolution than science and technology. Social, environmental, and behavioral determinants of health play a larger role in the well-being of most of us than do traditional medical care and our genomic profile. It's a startling and disappointing fact that in the United States the zip code in which a person lives is more predictive of his or her life expectancy than that person's genetics [12]. In the chapters that follow, I will highlight how some of those social, environmental, and behavioral determinants impact health as well as important work being done outside medicine that's promoting health and well-being.

One catalyst for launching Precision Health was the recognition that many of the outcomes from U.S. health care (broadly defined) have been disappointing. The United States spends more of its GDP on health care than any other country in the world. Yet the U.S. ranks below many of the most industrialized nations by standard outcome measures such as longevity [13] and infant mortality [14].

There are a variety of reasons for these outcomes, but the health care system certainly shoulders some of the blame. As I explain in the next chapter, the system is largely reactive, one-size-fits-all, fragmented, detached and disconnected from patients, and riddled with misguided incentives and opaque pricing. Precision Health can help remedy these shortcomings and ultimately deliver improved health outcomes.

ABOUT ME

Born in Little Rock, Arkansas, I grew up in a home that placed great emphasis on education. I attended all-white schools through the eighth grade, but as a part of a court-ordered desegregation plan, I was bused to a junior high school across town for ninth grade. This was a defining moment in my life. I immediately learned that what was billed as "separate but equal" was separate but certainly not equal. In the scarcely stocked library, books on the lower shelves had been damaged by rats. Banisters were missing from stairwells. Plaster was peeling from the walls. These were the bitter fruits of racial prejudice. It was eye-opening to see this injustice, and it had a profound effect on me. It kindled in me an interest in diversity and inclusion that continues to this day.

I attended the famously desegregated Little Rock Central High School where I was inspired by the elegance and rigor of math, physics, and chemistry. But I was also drawn to the challenges of bringing more quantitative approaches to biology. It was then that I first thought about the importance of using these disciplines to solve real-world problems and bring profound benefits to the lives of people. Becoming a physician-scientist was at the intersection of these interests.

While at Brown University for college and medical school, I took a bioengineering course as an undergraduate that sparked my interest in the physiology of the inner ear balance system (known as the vestibular system). The course focused on the use of mathematical and engineering models to study and understand physiological systems. The professor used the vestibular system, and the eye movements that depend upon input from it, as an example of how you could use relatively straightforward mathematical models to describe the way the system worked. Even more importantly, you could also state hypotheses, design experiments, and interpret data in the conceptual framework established by these models. This approach appealed to my fascination with how complex systems work, and I devoted my early career to understanding the vestibular system and treating disorders that result from its dysfunction.

My goals and my training as a scientist and clinician emphasized an understanding of the functional mechanisms of the system I was studying and the ways those mechanisms are altered in disease. As was the case for most of my generation of physician-scientists, I was firmly focused, in the parlance of this book, on the "cures" aspect of medicine. It was through my experiences as a scientist pursuing basic research directed towards understanding the intricate physiology of the vestibular system, and a clinician focused on the diagnosis and treatment of vestibular disorders, that I experienced first-hand the impact of discovery-focused research on health and medicine.

In the spring of 1995, two years after I had joined the faculty of the Department of Otolaryngology—Head and Neck Surgery at Johns Hopkins, a man came to my office and explained that he was suffering from a bizarre set of symptoms. For example, when he sang in the shower, he would see the shampoo bottle, the loofah, and the shower head moving in a circular motion.

Similarly, if he hummed a tone or heard certain loud noises in his right ear while looking in the mirror, he saw that his eyes were moving in conjunction with the sounds. When I tested him, I could clearly see that his eyes moved in a consistent pattern—upward and counterclockwise—and the pattern was tightly linked to the sound.

I suspected the problem stemmed from an opening in the bone that should cover the superior semicircular canal, which is one of the three tiny canals hidden deep within the inner ear. (These canals serve as part of the vestibular system, a set of inner-ear structures that provide input to the brain on motion, equilibrium, and spatial orientation.) I made this hypothesis because there is a well-recognized relationship between the orientation of individual semicircular canals and the eye movements evoked by stimulation of these canals (activation of a canal results in eye movements in the plane of the canal). An opening in the bone covering the superior canal would, I reasoned, make it responsive to sound and pressure stimuli because of the mechanical flow of fluids in the inner ear. Several years of studies on this and other patients with similar symptoms and signs accompanied by related basic research confirmed that this was, indeed, the mechanism.

I named this condition *superior canal dehiscence (SCD) syndrome*, and my colleagues and I at Johns Hopkins developed an operation to correct it. We published the first paper describing the disorder in 1998 and also showed that there were specific hearing abnormalities associated with it [15]. It's been extremely satisfying to know that hundreds of people have now had operations to treat SCD and that their everyday lives have been improved.

My point in mentioning this work here is that it was an understanding of the physiology of the vestibular system, informed by discovery-based research, that enabled this syndrome to be identified and subsequently treated. SCD as a disorder did not originate with the patients I initially saw in 1995. There had been reports in the medical literature over several previous decades describing people with symptoms that were almost certainly due to this disorder. But the association with a specific abnormality of the vestibular system had never been made because the scientific underpinnings had never been studied. There are many examples in this book of scientific advances that have led to improvements in human health that were not necessarily anticipated or planned.

A desire to impact research, education, and health systems on a broader level eventually led me to leadership positions in medicine and research universities, culminating in a position as dean of medicine at Stanford. I also came to realize that having a truly transformative impact on health and health care delivery requires much more emphasis on prediction and prevention than has been the case in the past.

Along the way, in my educational, training, and work experiences I have learned the values of listening carefully, acquiring and imparting rigorous scientific and technical training, and assessing the potential for systems errors that can lead to adverse consequences. In my own work and in the activities of others I have seen the value of persistent and diligent struggle in the face of uncertainty, complexity, and the risk of failure. I have come to appreciate the power inherent in the interface between technology and health. I also learned, firsthand, the importance of working within an environment rich in multiple complementary disciplines where ideas can cross-pollinate and expertise can be leveraged in new and creative ways.

I happily find myself in one of the few places where this vision of Precision Health can become a reality. At Stanford, we can draw on our world-class medicine, basic biological and physical sciences, engineering, and computer science, along with our renowned statisticians, educators, social scientists, ethicists, designers, economists, and business and legal scholars—not to mention our collaborative relationships with leading Silicon Valley innovators.

THE ORIGINS OF PRECISION HEALTH AT STANFORD

Having spent my professional life in and around research universities and academic medical centers, I—like many other health care professionals with experiences similar to mine—was full of opinions about how to improve care and how to make academic medical centers more effective. All of my education and work history helped to shape my approach to leading Stanford Medicine. But when it came to developing the Precision Health vision, there were three things in particular that influenced me: a conference, a speech, and a book.

The conference was hosted by the University of California, San Francisco (UCSF) in May 2013, just six months after I had become dean at Stanford. Susan Desmond-Hellman, then the chancellor at UCSF, brought together leaders from biomedical research, medical practice, government, and industry—the meeting featured the director of the NIH, the governor of California, and the CEO of Facebook, among others. We were all there to discuss how to move from one-size-fits-all treatments for diseases to medical care that is tailored to the distinctive features of each individual. This was billed as "precision medicine," and it was timely. There was already evidence of the impact of applying genomics and data science to the treatment of severe acute diseases such as breast cancer. No longer was the same treatment recommended to all women based simply upon the size of the tumor and presence or absence of distant metastatic disease. The development of specific antagonists, whose efficacy was determined based upon specific receptors present or absent in tumors, was having a major effect on improved survival (and those effects are even greater today).

The discussions were stimulating and thought provoking. And while the "precision" part of the event intrigued me, I was struck by the focus on "medicine." Everything on the agenda revolved around disease—almost as if it was inevitable. Curing disease is critical, of course, but *preventing* disease is even better.

Another influence on my thinking was a speech delivered by Elias Zerhouni, a former director of the NIH and later president of R&D for Sanofi. He spoke eloquently at a Stanford Medicine retreat in January 2014 about the need for a shift in the practice of medicine. While a focus on cures remained critically important, he recommended placing heightened emphasis on predicting and preventing disease. He also called for developing a better understanding of disease mechanisms. His talk built on a theme he had introduced during his time at NIH, which was for medicine to be predictive, personalized, preemptive, participatory.

The book that influenced my thinking was *The Decision Tree*, by Thomas Goetz, who at the time was executive editor of *Wired* magazine [16]. The "decision tree" of his title was a system that would help guide people toward the best decisions about their health—drawing on new science and new technologies, in particular. I found it to be an excellent overview of the different ways in which health and health care could be reoriented to focus more on prevention.

With all of that as a backdrop, in November 2014 I had breakfast at Buck's—a popular restaurant a few miles from Stanford—with two professors at the School of Medicine, Peter Kim and Steve Quake. I had asked them to meet with me because I wanted to brainstorm about some of the overarching themes for the work of the medical school, and I knew I could count on them for insightful and creative ideas.

My colleagues and I had recruited Peter to join the faculty—his previous positions included leading global R&D for Merck and serving as a professor at MIT's Whitehead Institute for Biomedical Research. Steve had developed a way of measuring and detecting cell-free DNA, which was one of the greatest diagnostic advances of the first decade of the 21st century. (I discuss it in more detail in chapter 5.)

We discussed several principles and topics—such as behavior, genomics, economics, measurement, prevention, and prediction. But the first two words I wrote in my notebook that morning were "precision" and "health." With Steve's background in diagnostics, we were able to talk about shifting the focus of health care so there would be more emphasis on the "health" part. The three of us agreed that Stanford was uniquely positioned to put forward a new vision, built around using prediction and prevention to advance health.

Our breakfast discussion led me to sketch out several ideas, which I presented in my closing remarks at a Stanford Medicine retreat in January 2015, at Fort Baker near San Francisco. I didn't go into great detail—I just wanted people to hear some of my preliminary thoughts about Precision Health and I wanted their feedback. I was pleased that my thoughts seemed to strike a chord with many of those in attendance. In particular, the theme and the message resonated strongly with the then leaders of the two hospitals that are a part of Stanford Medicine: Amir Rubin, president and CEO of Stanford Health Care (SHC), and Christopher Dawes, president and CEO of Lucile Packard Children's Hospital Stanford (LPCH). Since coming to Stanford, I had been searching for a theme that would bring the three entities of Stanford Medicine (School of Medicine, SHC, and LPCH) closer together: a theme that could help unite the different components of Stanford Medicine and advance its mission. We all agreed that Precision Health was exactly that theme.

Just a few weeks after our retreat, we were pleasantly surprised when President Obama held an event at the White House to announce a federal government initiative devoted to "precision medicine." The objective, he said, would be "delivering the right treatments, at the right time, every time, to the right person" [17]. The initiative had five parts:

- Using the federal government's National Cancer Institute to help expand and improve research into cancer treatments
- Working with the NIH to create a research group of one million people, known as "All of Us," and using the data from that cohort to discover the causes—and eventually the cures—of deadly diseases
- Modernizing regulation, with a focus on developing a new approach to evaluating next-generation genetic tests
- Expanding public-private partnerships to enable development of the infrastructure needed for the cancer treatment research and the "All of Us" initiative
- Protecting patient privacy

To help put precision medicine in perspective, the director of the NIH, Francis Collins, and the director of the National Cancer Institute, Harold Varmus, published an article on the website of the *New England Journal of Medicine*. They pointed out that it was now possible to bring more precision to medicine thanks to developments like biological databases (such as the human genome sequence), new forms of characterizing patients (such as proteomics and metabolomics), and new computational tools to analyze large data sets [18].

The Obama administration's focus on "medicine" (treatment of diseases after they occur) contrasted with our focus on "health" (with more emphasis on prediction and prevention of diseases), but we interpreted the shared focus on "precision" as a signal that we were on the right track. We soon organized a faculty working group, led by the Department of Medicine chairman Bob Harrington, and including faculty and staff from the School of Medicine as well as from SHC and LPCH. That group spent more than a year developing the ideas that would define Precision Health. Their expert work led to the development of a comprehensive plan for Precision Health. The working group released its findings in October 2016, and since then we have been working to instill the Precision Health plan throughout the School of Medicine, SHC, and LPCH.

It's been gratifying to see broad adoption of the theme and components of Precision Health throughout our enterprise. David Entwistle, who began as president and CEO of SHC in July 2016, and Paul King, who began as president and CEO of Lucile Packard Children's Hospital and Stanford Children's Health in February 2019, have firmly embraced the vision. After David's arrival, we were able, for the first time, to develop a truly integrated strategic plan for Stanford Medicine, with Precision Health being the unifying principle. Marc Tessier-Lavigne, who became Stanford's 11th president on September 1, 2016, and who has previously worked as a neuroscientist, biotechnology executive, and president of a biomedical research university, has endorsed Population and Precision Health as an important strategic objective for Stanford University's research community.

It has also been reaffirming to see that several other institutions have recently adopted Precision Health as a strategic theme. These include Cedars-Sinai, Geisinger Health System, Indiana University, UCLA, the University of Chicago, the University of Michigan, and the University of Texas.

ABOUT THE BOOK

I was determined to write this book to provide an overview of the Precision Health vision. But I also wanted to help reorient how health and medicine are viewed in the United States, and even throughout the world. While you'll see that Stanford professors feature prominently, as do several companies operating near Stanford, the vision I'm putting forward is universally applicable. My inclusion of the companies is intended to provide an overview of the wide-ranging approaches and technologies that have the goal of improving health and health care. This overview of commercial activity is not intended to be comprehensive, nor does the inclusion of a company in any way reflect an endorsement of its approach or likelihood of success [19].

Virtually any institution, or any individual, can embrace the tenets of Precision Health and begin working toward achieving better health outcomes. And all communities—regardless of income levels and ethnic, racial, or religious composition—can benefit from Precision Health. Indeed, while Silicon Valley is seen as a cradle of wealth, it's also home to several jurisdictions where incomes are well below the national average, and where public health indicators paint a picture of distress. We are working in these communities with as much or more determination as we are in other communities with wealthier and healthier profiles.

To showcase the importance of Precision Health, chapter 1 is devoted to the state of health in the United States, as well as the health care delivery system. While there are gains to report on both fronts, it's also clear that there's considerable room for improvement and reform. In chapter 2, I address a fact that gets overlooked in most discussions of health: medical care plays only a small role in determining our health outcomes. Much more important are environmental, social, and behavioral factors, and I explore some of the reasons why they have been so difficult to address and why I believe components of Precision Health, such as the revolution in digital health, offer promising new hope.

Progress in medicine is enabled by pushing the bounds of conventional thinking in pursuit of a better way of treating diseases and other medical conditions. Chapter 3 features some of the innovations and disruptions—past, present, and hopefully future—found across health and medicine. I also describe the environments that are most likely to give rise to innovation.

In chapter 4, I focus on the importance of basic science and its role in discovery. As much as we know about the human body and how it functions, we get daily reminders that there is still much more to learn. Only by advancing our under-standing will it be possible to develop the therapies that can improve health and well-being. In this chapter I profile several trailblazers whose breakthroughs rest on a foundation of basic science.

The chapters that follow are dedicated to the three main pillars of Precision Health. In chapter 5, I discuss the many different ways in which it's possible to preemptively identify deviations in health that may become debilitating, which makes it possible for individuals—acting alone and/or with health care profes-sionals—to focus on interventions that will increase the likelihood of staying healthy. In chapter 6, I show how a range of tools—from smartphone technology to genome sequencing—are helping to avert illness and promote health and well-ness. In chapter 7, I document a range of breakthroughs—particularly in the can-cer field—that are being applied to help people recover from illness or disease. In the conclusion, I look at how health and medicine have evolved over the past century and how they may continue to evolve in the future.

For anyone with an interest in issues related to health and medicine, this is an exciting moment. We are learning more and more about what contributes to human health, and the different ways in which individuals can empower them-selves to lead healthier lives. We are on the brink of an amazing transformation in the practice of medicine.

I hope this book will help you understand the dynamic future that lies ahead. I also hope it will inspire you to work with others—whether family, friends, or your broader community—to help ensure that the Precision Health vision can become a reality for people in the United States and throughout the world.

CHAPTER 1

THE STATE OF U.S. HEALTH AND HEALTH CARE DELIVERY

One of the motivations for launching Precision Health was to confront an uncomfortable reality: in the United States, there's a lot about health conditions, and our health care system, that's unsatisfactory. To be sure, the United States can be the very best place in the world to obtain the latest, most scientifically advanced treatments for severe diseases for those who have access to these services. But there are dramatic disparities in health and in access to high-quality health care, based on factors such as income and geography. There are also shortcomings embedded in the U.S. health care system, which is one reason why we spend more on health care, on a per-capita basis, than any other country, but our health indicators (such as life expectancy) put us on par with countries that spend less—*much* less. In this chapter, I examine both U.S. health conditions and U.S. health care, and show how millions of Americans are not seeing the health benefits that are typically associated with living in a high-income country such as the United States.

THE HEALTH PARADOX

Health conditions in the United States are heavily bifurcated, with certain segments of the population seeing great progress while others see their health eroding.

The backdrop to the progress is the revolution in health that's unfolding, with much of it happening in and around Silicon Valley. It's clear that we're living in a time of unprecedented possibilities, with new knowledge and technologies accelerating the pace of biomedical discovery. In the area of biomedicine, there's a convergence of different fields and ideas and approaches underway.

One small but revealing symbol of the potential for progress is the research being conducted by Stanford faculty. Approximately two-thirds of the professors in the chemistry department are doing biologically focused research. So are about

Discovering Precision Health: Predict, Prevent, and Cure to Advance Health and Well-Being, First Edition. Lloyd Minor and Matthew Rees.
© 2020 John Wiley & Sons Ltd. Published 2020 by John Wiley & Sons Ltd.

30 percent of those in Stanford's engineering school. Several factors account for this shift in focus to research questions and opportunities in biomedicine by experts in other disciplines. The fields of biology and medicine have become quantitative endeavors. Gone are the days when the scientific inquiry in biomedicine was driven principally by qualitative description. The same analytical methods and approaches that have fueled advances in the physical sciences and technology for many decades are now being applied with enormous success in biomedicine. The questions being addressed and the discoveries being made, thanks to these quantitative approaches, are having a tremendous impact.

There are many examples of the transformation in biomedicine that is occurring because of the adoption of quantitative approaches. Mapping of the human genome and the subsequent advances in sequencing technology have changed the landscape of genetics. These advances—exciting as they are—increasingly seem modest compared with the impact of more sophisticated algorithms focused on identification of the relationships between the genome and diseases as well as the interactions between the genome and other nongenetic risk factors for disease. These same transformations are having an impact on fundamental, discovery-focused science.

The cell atlas initiative of the Chan Zuckerberg Biohub focuses on building a repository of all the different cell types in the human body—something that is currently unknown. Understanding all the different cell types is crucial, points out Steve Quake, a Stanford professor and co-president of the Chan Zuckerberg Biohub: "Having this knowledge will lead to greater understanding of the basic biology of human beings as well as what goes wrong and causes disease" [1]. It will be enabled by exciting new technologies such as CRISPR ("Clustered Regularly Interspaced Short Palindromic Repeats"), a gene-editing tool that will be used for experiments exploring whether certain combinations of genes can halt the progression of a disease—or even reverse it. The findings can be the basis for new medicines and new tests that are focused on combating specific diseases.

As breakthroughs like these are pursued, we are seeing the adoption of various technology-based products that are enabling people to become more engaged with their health and, ultimately, to live longer, healthier lives.

But set against this hopeful environment is an altogether different reality: certain segments of the U.S. population are experiencing a decline in basic indicators of good health. There are many ways to illustrate this decline, but life expectancy is perhaps the easiest to understand.

At the beginning of the 20th century, U.S. life expectancy was just 47.3 years. That figure rose steadily in the decades that followed, thanks in large part to medical advances, and by the start of the 21st century U.S. life expectancy was 76.8 years [2]. For the next 14 years, the incremental gains continued. But then something happened.

In 2015, life expectancy declined. Then it happened again in 2016, and again in 2017. This was the first decline in U.S. life expectancy over three consecutive years since the period coinciding with the end of World War I and the Spanish influenza. While the declines were quite modest, they did help illuminate the U.S. health challenges. The declines were also a reminder that the United States fares poorly in international comparisons. U.S. life expectancy is now only the 43rd highest in the world [3]—in 1960, the U.S. ranked 13th [4].

The U.S. average masks wide disparities. For example, there is a six-year difference in life expectancy between the residents of Hawaii and Mississippi, according to a study published in the *Journal of the American Medical Association* in 2017. There is a *20-year* difference between one county in Colorado and one in South Dakota [5].

There is also a large life expectancy gap based on income. Men with earnings in the top 1 percent of the population live 14.6 years longer than men in the bottom 1 percent (among women, the gap is 10.1 years), according to a 2016 study coauthored by economist Raj Chetty [6]. While men in the top 5 percent of the income distribution saw their life expectancy increase by 2.3 years between 2001 and 2014, it only grew 0.32 years for those in the bottom 5 percent. The gap was even larger among women—2.91 years and 0.04 years, respectively [7].

The gap is not just between the very rich and the very poor. In recent years, the mortality rate for men ages 65–79 in the top 1 percent of wealth distribution has been 40 percent lower than the average mortality rates for all tax filers in that age bracket, according to UC Berkeley economists Emmanuel Saez and Gabriel Zucman. From 1979 to 1983, the difference between the top 1 percent and everyone else was just 10 percent [8].

A study conducted by seven professors at the Stanford School of Medicine, led by Latha Palaniappan, documented the persistence of U.S. health disparities from 2003 to 2015. The study, which was published in November 2018, showed that while the age- and sex-adjusted mortality rates decreased by 12 percent in the total population, high-income counties experienced a 15 percent decline, while in low-income counties the decline was only 7 percent. Similarly, adjusted mortality rates for heart disease declined 30 percent in high-income counties, but 22 percent in low-income counties. The study also showed that African Americans have a higher mortality rate than other groups (Asian Americans, Hispanics, non-Hispanic whites, and American Indians/Alaska Natives) [9].

These disparities highlight the need for remedies that will help those who are falling behind. One of the most disturbing facts about U.S. health is the number of people who die prematurely each year and the causes of those deaths. The authors of a 2013 report sponsored by the National Institutes of Health wrote that "Americans are dying and suffering from illness and injury at rates that are demonstrably unnecessary" [10].

The causes of those deaths were spelled out in another comprehensive study, which was published in 2013 in the *Journal of the American Medical Association*. The researchers found that the primary causes of U.S. morbidity and mortality were poor diet, obesity, smoking, and high blood pressure [11]. The study has continued to be updated, and there is extensive data comparing current trends with those that existed in 1990. Some of the news is encouraging: the number of people dying from ischemic heart disease declined by nearly 100,000. On the other hand, heart disease was still responsible for nearly 545,000 deaths—well more than twice the number of deaths from any other condition. (The second-biggest killer in 2016 was Alzheimer's and other dementias, which were responsible for close to 239,000 deaths [12].)

When deaths were broken out by causes, and not specific diseases, one factor stood out from the rest: diet. The researchers found that "dietary risks" accounted for close to 530,000 deaths in 2016. Nearly 84 percent of the deaths stemmed from cardiovascular diseases, and the rest stemmed from a combination of neoplasms and diabetes, as well as urogenital, blood, and endocrine diseases [13].

The dietary risks are reflected in the expanding waistlines of the American people. Today, nearly 40 percent of American adults qualify as obese (meaning a body mass index of 30 or higher), as do 18.5 percent of children 19 and under [14]. The only countries with higher obesity rates (not counting a number of tiny Pacific and Caribbean islands) are Kuwait, Belize, Qatar, and Egypt.

What's striking is how quickly the profile of the American population changed. As recently as 1980, just 10 percent of the U.S. population was obese. Although obesity rates have been rising globally—there's been a tenfold increase in childhood obesity over the past 40 years [15]—the percentage point increase in American obesity since 1980 has been greater than in any other country in the world, according to a study published in 2017 in the *New England Journal of Medicine* [16].

The reasons for this decline in health are varied, and they speak to the need for new approaches to health—particularly focused on prediction and prevention. In later chapters, I highlight how select initiatives can not only treat obesity but try to prevent it (particularly in children) by emphasizing the value of both a healthy diet and regular physical activity.

THE U.S. HEALTH CARE CONUNDRUM

Health care is one of the most debated subjects in the United States. Consider the passionate feelings about the Affordable Care Act—better known as Obamacare—and whether to preserve it, reform it, or repeal it. What's striking about U.S. public opinion related to health care is not the divide between Republicans and Democrats but rather the differences in how people feel about the care they receive versus the system that provides that care.

In November 2017, the Gallup organization asked more than 1,000 people to rate the quality of care that they received, and 77 percent said it was "excellent" or "good." There's been little fluctuation in that number dating back to 2001 [17]. But when people were asked to describe the state of the U.S. health care system, 71 percent said it was "in a state of crisis"—a sentiment that has not changed much since 2008 [18].

Although I will emphasize health care in later chapters, I want to focus here on the *health care system* and touch on some of the features that people find unsatisfactory. I am certainly familiar with the system's inadequacies and will start with something that reflects those inadequacies: how it has been insulated from the technology disruptions that have shaken up countless other industries.

One way to gauge the slow pace of innovation in how the health care system operates is the absence of any game-changing products or companies akin to, say, Google, Uber, Airbnb, Amazon, etc. I certainly recognize the obstacles to disruption, such as extremely complex billing systems, restrictive government regulations, and the high stakes associated with any innovation that involves the care and treatment of human lives. Nonetheless, the effect is striking: how health care is delivered, and the environments in which medicine is practiced, have not changed much since I graduated from medical school in 1982. Yes, there have been some modifications, such as the adoption of electronic health records (which have brought their own set of issues, as I describe below), but the foundation of the system remains the same. That's problematic for everyone involved, but primarily for patients and the health care professionals who serve them.

THE "SOPHISTICATED" TECHNOLOGY IN DOCTORS' OFFICES

Emblematic of the lack of innovation is the fact that many (if not most) physicians' offices still rely on a device that disappeared in just about every other industry two decades ago: the fax machine. "It's been the most sophisticated piece of technology in many doctors' offices for decades," points out Bill Evans, CEO of the venture capital firm Rock Health. Here's how one journalist, Sarah Kliff, writing in 2017, described the situation:

> In the medical sector, the fax is as dominant as ever. It is the cockroach of American medicine: hated by doctors and medical professionals but able to survive—even thrive—in a hostile environment. By one private firm's estimate, the fax accounts for about 75 percent of all medical communication. It frustrates doctors, nurses, researchers, and entire hospitals, but a solution is evasive.

Kliff goes on to point out that one of the reasons fax-based communications endure in the medical field is that hospitals don't necessarily want to share patient information with each other:

> While patients might *want* one hospital to exchange information with another hospital, those institutions have little incentive to do so. A shared medical record, after all, makes it easier to see a different doctor. A walled garden—where records only get traded within one hospital system—can encourage patients to stick with those providers [19].

The persistence of the fax machine (and the paper that accompanies it) demonstrates how technology has often been treated as a cost of doing business and not a tool for progress (as it has been in just about every other industry). The fax machine is also an administrative headache that saps the productivity of all health care professionals who are subject to it. Today, about one-third of physician practices insist on doing business with paper forms and fax machines. It is often used when a physician's office fills out a claims form on paper and faxes it to the payer, who pays someone to transcribe it into their system. Then the payer identifies information that is missing in the form but is needed to process a claim. The form gets faxed back to the doctor's office, which amends it and faxes it back. The payer then must pay someone to transcribe the information into the system.

These kinds of inefficiencies drive up the cost of transactions. There are also health consequences. The absence of shared medical records makes it nearly impossible to get a longitudinal view of a patient's health care history. This is striking, particularly when compared with other products, such as one's car, where a comprehensive maintenance history is often easily accessible.

THE UNFULFILLED POTENTIAL OF ELECTRONIC HEALTH RECORDS

During my time as a resident, I remember far too many nights when I was on call and would need to contact hospital security in the middle of the night. The reason? I needed them to open the door to the office of a faculty member so that I could track down a chart or a radiology study on a patient who was having surgery at 7 a.m. I also remember taking care of patients in the Emergency Department who had received all their care in the health system in which I was training, but I did not have the benefit of any of this information because the chart with their medical history could not be located.

My experience was much more the rule than the exception in U.S. health care. Indeed, as recently as 2008, only 10 percent of doctors kept digital records on their patients. The other 90 percent made notes on paper and stored them in manila folders on shelves and in filing cabinets. Paper records had some obvious disadvantages. They took up space, and they were difficult to share with other physicians, hospitals, and insurance companies. Patients switching doctors, hospitals, or places of residence could not easily bring their records with them.

In 2009, in the wake of the financial crisis, the federal government acted to remedy this situation. The Health Information Technology for Economic and Clinical Health (HITECH) Act set aside $27 billion of federal funds to encourage health care providers to adopt electronic health records (EHR) systems, and more money was subsequently made available for training and assistance. All told, the federal government spent about $35 billion on bringing the U.S. health care industry into the electronic age. The program was highly successful in that it made EHRs commonplace. Today, nine in 10 doctors have adopted them. We have made a colossal transformation in a relatively short period of time.

It is also true that the potential benefits of the data that exist in electronic health records have not been realized. But with some changes in technology, regulations, and attention to training, EHRs may soon serve as the backbone of an information revolution in health care—one that will transform health care the way digital technologies are changing banking, finance, transportation, navigation, internet search, retail, and other industries. Regulations are being implemented that will put patients in control of their own health records and facilitate the sharing of data among health care organizations. Engineers are developing artificial intelligence technology that can take notes for physicians, summarize the important points from a patient's record, and assist in medical decision-making. Apple's recent app for medical information, which gives third-party developers the ability to pull information from health records, is expected to be the first of many developments that bring health care data to patients' fingertips. There are a lot of reasons to be optimistic that we will be able to have both high-tech and high-touch medicine.

Despite these obvious benefits of EHRs, their true potential to improve the way health care is delivered has not been realized. As implemented today, EHRs have too many of the drawbacks of paper records. The promise of being able to send them easily from one office to the next has been hampered by a lack of standards and perverse incentives in the health care marketplace to hoard information. Worse, EHRs, with their cumbersome user interfaces and onerous billing requirements, have become a burden to doctors and nurses, contributing to burnout and information overload among physicians and degrading patient care. "A clinician will make roughly 4,000 keyboard clicks during a busy 10-hour emergency-room shift," writes Abraham Verghese, professor for the theory and practice of medicine at Stanford. "In the process, our daily progress notes have become bloated cut-and-paste monsters that are inaccurate and hard to wade through" [20].

While the design of EHRs is a topic of considerable criticism from physicians, much of the data entry is driven by regulatory considerations. The authors of a 2018 article published in the *Annals of Internal Medicine* described their experience of helping to launch EHR software (Epic Systems) in health systems throughout the world. (The same software is used widely in the United States.)

> We noted a significantly different interpretation of the EHR abroad: Physicians were more likely to report satisfaction with its use and cite it as a tool that improved efficiency. We also found that clinical documentation differs from that in the United States. In other countries, it tends to be far briefer, containing only essential clinical information; it omits much of the compliance and reimbursement documentation that commonly bloats the American clinical note. In fact, across this same EHR, clinical notes in the United States are nearly 4 times longer on average than those in other countries.

The authors also noted that since enactment of the 2009 HITECH Act, clinical notes in the United States have doubled in length, thus supporting their conclusion that simplifying regulations "would benefit the health care system and patients alike" [21].

It's clear that transforming EHRs into sophisticated clinical tools depends on reforming the technology that underlies them and the regulations that govern them. But it's also clear that radical changes will be required at many different levels, and physicians in particular are going to need to reexamine their role in shaping the future. In 2018, Stanford Medicine published a white paper that contained several recommendations (*see box on next page*) [22]. A long-form article in the April 2019 issue of *Fortune* also provides a detailed overview [23].

WHAT HANDICAPS THE U.S. HEALTH CARE SYSTEM

Fax machines and electronic health records are far from the biggest issues facing U.S. health care, but their prominence in the health care system is a painful reminder of the system's many shortcomings. Many thoughtful and often provocative books have been written documenting those shortcomings, such as *The Innovators Prescription: A Disruptive Solution for Health Care*, by Clayton Christensen and Jerome Grossman; *The American Health Care Paradox: Why Spending More Is Getting Us Less*, by Elizabeth Bradley and Harvey V. Fineberg; *More Than Medicine: The Broken Promise of American Health*, by Robert M. Kaplan; and *An American Sickness: How Healthcare Became Big Business and How You Can Take It Back*, by Elisabeth Rosenthal. My intent here is to briefly highlight a few of the fundamental problems that handicap the system, since they underscore the need for the kinds of new approaches represented by Precision Health.

Reactive

In the United States, the term *health care*, as it's commonly thought of, is a misnomer. It's really *sick care*—people tend not to use health care unless they are responding to an injury, illness, or disease diagnosis—and there are few financial incentives in the system for providers to focus on prevention.

One Size Fits All

Every person with a given diagnosis tends to receive the same treatment, regardless of his or her age, sex, and other medical conditions, even though all those variables dramatically influence the responses to treatment.

Fragmented

When an individual enters the medical system, there is often very little coordination among all the different health care providers. Their communication can be haphazard, and they may not have access to the same pieces of patient information, which can lead to inadequate or incorrect treatments.

Medical Practices

- Invest in adequate EHR training when onboarding clinicians and bring them up to speed when incremental changes are made.
- Enlist clinicians to help prioritize EHR development tasks and to design clinical workflows that take advantage of EHR capabilities (e.g., the Sprint team model).
  - Tailor the size and makeup of clinician development teams, taking into account the clinical resources available.
- Deliver EHR development projects soon after clinicians ask for them.
- Establish an EHR governance process that gives the clinical organization nimbleness in responding to health emergencies and crisis scenarios.
- Make analytics data available to clinicians—presented in a way that is intuitive at the point of care.
- Shift nonessential EHR data entry to ancillary staff. In the near term, consider increasing the number of medical assistants to act as "digital scribes" (though this option is expensive). In the long term, seek automated solutions to eliminate manual EHR documentation.
- Reevaluate your organization's interpretation of privacy rules.
- Create opportunities for patients to digitally maintain their records (providing family history, medical history, medications, health monitoring data, etc.).
- Junk the fax machine (if you still have one) and embrace electronic communications.
- Start accepting electronic payments, if you don't already.

For Payers

- EHRs reflect the current fee-for-service payment paradigm. Commit to value-based care and provide adequate support to clinicians under this model, including greater reimbursement for preventive care services and the use of digital health to engage patients.
- Create common standards for billing and quality reporting across payers.
- Streamline preauthorization procedures.
- Make claims data more accessible to physicians to enable a longitudinal view of their patients.

For Regulators

- Affirm commitment to value-based care and move away from requiring literal documentation of patient-doctor interactions.
- Create more flexibility around who needs to enter data into the EHR, as many tasks do not require the expertise of a highly trained clinician.
- Clarify information-blocking rules to encourage open APIs and eliminate perverse incentives to hoard information.

For Technologists

- Clarify definitions of interoperability—in collaboration with other stakeholder groups—and adopt common technical standards to support them.

- Develop systems and product updates in partnership with your end users—less than half of U.S. physicians believe EHR developers are responsive to their feedback.
- Embrace open APIs and nurture a community of developers to enable an app-based ecosystem that puts the patient in control.
- Develop and market an ecosystem of third-party apps that put patients in control of their own health data.
- Focus on eliminating the manual entry of data into the EHR by recruiting AI, natural language processing, and other emerging technologies.
- Develop AI to increase the intelligence of clinical information systems, enabling them to

  1. Synthesize relevant information in the EHR before each patient encounter and present the physician with a pithy summary.
  2. Combine patient complaint information with EHR databases and the latest medical literature to support medical decision-making.
  3. Deliver current and contextualized information to each member of a patient care team (i.e., enable intelligent "care traffic control").

Detached and Disconnected from Patients

Much of the health care system is defined by one-way transactions: patients are diagnosed and receive treatment, but there's often little communication with the patients and their families about their preferences, their family history, or their financial circumstances. This can lead to ill-advised decisions about what treatments to provide.

Low Value

The health outcomes in the United States are not what they should be, particularly given the level of spending. In 2016, the United States devoted $3.3 trillion to health care, which was 17.9 percent of the country's gross domestic product [24]. Other developed economies spend less—a lot less. Among the members of the Organization for Economic Cooperation and Development—a group of developed countries—the second-highest level of spending in 2016, as a share of GDP, was 12.4 percent (Switzerland) [25]. The U.S. figure was also twice as high as the average of other comparable countries [26]. Yet U.S. health outcomes are typically no better—and often worse—than those found in other developed countries.

Misguided Incentives

Much of the U.S. health care system is based on a reimbursement model that rewards volume of care rather than outcomes of care. As a result, there's little incentive for physicians or hospitals to focus on whether specific treatments are successful, or on the costs of post-acute care.

Opaque Pricing

Few people outside the health care industry have a comprehensive understanding of the interplay between health care delivery and the fees charged and the payments made. "Imagine if you paid for an airplane ticket and then got separate and inscrutable bills from the airline, the pilot, the copilot, and the flight attendants," writes Elisabeth Rosenthal, a Harvard-trained physician and former *New York Times* reporter. "That's how the healthcare market works" [27].

To further illustrate this point, consider a story from Alex Azar, the current U.S. secretary of health and human services. In a March 2018 speech, he recounted his own battle with opaque pricing in a hospital:

> A few years ago, my doctor back in Indiana wanted me to do a routine echo-cardio stress test. I figured this could occur within the scope of his practice, which was connected to a major medical center. Instead, I was sent a few floors down, where I was told to start handing over all sorts of information to a receptionist. Soon enough, I have a plastic wristband slapped on me, and, to my surprise, what I thought would be a simple test in the room next door had resulted in my being admitted to the hospital.
>
> Now, I had a high-deductible plan, so I would be paying for this test out of pocket. As someone who works in healthcare, I knew that the sticker price on the test had just jumped dramatically by my receiving it within a hospital—something that might never occur to most healthcare consumers. So I asked how much the test was going to cost, and was told that information wasn't available. Fortunately, I didn't just fall off the turnip truck, so I persisted, and, eventually the manager of the clinic appeared and gave me the answer. The list price was $5,500.
>
> I knew that wasn't the right answer either. The key piece of information was what my insurer would pay as a negotiated rate, or what I'd pay with cash. That information didn't come easily, but eventually, I was told it would be $3,500.
>
> I happened to know of a website where you could search typical prices for such procedures, so I looked up what it would have been if I'd received it outside of the hospital, in a doctor's office. The answer was $550.
>
> Now, there I was, the former deputy secretary of Health and Human Services, and that is the kind of effort it took to find out how much I would owe for a procedure. What if I had been a grandmother? Or a 20-something with a high-deductible plan [28]?

The opaque pricing Azar describes is a source of exasperation for countless individuals, but it also points to the inefficiencies in the system and a reason why health care spending over the past decade has been rising five times faster than the inflation rate.

Overlooking the Biggest Determinants of Health

The U.S. health care system is primarily devoted to the treatment of diseases after they occur. That has led to the creation of a health care delivery system that often provides leading-edge treatments for a range of conditions and diseases. But medical care directed toward treating disease plays only a small role in determining our health outcomes. Much more important are behavioral, environmental, and social factors. Those factors are largely overlooked within the U.S. health care system—something I explore in detail in the next chapter.

Physician Burnout

There's one other key contributor to dysfunction in the delivery of health care: physicians. More specifically, physicians who are burned out. That was the conclusion of a 2018 paper by Tait Shanafelt, director of the WellMD Center at Stanford, and Daniel Tawfik, an instructor in pediatric critical care medicine at Stanford. As part of the study, they sent surveys to physicians throughout the United States. Nearly 6,700 responded—and 10 percent declared that they had been responsible for at least one major medical error in just the previous three months. The survey also revealed that physicians who reported burnout were more than twice as likely to commit a medical error than physicians who were not burned out [29]. Those errors included mistakes in medical judgment, mistakes in diagnosing illnesses, and technical mistakes during procedures.

The frequency of mistakes is even more worrisome given the prevalence of physician burnout. The same study revealed that 55 percent of physicians were experiencing symptoms of burnout, which can stem from many different factors. While we need to be focused on the well-being of all health care professionals, a 2017 article coauthored by Bryan Bohman, a Stanford professor and founder of our physician wellness committee, highlighted a few reasons to be focused on physicians:

> First, physicians have been hard-hit by the organizational transformation of the health care system, resulting in an epidemic of burnout and declining professional fulfillment. They have suffered a reduction in their sense of professional autonomy, have experienced a significant increase in clerical duties, and are beholden to a growing array of imperfect and inconsistent quality and productivity metrics. Second, medical training has historically acculturated physicians to deny their own self-care in the service of others [30].

Another contributor to burnout is the documentation demands associated with electronic health records. Studies show that physicians devote 34 to 55 percent of their workday to EHR-related tasks. Steven Lin, the medical director at Stanford Family Medicine, points out that while some of this time bolsters ongoing care, "much of it instead serves billing documentation, defense against litigation risk, and regulatory compliance."

I don't think many people become doctors because they love doing documentation. While documentation is part of the medical school curriculum at Stanford, for many aspiring physicians it's something they must figure out as they go through their clerkships and residency training. Then, when they start to practice, the burdens are likely to grow: EHR record-keeping, inbox management, digital messages from patients, managing providers, etc. "It's a huge shock to a lot of the younger trainees, as well as older, experienced physicians," says Lin. "Across the age and experience spectrum, many doctors are just deciding not to go to EHRs and risk the penalties surrounding meaningful use, or to leave medicine altogether. It's a big problem." Indeed, a 2017 study commissioned by the Association of American Medical Colleges predicted that by 2030, the United States will face a shortage of between 40,800 and 104,900 physicians [31].

Studies show that physicians who use medical assistants to act as digital scribes and record the content of the patient-doctor interaction show far more satisfaction and lower rates of burnout. University of Colorado Health experimented with increasing the ratio of medical assistants (MAs) to physicians, from 0.4 MA per physician to nearly two. Before the physician enters the room, an MA has spent 20 minutes talking with the patient, updating the medical records, and handling minor medical issues, such as vaccines and screenings. When the physician walks in, the MA stays in the room, acting as a scribe during the exam. They found that over the course of a year, this approach went a long way toward relieving physician burnout: the metric they use to measure physician burnout declined from 55 percent to 14 percent. Assigning two people for each physician to act as scribe may not be a cost-effective solution, however.

AI researchers are working on automating the job of the scribe. Google and Stanford Medicine have been collaborating on a digital scribe project that would listen to the dialogue in a patient visit and take notes. The idea is not merely to take a transcription, but rather to knit the dialogue into a narrative. In the study, each doctor wears a microphone to capture conversations with patients, which are used to train machine-learning algorithms in getting the gist of a doctor-patient interaction. The goal is to train the algorithm to generate a pithy progress note. Google researchers say that its scribe can capture complex conversations typical of a patient-doctor conference even when family members and other practitioners are present in a noisy environment.

Scribes—whether live or automated—can play a valuable role and hopefully help remedy doctor burnout. In the meantime, there are significant expenses for health systems when physicians leave medicine. The process of identifying and recruiting replacements can involve costs from $268,000 to $957,000, according to a study published in 2017 by Stanford's Maryam Hamidi [32].

I see the manifestations and the consequences of physician burnout. From the colleagues who leave the medical profession at relatively early stages of their career to colleagues whose personal and professional lives are disrupted by stress and anger, the manifestations of burnout are hauntingly tragic. Shortly after I arrived at Stanford in the fall of 2012, a group of clinical faculty in the School of

Medicine came to see me to discuss the problem of physician burnout within our own academic medical center and nationally. These faculty wanted to do something about burnout, and they wanted Stanford Medicine to take the lead in proactively and constructively addressing the problem.

To help address these issues, in 2017 Stanford's School of Medicine hired a chief physician wellness officer, Tait Shanafelt, making us one of the first academic medical centers in the United States to hire someone for such a position. As mentioned above, he is the director of the Stanford Medicine WellMD Center, which is focused on improving the health and professional fulfillment of physicians.

Shanafelt's interest in the issue stems from observations during his residency at the University of Washington, when he saw the extraordinary demands being placed on interns he was supervising. He subsequently helped design and lead a study to examine the nexus between burnout and quality of care. The study, which was published in the *Annals of Internal Medicine* in 2002, revealed a close response relationship between burnout and suboptimal patient care: the higher the burnout score, the greater the frequency of residents reporting errors or providing suboptimal care to patients. Among residents with a high burnout score, 53 percent indicated that they had provided sub-optimal care at least once in the previous month, a rate markedly higher than those without high burnout scores [33]. Shanafelt also spent over a decade at the highly respected Mayo Clinic in Minnesota, where he conducted studies of physician well-being.

Today, as the head of the WellMD Center, Shanafelt is focusing on several issues. One is building safety nets for physicians who are in distress. Another is helping physicians and leaders create a culture where physicians support each other and create a practice environment that makes it easy for physicians to provide patients the care they need. He is also creating operational metrics that define whether the practice environment is a source of frustration or facilitates efficient delivery of the care patients need and promotes professional fulfillment. As Shanafelt has remarked,

> It's amazing to me that administrative leaders can create spreadsheets with detail to three decimal places for metrics such as how many patients are seen per room per day, how often a clinic runs late, and other operational aspects of the practice environment. But they rarely have categories for things like the consistency of an operating room team working together or how many minutes per night primary care doctors are logged in from home charting in the EHR as dimensions they should be optimizing.

To address this, Stanford has created new metrics—including time spent charting in EHRs during personal time—and is working with administrative leaders to track and improve them by providing physicians additional assistance in the clinic, redesign of work flows, and better team-based care. Another important intervention has been for every department chair to appoint a director who works with WellMD to improve professional fulfillment for physicians in the department. In collaboration with the clinical and improvement leaders in their departments, these individuals are tasked with addressing the local irritation and friction points unique to their department/specialty or local practice. Larger-scale efforts with operations and improvement leaders are designed to improve operational metrics on the efficiency of the practice environment (time spent on clinical documentation at home, operating room turnaround time, time per week more broadly).

The center has also been working on organization-wide efforts to improve dimensions with broad relevance independent of specialty, such as the following:

- Cultivation of community and connection between colleagues by helping physicians connect with a small group of colleagues regularly to provide support for the unique personal and professional challenges of a career in medicine—a strategy found effective in two randomized controlled trials that Shanafelt helped lead at the Mayo Clinic [34].

- Development and testing of strategies to improve self-valuation (studies demonstrate that low self-valuation is a critical driver of burnout in physicians).

- Development and testing of strategies to encourage leadership behaviors among division chiefs that cultivate professional fulfillment among those they lead.

- Creation of a formal peer support program to serve as a safety net for physicians experiencing distress related to the professional (medical error, friction with a supervisor or coworker, dealing with a malpractice suit) or the personal (relationship issues, problems with work-life integration).

Stanford has also been at the forefront of developing an organizational model that illustrates how the quest to cultivate professional fulfillment among physicians is about far more than personal resilience and requires structural, system-level changes in the organization and practice environment. This model has now been used around the country to heighten awareness of physician burnout among those who are able to do something about it, such as administrative leaders and people who serve on hospital boards. A 2018 paper coauthored by several Stanford officials highlighted seven ideas that should motivate board members around the country to focus on making this issue a priority for their organization:

- Burnout is prevalent among physicians and other health care professionals.
- The well-being of health care professionals affects the quality of care.
- Distress among health care professionals has a tangible fiscal cost to organizations.
- Greater personal resilience is not the solution.
- Different occupations and disciplines have different needs.
- Approaches to remedy the problem have been developed.
- Interventions have been shown to work [35].

I've been encouraged by other institutions joining our efforts. As of January 2019, 16 academic or academic-affiliated medical center members (including Stanford Medicine) had become part of a Physician Wellness Academic Consortium (PWAC), which is focused on driving innovative advancement of physician well-being. The consortium is taking the following steps:

- Applying common measures for longitudinal assessment of physician well-being and the primary drivers of well-being.
- Developing and testing innovative strategies to improve physician well-being.
- Meeting at regular intervals to share innovative best practices to improve physician well-being.
- Implementing evidence-based/best-practice strategies to improve physician well-being.

We're also seeing interest by leaders of the medical establishment. In the fall of 2018, Shanafelt and I were among the authors of a *Health Affairs* blog posting that made the case for health systems to hire a chief wellness officer (CWO) to support the well-being of clinicians [36]. The other coauthors included the president and CEO of the Association of American Medical Colleges, the presidents of the National Academy of Medicine and the American Nurses Association, and the CEO of the Accreditation Council of Graduate Medical Education. The role of a CWO is to help lead all aspects of organizational change necessary to reduce burnout and cultivate professional fulfillment. The CWO is a senior leader who plays a role analogous to that of the chief medical officer or chief quality officer. The key responsibilities of the CWO include evaluating the scope of the problem within the organization, reporting the results to senior leaders (e.g., the hospital board, dean, department chairs, operational leaders), developing an organization-wide strategy to drive improvement, and overseeing broad system-level efforts to make progress in the dimensions most relevant to the local organization.

Once again, these efforts primarily focus on system-level improvements addressing dimensions of organizational culture and inefficiency in the practice environment. CWOs should also have expertise in tactics and strategies to support local unit-level efforts to address unit-specific issues. They must be effective in engaging other leaders (chief quality officer, chief medical officer, chief medical information officer, and human resources officer), partnering with them to drive necessary change and measuring the progress.

While change comes slowly in medicine and health care, as I will explain in more detail later, I am encouraged by the speed with which this issue has become a priority for many individuals and institutions. A lot more still needs to happen, and when it does, physicians *and* their patients will see the benefits.

* * *

One incontrovertible fact applies to U.S. health and the U.S. health care system: there's a clear need for improvements to both. Declining life expectancy, coupled with large life-expectancy gaps based on geography and income, is a tragedy at a moment when there are extraordinary new tools to enable healthy living. Similarly, the multiple flaws embedded in the U.S. health care system are imposing great costs on the United States—in outright spending (with low returns on that spending) and the care and treatment of patients.

I am confident that changes inspired by Precision Health approaches could help reverse the gloomy state of affairs I've just described. But first, I will explore the determinants of health that are largely overlooked by the U.S. health care system.

CHAPTER 2

THERE'S MORE TO "HEALTH" THAN HEALTH CARE

One of the essential ideas underpinning Precision Health is that medical care plays only a small role in determining our health outcomes. For too long, "health" has been equated with the amount and quality of medical care that's delivered. Doctors have focused their work primarily on treating disease. That's how they've been trained, how they've practiced, and how they've thought for as long as the medical profession has existed. The gold standard of medicine has always been to find treatments that work for large numbers of people and match them appropriately to the conditions facing their patients.

But this is an incomplete and flawed approach, in a few different ways. It's reactive—it focuses on people only after they're sick. More fundamentally, it doesn't take account of the factors outside medical care and genetics that drive human health. While every individual is different, the key areas below show approximations of what are typically the key drivers of health outcomes, and the importance of each one relative to the others:

- Environmental and social factors: 40 percent
- Behavioral factors: 30 percent
- Genetics and biology: 20 percent
- Clinical care: 10 percent

The relative weighting of these categories is likely to change as our knowledge of human genetics and biology increases and as we can translate this knowledge into more effective approaches to prediction and prevention. As discussed in the vignette at the beginning of the introduction, more-precise tests that screen for risk factors and enable diagnosis of disease at a much earlier stage are on the way. Although the specific percentages for each area vary among studies [1], the categories are not isolated—they clearly interact with each other. We know, for example, that the environment in which a person lives can have a profound influence on individual behavior. In the United States, for example, obesity [2] and

---

Discovering Precision Health: Predict, Prevent, and Cure to Advance Health and Well-Being,
First Edition. Lloyd Minor and Matthew Rees.
© 2020 John Wiley & Sons Ltd. Published 2020 by John Wiley & Sons Ltd.

the use of tobacco [3] tend to be more concentrated among people with low incomes. But the universal conclusion from all studies that have addressed this topic is that social, environmental, and behavioral factors are highly significant determinants of health. Recently, Robert M. Kaplan and Arnold Milstein, both of Stanford, reviewed the contributions of medical care to health outcomes, drawing on the conclusions reached in four major studies. They stated, "Healthcare has modest effects on the extension of U.S. life expectancy, while behavioral and social determinants may have larger effects" [4].

There are many reasons why behavioral and social determinants have received far less attention, particularly in the community of academic medicine, compared with genetics and medical care. These reasons include cultural expectations (physicians being identified with the *treatment* rather than the *prevention* of disease), perverse incentives in payment systems (reimbursements for care delivered and procedures performed that are not necessarily linked to outcomes), and the sheer complexity of these factors. The net effect has been a relative paucity of studies and actionable changes in social, environmental, and behavioral determinants.

But the future, as I will describe in the pages that follow, offers tremendous opportunities to transform health by moving from reactive medical care to proactive health care. We are living amid a biomedical revolution. Our understanding of the mechanisms of disease is growing in ways that enable us to prevent diseases altogether or diagnose them, and therefore treat them, much earlier and more effectively. New technologies applied to the monitoring of health will play an important role. Finally, the engagement of each of us in our health and well-being, enabled by the information we have about our health, can be transformative.

PRECISION HEALTH AND POPULATION HEALTH

This chapter highlights some population-level health challenges, such as obesity and poor nutrition. The wide-ranging remedies that are typically utilized to help meet such broad challenges contrast with the Precision Health approaches, which are tailored to specific individuals. But the two are not in conflict. In fact, they can complement each other, thanks to the explosion of data generated from sources such as wearable devices, electronic health records, insurance claims, and clinical trials. These data, when coupled with the technology to manage and analyze them, make it possible to target emerging diseases with precise interventions at the level of the individual *and* at the level of the population as a whole. For example, as we further explore the roles of diet and exercise in preventing cardiovascular disease and cancer, we are likely to discover optimal combinations of certain behaviors for certain genotypes and phenotypes, leading to precise approaches to prevention rather than the one-size-fits-all public guidance that has long characterized our approach.

The intersection of population health and Precision Health has also enabled the creation of new scientific approaches to meet health challenges. That was part of the impetus for Stanford establishing the Center for Population Health Sciences in 2015. The center is focused on improving individual and population health by fostering collaboration across diverse disciplines and data, with the goal of understanding and addressing social, environmental, behavioral, and biological factors on a domestic and global scale. It has more than 750 members, more than 230 research trainees, 42 community partners, and research in 24 countries. Its research initiatives span a wide variety of topics, including community resilience and socioeconomic equity, gender, and healthy aging. The center's work emphasizes linking the precise determinants of an individual's health to the underlying drivers of population health—encompassing lifestyle choices, social factors, the environment, infectious agents, medical care, and genetics.

By applying Precision Health solutions to improve population health, especially in underserved populations, and by using lessons learned from large populations to predict, prevent, and cure more precisely, we can maximize wellness for all individuals and impact millions of lives.

GENES ARE ONE PIECE OF THE HEALTH PUZZLE

The belief that genetics is the overwhelmingly dominant determinant of health is, in many respects, unfortunate. This is not to say that genetic determinants of disease are unimportant—quite to the contrary. But it is also incorrect for people to believe they are at the mercy of their genes and medical care, and thus their individual behaviors don't have significant impact. The reality is dramatically different. As Cashell Jaquish, a genetic epidemiologist at the National Heart, Lung, and Blood Institute, has said, even a genetic predisposition to heart disease (the leading cause of death among Americans) "doesn't mean you are fated to have [it]. Other factors, like not smoking, diet and exercise, can have a very large effect. Family history does increase your risk slightly, but not as much as [not doing] these other things" [5].

The nexus between genes and many chronic conditions can also be overcome with smart behavioral patterns. Consider obesity. "I like to say that obesity is 80 percent genetic and 100 percent environmental," Philip F. Smith, codirector of the office of obesity research at the National Institute of Diabetes and Digestive and Kidney Diseases, told the *Washington Post*. "You won't become obese unless you overeat." He added, "For most people, I can say unequivocally that genes are not your destiny. They can predispose you to obesity, but only if you consume more calories than you burn off" [6].

Further proof of that comes from a 2007 study, published in the *New England Journal of Medicine,* based on people who were part of the landmark Framingham Heart Study. Although the study found that obesity was 40 percent more likely if one's sibling had already become obese, it was 57 percent more likely if someone's friend had become obese, and 171 percent more likely among close mutual friends [7]. One of the study's coauthors pointed out, "What appears to be happening is that a person becoming obese most likely causes a change of norms about what counts as an appropriate body size. People come to think that it is okay to be bigger since those around them are bigger, and this sensibility spreads" [8]. A related issue is that close friends eat together and end up taking cues from each other about what's customary when it comes to the types of foods to eat and how much.

Physical activity can help neutralize the impact of a genetic predisposition to obesity. A study published in 2011, involving more than 200,000 adults, found that although a certain gene variant (FTO) increased the risk of obesity by 23 percent, those with the variant who were physically active had a risk of obesity 27 percent lower than that of inactive adults [9].

While genes are not the exclusive drivers of health, the environment in which one lives—both the social and physical dimensions—is a critical influence. That influence takes several different forms, but it starts with something basic: social connections. "People who feel more connected to others have lower levels of anxiety and depression," says Emma Seppälä, science director of the Stanford Center for Compassion and Altruism Research and Education and the author of *The Happiness Track: How to Apply the Science of Happiness to Accelerate Your Success.* She also points to studies showing that connected people have higher self-esteem and greater empathy for others. They are also more trusting and cooperative, and as a consequence, she says, "others are more open to trusting and cooperating with them. ... In other words, social connectedness generates a positive feedback loop of social, emotional and physical well-being."

A few years ago, trained interviewers met with 100 people from Santa Clara County (the county that encompasses most of Stanford) as part of a project launched by the Stanford Prevention Research Center. The questions during the one-on-one sessions revolved around wellness: what contributed to it, what detracted from it, etc. Following the interviews, researchers working on the project identified the 10 markers of wellness that were mentioned most often. The most important? The existence of a social network, which provided opportunities to receive support and companionship, to feel loved, and to have a sense of belonging [10].

As important as social networks and connections are, there are many other factors that influence health, and for many people—particularly children—there are multiple social determinants of health. This refers to the circumstances, outside of medical care and genetics, that influence health and well-being. In challenging living conditions, for example, infants can be born with what's known as a *thrifty phenotype.* It is supposed to help children adapt to the conditions in which they may be living. But the existence of this phenotype has also been linked to adverse health outcomes [11].

Health and life expectancy are often correlated with income, as I noted in the previous chapter. Consider that those with low incomes often live in so-called food deserts, where there is little access to grocery stores selling a wide variety of healthy foods (particularly fresh fruits and vegetables). Similarly, those with low incomes may not have the time or resources to travel to neighborhoods offering healthy food options, and they may also lack access to quality health care services. For people living with those circumstances, and others like them, health outcomes are often much worse than those found in higher-income communities.

Lisa Chamberlain, an associate professor of pediatrics at Stanford's School of Medicine, has been active in highlighting health disparities and trying to remedy them. "So much of our health is generated by our environments and the choices that we have," says Chamberlain.

> It's often thought that choices are simple. For example, do you choose to exercise or not exercise? Do you choose to eat healthy foods or unhealthy foods? People know they should be eating healthy and exercising regularly. But they are making logical choices based on their income level and where they live. That's why health is often driven more by a person's zip code than their genetic code. And that's why you can see the health profile of entire neighborhoods decline. It's not because they have the same genes—it's because they all face the same choices.

She believes the most influential social determinant of health is education. For many children, that means they've already fallen behind in both categories by the time they enter kindergarten. "They're set up to fail," she says. "Many children from low-income families don't end up attending preschool because it costs $20 per hour, while the free federal program, Head Start, has huge waiting lists."

Chamberlain also works as a physician at the Gardner Packard Children's Health Center, a community-based clinic serving primarily low-income families. (Her work at Gardner followed 14 years of seeing patients at Ravenswood, a family health center in East Palo Alto.) When she sees children who are starting kindergarten, she ensures that they have the required immunizations and tests their vision and hearing. She also screens them developmentally to check their school readiness skills: Do they know their colors? Can they write their name? In one recent year, she and her colleagues evaluated five-year-old children in the clinic, and just 13 percent were ready for kindergarten. (The comparable figure for children attending Palo Alto schools, just a few miles away, is typically 85 to 90 percent.) "Not only are these children starting kindergarten behind," says Chamberlain, "they're being set up to fail."

Among the many health challenges faced by low-income children are the meals they're served at school. These meals—which include lunch and sometimes breakfast—often have little or no nutritional value, thus setting the children on a path to weight gain and, potentially, obesity. Low-quality food is a longstanding problem at schools, but there are entities trying to make a difference. Revolution Foods, for example, works with more than 1,500 schools, spread across 16 states and Washington, DC, and it is focused on providing healthy foods, such as fruits and vegetables.

But bringing healthy food into schools often faces significant obstacles. Chamberlain, for example, tried to get a low-income district to drop its existing food provider and switch to Revolution. But the existing provider—a national company that provides meals to schools throughout the country—was able to come in at a lower cost, as it provided something that Revolution did not: cafeteria workers. Dropping the national company would lead to the district incurring unsustainable fiscal deficits. The superintendent told Chamberlain, in so many words, "I know these kids need healthier food. But what am I supposed to do? I have enough trouble focusing on academics and everything else. I can't take on food as well."

That story is emblematic of the challenges we face in improving the diets of all people, and it's a potent reminder of how the environment in which you live can have a major influence on your health. There's considerable evidence that attention to and improvements in the environment and social and behavioral factors lead to better health. Consider Los Angeles in the 1990s. The air quality was poor; now, it's much improved. A study by investigators at the University of Southern California showed gains in lung function in children that paralleled improvement in air quality in Los Angeles. In 1998, 7.9 percent of 15-year-olds had significant lung defects. In 2011, the percentage of 15-year-olds with these lung defects had fallen to 3.6 percent [12].

While health challenges are often more pronounced for those with lower incomes, the challenges are embedded in the way most Americans live their lives. We tend to drive much more than we walk. We eat processed food rather than cooking fresh food. We sit in chairs for much of the day, staring at a screen. Increasingly, we do our shopping and get our entertainment without even leaving our homes. While these conveniences certainly have benefits, there are also trade-offs. One of them is that many researchers believe we now have a culture that is obesogenic (i.e., it contributes to obesity). "Our whole economy is driven toward convenience," says Abby King, a professor of health research and policy and of medicine at the Stanford School of Medicine, "and convenience often goes hand-in-hand with poorer choices in terms of health."

King is working to remedy this—not by eliminating the conveniences of modern life, but rather by spurring changes to local communities that can contribute to the health of people living in those communities. She and her team are doing this through empowering and activating residents themselves to be part of positive change in their local neighborhoods and communities. The global initiative that she leads, called Our Voice, has completed a range of projects, such as promoting better food and physical activity environments in low-income sections of California's San Mateo County [13], increasing the community's understanding of the variety of foods being offered at farmers' markets in Arizona [14], and investigating the walkability of higher- and lower-income neighborhoods in Mexico [15]. "We focus on monitoring, nudging, and activating residents to not just change their own behaviors, but also to change the context in which they and their neighbors live," says King [16].

They describe their efforts as "citizen science by the people," and the community engagement process begins with a mobile app called the Stanford Healthy Neighborhood Discovery Tool [17]. Using this app, residents walk around their environments and narrate what helps or hinders their health. They then meet with other residents to talk about what they've seen and learned, and then learn how to communicate this information and advocate for healthier neighborhoods with local decision makers. "People love to be engaged in this way," says King, "and see their neighborhood from a different perspective." Harnessing technology, she says, can help advance the ultimate goal: for everyone to lead healthy, active lives.

King and others are helping us understand the social, environmental, and behavioral determinants of health. This is vitally important, but it is not enough. We must also understand health in its entirety. William Osler, whom I mentioned in the introduction, moved medicine forward with his studies of the natural histories of diseases. Today's challenge is to understand the natural history of health. To begin to create such a history, researchers from Stanford Medicine and Verily are studying biological markers and recording health data from devices that will be worn by thousands of people. This data is enabling us to understand markers of health trajectories better than ever before.

We are also working to expand the understanding of wellness and well-being in a larger sense, with a focus on identifying what factors help people maintain health and wellness, in order to develop techniques that will help people to change their lifestyles. The Stanford Prevention Research Center, which I mentioned earlier, is on the frontlines of this effort. John Ioannidis, a professor of medicine at Stanford, is forthright about what he wants to achieve. "This is an effort to change the world of medicine and health," he says. "I see this as a way to refocus the key priorities of biomedical research."

> The vast majority of biomedical research has focused on treating diseases. A much smaller part has focused on maintaining health and maybe some prevention efforts. But there's very, very little research that has tried to look at the big picture—what makes people happy, resilient, creative, fully exploring their potential and living not only healthy, but more-than-healthy lives [18].

The center's research has involved enrolling 40,000 people—10,000 each in the United States, China, Taiwan, and Singapore, and possibly also other countries downstream—and asking them 76 questions that are connected to 10 different dimensions of well-being. Blood samples, as well as other biological samples collected from participants in most sites, will be available to be studied. These analyses, says Ioannidis, may reveal biological markers for wellness and well-being. "Just as we can monitor diabetes by looking at blood sugar levels, is there some biomarker that can tell us something about how one feels about one's life? Are there biomarkers that indicate levels of wellness and well-being and that change as people's levels of well-being increase or decrease?"

BEHAVIORS CAN CHANGE—AND DO CHANGE

I recognize that encouraging health-promoting choices is not an easy task—I once heard a Silicon Valley venture capitalist say he would never invest in a company that was trying to change human behavior, no matter how promising. But I believe that while it's certainly not easy, it can be done. Stanford Medicine research has already demonstrated how.

Abby King, whom I mentioned earlier, has spent her career studying how to encourage health-related behavior change, particularly among older adults and those living in disadvantaged communities. Again and again, she has found that motivationally targeted mobile apps significantly increase key health-promoting behaviors such as physical activity and spending less time sitting throughout the day. Analytical facts-and-figures approaches, which include personalized goal setting and self-monitoring, are effective, and so are social approaches, which include social comparisons, norms, and support.

The demand for diagnostic and motivational tools is growing. In March 2015, Stanford researchers introduced MyHeart Counts, a mobile health app developed by Stanford Medicine faculty that runs on Apple's ResearchKit platform. Just six months later, nearly 50,000 people had agreed to participate in a cardiovascular study connected to the app [19]. Its users can monitor their daily activities and risk factors for cardiovascular disease and then share this data with researchers. Though most people visit their doctor only a few times a year, their phone is almost always at hand. With MyHeart Counts, they can get continual feedback about their behaviors and how to improve those behaviors in a way that promotes heart health.

There are many other such tools, and they are helping to reorient health and health care throughout the world. One of them, a mobile app called reSET, manufactured by Novartis, is used to treat substance disorders. It was approved by the Food and Drug Administration in September 2017, and Novartis launched it in November 2018. The app is intended to be used as part of a 90-day prescription that also includes outpatient clinician-delivered care.

While digital technology can help drive behavioral change, the proliferation of this technology can contribute to an always-on environment, which leads many people to never quite disconnect. That interferes with activities like meals, exercise, social engagements, and sleep. It's a toxic combination that contributes to a variety of social maladies.

The writer and entrepreneur Arianna Huffington knows the cycle all too well: one day in 2007, she collapsed from exhaustion and broke her cheekbone in the process. She was diagnosed with acute burnout, and she says that as a result of the episode, "I made changes in my life, including renewing my estranged relationship with sleep and redefining my idea of success" [20]. Today, she's the leader of Thrive Global, which declares that its mission is "to end the epidemic of stress and burnout by changing the way we work and live."

The company is strongly focused on advancing prevention by changing behaviors. Huffington talks about "going upstream ... identifying and addressing stress triggers before they become symptoms." She believes that health outcomes can be changed "by focusing not just on the root causes of chronic and stress-related illnesses, but also on how well-being enhances performance."

Thrive Global emphasizes "Microsteps," which are small changes in behavior that eventually lead to healthier habits. They take many different forms: leaving electronic devices outside the bedroom (to foster better sleep), sitting down to eat (to promote more mindful consumption), holding meetings while walking (to promote exercise), responding to email only at certain times (to reduce distractions).

Huffington is a fan of B. J. Fogg, who is director of the Persuasive Tech Lab at Stanford. He talks about changing behavior through simplifying it. "The more you succeed, the more capable you get at succeeding in the future," Fogg says. "So you don't start with the hardest behaviors first, you start with the ones you want to do and you can do and you persist" [21].

* * *

There is a clear need for new ways of thinking across the entire health care community. The focus of medicine today is still on the clinical signs and symptoms that we can easily see and measure, such as an elevated blood-pressure reading or a patient's reports of fatigue. Rarely addressed are the factors that matter most and would yield rich insights into why the disease occurred in the first place.

Fundamental to the new thinking must be a recognition that medicine should not be seen as a game of catch-up—a matter of reactive, after-the-fact treatment. Instead, we must commit to not only curing disease definitively when it strikes but keeping people from getting sick altogether. This means transforming the societal view of health from negative ("We have it and then lose it") to positive ("We can optimize and enhance at any stage").

The encouraging news is that we are increasingly able to quantify the factors that affect our health and untangle the relationships among the four factors listed at the start of this chapter, thanks to data from electronic medical records, genomic sequences, biospecimen repositories, insurance records, and wearable sensors. We can now start to answer such questions as: How does our behavior affect our genes? How do our genes affect our social status? How does our socioeconomic status affect our behavior?

The more precisely we can answer these questions, the more we will be able to tailor treatment for that disease and, best of all, predict and prevent other diseases altogether.

CHAPTER 3

THE INNOVATION AND DISRUPTION POWERING PROGRESS IN HEALTH

Living in Silicon Valley for the past seven years has allowed me to meet countless individuals who are on the cutting edge of innovation, across multiple industries. Predictably, I'm often attracted to the latest and greatest innovations connected to biomedicine and health care, but innovations in other sectors are frequently of equal interest. Indeed, it is hard to imagine an area of innovation that one day won't have an impact on health and health care. I've included "Disruption" in the chapter title because certain innovations yield more than incremental changes— they disrupt entire industries. Think of Uber and Lyft relative to the transportation industry, or Airbnb with the lodging industry.

My interest in innovation reflects my intellectual curiosity, but it's much more than that. When I get daily reminders of all the ways in which there's significant room for improvement in both the U.S. health care system and the health conditions of the U.S. population, as I discussed in chapter 1, I get excited about the potential for new products and new ideas to deliver progress.

Much of the innovation and disruption featured in this chapter has happened at Stanford—a setting I always find intellectually stimulating, given that I regularly work with faculty members who think outside the box. (Or, as described by Lucy Shapiro, who is profiled below, "At Stanford, we don't just think outside the box. We don't even know there is a box.") This chapter includes examples of innovation and disruption because both are central to transforming health and health care delivery. Realizing the full benefit of innovation and disruption ultimately depends on commercialization. Although industry plays a critical role in that process, research universities and academic medical centers can and do as well. Indeed, the process of innovation, disruption, and commercialization can be accelerated when industry and academia work as partners. In this chapter, I describe how Stanford has encouraged that partnership and give examples of Stanford professors commercializing their research. I also provide examples of companies that are providing innovations and disruptions in health and the delivery of health care.

Discovering Precision Health: Predict, Prevent, and Cure to Advance Health and Well-Being, First Edition. Lloyd Minor and Matthew Rees.

COMMERCIALIZATION OF SCIENTIFIC AND TECHNOLOGICAL ADVANCES AND THE RELATIONSHIP BETWEEN ACADEMIA AND INDUSTRY

Countless scientific and technological advances that have led to broad-reaching improvements in health care can be traced back to research that began in academia. One recent example is cancer immunotherapy. Among the many different individuals who contributed to new insights about the pioneering treatment, two of the most important were James Allison and Tasuku Honjo. Their work led them both to receive the Nobel Prize for Physiology or Medicine in 2018, and both are based in academia. Allison is a professor at the MD Anderson Cancer Center, which is part of the University of Texas, and Honjo is a professor at Kyoto University in Japan. The knowledge they uncovered helped pharmaceutical companies develop drugs known as *checkpoint inhibitors*, which help the body's immune system ward off cancer.

Cooperation between academic institutions and industry often leads to concern about conflicts of interest. For example, patients may wonder if they are being prescribed a certain drug because the physician has a financial incentive to do so. This area has complex overtones of ethics, transparency, and integrity.

Management of conflict of interest requires a rigorous, nuanced approach that is rooted in strong institutional principles. Academic institutions such as Stanford University must remain trusted centers of discovery, innovation, and care delivery. We must have unbiased and ethical dedication to the best treatment available for our patients and to the preeminent pursuit of knowledge.

We also recognize that achieving the maximal impact of our scientific and technological advances requires commercialization. As will be evident from examples given in this chapter, the scaling and full translation of amazing advances made by our faculty is rarely possible within our institution, nor would such scaling be within the scope and intent of academic centers. An example is the screening of the many thousands of potential chemical compounds—not something academia is focused on doing—that could optimally reach a cellular target discovered in one of our laboratories. Correspondingly, the structure and organization of industries makes it difficult to achieve early-stage as well as fundamental, discovery-based lines of research. For these reasons, we work closely with the private sector, combining our expertise with theirs and working toward common goals, all while striking a delicate balance to avoid conflicts that could derail the important role of academic institutions in the pursuit of discovery and transformation.

Stanford carefully scrutinizes the relationships and financial arrangements between faculty, staff, and students with commercial entities. The fundamental underpinning of our policies governing conflict of interest is transparency. All individuals are required to formally disclose relationships with the private sector in an annual reporting process. These interactions are reviewed and monitored for potential conflicts. In addition to this annual reporting, a variety of mechanisms exist to provide oversight during the normal course of business. Examples of such oversight include contract negotiations, purchasing decisions, scientific presentations, clinical treatment decisions, development of new inventions, and patent filings.

Stanford takes strong measures to ensure that it remains true to its academic missions of objectivity, openness in science, and impartiality. With a few exceptions, technologies are licensed either nonexclusively or exclusively within a limited field of use. Stanford seeks a licensing strategy for each technology that will result in the broadest possible commercial application and that will maximize and accelerate societal benefit. Personal gifts are banned, and even student summer internships are reviewed to ensure that they don't bring the institution into conflict. In the care delivery setting, strong precautions are in place to avoid the emergence of incentives that could have an impact on decisions being made by physicians. Individual faculty members generally cannot be involved in a clinical trial of drugs they have had a role in developing, for example, and review and management processes are in place if financial conflicts of interest are identified.

At Stanford, oversight for these functions ultimately rests with me, as the dean of medicine, and with the dean of research at Stanford, along with the senior associate dean for clinical affairs and the senior associate dean for research. "Our ability to take a rigorous and nuanced approach to conflicts of interest is vital to keeping the engine of innovation running," says Michael Halaas, associate dean for industry relations and digital health.

HOW DIGITAL HEALTH CAN DRIVE DISRUPTION AND INNOVATION

One of the key drivers of innovation and disruption in health and health care is the burgeoning digital health sector. As I describe in more detail in chapter 5, there are many different digital health devices and tools, but they typically (1) feature consumer-focused devices and technologies and (2) involve artificial intelligence (AI) and data science to improve the delivery of health care. The two categories are intertwined, since the consumer-focused devices and tools typically generate data—data that may be interpreted by analytical approaches and methods.

In 2018, nearly $8.1 billion was invested in digital health startups—up from $5.7 billion in 2017 (which had been a record high) and just $1.1 billion in 2011. Rock Health, a venture capital firm, projects that the digital health market should grow to $120 billion in the next four to six years [1].

The optimism reflects an array of macro conditions: high penetration of mobile devices, expanding computing and storage power, data analytics, and advances in artificial intelligence. Specific to health care, greater understanding of the human genome, coupled with breakthroughs such as CRISPR, open vast new possibilities. These were some of the factors that led the celebrated internet analyst and investor Mary Meeker to observe in her 2017 "Internet Trends Report" that health care is at a "digital inflection point" [2]. (She also highlighted digital health adoption across generations, more hospitals enabling digital patient access, and growth in the number of personalized medicines.)

"There has never been a better time to be a digital health entrepreneur," says Ursheet Parikh, a health care investor at Mayfield, a Silicon Valley venture capital firm. But in order to succeed, says Parikh, companies in the digital health space must do four things in particular:

- Solve a truly hard health problem (such as detecting cancer early)
- Deliver a delightful user experience that results in sustained user engagement and behavioral change
- Be great enterprise entrepreneurs and navigate the complex health care ecosystem
- Create and own their own category and movement

None of those is simple, of course, and even amid the favorable conditions it's still very difficult for health-focused entrepreneurs (digital or otherwise) to succeed. Investors in health care understand this as well as anybody, and they are quick to name an array of challenges. One such challenge is the "significant informational asymmetries in health care," says Bill Evans, CEO of Rock Health.

> Not all participants share a common understanding or knowledge about how the market functions. That creates dislocations where supply signals and demand signals don't come together in an efficient market for new services—or even existing services.

Another challenge is how technology has been treated in health care, points out Hemant Taneja of General Catalyst, a venture capital firm based in Palo Alto.

> Technology hasn't really been the leverage point in how we deliver care inside of health systems, even though billions of dollars have been spent on digitization across the industry over the past 15 years. One result of this digitization has been that health systems have become less productive and they've had to hire more people. That's not what technology is supposed to do. The core issue is that health care is not an open innovation ecosystem, and it doesn't embrace a lot of the advances in technology that we see in other sectors. That's a function of how the health care–specific software companies have grown up. They have been very monolithic and closed, much like the mobile telephone carriers were 20 years ago.

These challenges underscore that one of the keys to succeeding in health care starts with something basic: understanding how the health care system works. "Those who are working in health care know the workflows, and they have the doctors, and they have the ability to really integrate and influence innovative tools," points out Sumbul Desai, a physician who serves as vice president of health at Apple, and who previously launched Stanford's first digital primary care clinic. "But then they're so caught up in the day-to-day of delivery and care that it's hard to make time to do that."

A related issue, notes Parikh, is the extraordinary complexity of the system.

In the United States, 70 percent of the hospitals are nonprofits, with the government accounting for 40 percent of expenditures. Entrepreneurs too often don't understand how selling to a nonprofit is different, and how the process and needs of this customer are different. Every sector has its share of regulations to deal with, and healthcare is more regulated than most. And yet despite that regulation, it's far from transparent: bureaucracies are opaque, and patients rarely actually see the costs that are being accrued. Most of the decision-makers for technology products here are not technologists and most users of the solutions are also not technologists. This is a special kind of playing field, and entrepreneurs need to learn the terrain [3].

Parikh adds that for innovators, another key to success is to "follow the money."

Tech businesses talk about "ecosystems" a lot, but it's especially true with healthcare: a health startup will exist as part of a large, complex system that at times will seem ossified. A lot of startups have gone belly-up by thinking they could somehow bypass all of this and sell directly to the consumer. You have to understand the money flow: who is the user, who is paying for it, and who has the incentive [4]?

Given these challenges, I recognize that change is always going to be incremental. The health care system is simply too multifaceted for there to be a rapid, wholesale disruption. But change is coming, and in this chapter I profile several different individuals and companies. Some are already having a disruptive impact within their sectors; others exhibit the kind of innovative thinking that I believe will ultimately drive medical progress—and advance the Precision Health vision along the way. This list of those profiled is not intended to be exhaustive, and I am certain that there are many outstanding companies and innovations not covered here.

THE ENVIRONMENTS THAT FOSTER INNOVATION

One of the keys to innovation is giving people the freedom and autonomy to take big chances and, ultimately, make big discoveries. That can mean going down paths that are both wrongheaded and expensive to correct. It also means allowing redundancies and inefficiencies to proliferate. But the blessing of a chaotic system is that it is so diverse that no approach can automatically be excluded. Over the long term, experimentation and innovation are the key ingredients needed to allow us to address challenges and seize opportunities.

In the environment I've just described, trial and error are fundamental, and there are more false starts and errors than successes. Those who are doing the experimentation not only need to be learning throughout this process; they also need to be able to unlearn. By that I mean they must be willing to put aside preconceived notions of what is "right," because those notions—and the knowledge that underpins them—can stifle creativity.

An example comes from Johns Hopkins University. In 1942, physicists there came together to form an organization called the Applied Physics Laboratory. During World War II, they developed a device that became known as a "proximity fuze." It was part of anti-aircraft shells and was programmed to detonate once it was close enough to the intended target. It's been described as "the real secret weapon of World War II" [5], and one factor behind its creation was the relative inexperience of those working on it. As the one-time director of the effort once observed, "It was lucky that they didn't understand engineering very well because they would never have attempted to build a little radio in the nose of an artillery shell accelerated at twenty thousand times the force of gravity. The Germans and the British both started to develop such a fuze but gave it up" [6].

A more recent example of inexperience contributing to a breakthrough was Steve Quake's invention of a blood test for pregnant women, as a substitute for the risky amniocentesis procedure—something I describe in more detail in chapter 5. His insight was not a byproduct of decades of research and experimentation. Instead, it was enabled by looking at the issue through a different lens than biologists and physicians who are focused on maternal and fetal health. As Quake has explained,

> At some level the blood test was such a simple idea, I'm shocked that nobody had thought of it. But one reason why is that in order for it to work, it required a much different perspective about DNA measurement. And the way people in biology have normally thought about measuring DNA just didn't work in this situation. But for me, coming from a physics background and having developed sequencers and having a deep understanding of how they work, I knew how to approach this sort of measurement. Coming from another field was critical to getting to the solution.

Quake's experience as an "outsider" affirms a key underpinning of innovation: diversity. This means diversity in all its forms—encompassing people from different professional disciplines, as well as people from different racial and socioeconomic backgrounds. Studying people from all backgrounds in research provides a more complete understanding of what causes disease and how to prevent it. Including people from various ethnic backgrounds in genomic studies and clinical trials is especially important when we consider the critical role of social, behavioral, and environmental factors on health outcomes and how policies and societal structures can place uneven and unjust physical and psychological burdens on certain groups.

Just as diversity drives innovation, I've also seen three other factors play important roles. I call them the three C's: combination, collaboration, and chance.

By combination I mean the complex and often unpredictable mix of phenomena, facts, concepts, variables, constants, techniques, theories, laws, questions, goals, and criteria. Elvis's rock and roll combined gospel music with rhythm and blues. Gutenberg's movable type borrowed from Chinese playing cards and wine presses. In medicine, combination often means drawing on insights and expertise from people who may not have medical backgrounds, such as engineers.

Collaboration is also fundamental to innovation. While pop history about invention and innovation often involves the stories of individual innovators, the reality is that even the greatest scientists—Isaac Newton, Charles Darwin, Albert Einstein, Thomas Edison—were always engaged in important and fundamental collaboration with their contemporaries. In medicine, collaboration is a cornerstone of research, and innovations are almost always a product of teams of people working together to develop new drugs, procedures, or products.

Finally, innovation depends on chance. The annals of science are full of serendipitous inventions or discoveries: the New World, ozone, dynamite, the phonograph, vaccination, X-rays, radioactivity, classical conditioning, penicillin, sulfa drugs, Teflon, Velcro, superglue, microwave ovens, and even Viagra, which was originally designed as a drug to reduce blood pressure. As 19th-century French biologist Louis Pasteur said, however, chance favors the prepared mind.

The three C's certainly came together with my own discovery in 1998 of superior canal dehiscence, which I described in the introduction. Understanding this debilitating disorder, characterized by sound- and pressure-induced dizziness, required a combination of basic research and clinical investigation, as well as mathematics, neurophysiology, biomedical engineering, and imaging science. I also benefited from the collaboration of colleagues in multiple settings, from conception of the problem to the development of the surgical solution. Chance played a role, too, as the discovery was made possible by patients who sought my care and was enabled by my observation that the eyes of these patients did not move randomly when they were exposed to loud noises or changes in pressure. Instead, they moved in the plane of one of the inner ear balance canals.

The three C's also appear in different forms in the work of today's innovators—individuals working in a diverse set of fields, who are united by their push to discover new therapies and new treatments, or just more reliable research, that will lead to improvements in human health.

HOW THE ARTS HELPED ADVANCE ANTIMICROBIAL THERAPY

Lucy Shapiro is a scientific pioneer. The Virginia and D. K. Ludwig Professor in the Department of Developmental Biology at Stanford, she has a long list of achievements. Very long. She has founded multiple companies. She's one of the creators of a field known as *systems biology*, making the landmark discovery that cells are controlled as an integrated genetic circuit that uses the three-dimensional structure of the cell to regulate all its functions. She has also developed entirely new small molecule approaches to antimicrobial therapy. In 2013, President Obama awarded her the National Medal of Science.

Creative thinking, underpinned by scientific rigor, has been a key ingredient in her recipe for success. In college, she had an unorthodox double major: biology and fine arts. She's pointed to her undergraduate organic chemistry class as having "changed my whole life … it was the impetus for my becoming a scientist." (Shapiro talked her way into the class—it was an honors course and she had no chemistry background.) The fascination stemmed, in part, from her background as a painter. She said it gave her an ability to visualize organic molecules in three dimensions, which is the fundamental basis by which molecules in the living cell talk to each other [7].

A distinguished career followed—Shapiro earned a PhD at the Albert Einstein College of Medicine and then spent nearly 20 years there as a professor. She came to Stanford from Columbia University in 1989, as the founder of the Department of Developmental Biology in the medical school. A 2018 profile published in *The Scientist* described her as "a unique thinker from the start of her scientific career. … Over a span of 50 years, she has continued to conduct research that has revealed how the genetics of a cell dictates its spatial dynamics and how this relationship feeds back to modulate genetic regulatory pathways" [8].

Emblematic of Shapiro's unique thinking was how she approached antimicrobial therapy. Unlike most others in the field, she didn't rely on known mechanisms of antibiotic therapy, and in some cases she didn't even rely on biological compounds. Her creative thinking proved useful when she was serving on a scientific advisory board for SmithKline Beecham, a pharmaceutical company. She and another member of the advisory board, Penn State chemist Steve Benkovic, were distressed that pharmaceutical companies were stalled in their development of new antibiotics. She told him, "We should be able to do this." In 1999, they set out to create an entirely new chemical space, by focusing on boron.

> It's just below carbon on the periodic table. It appears in nature. And nobody had ever made it druggable. So we decided to make a whole series of small compounds with boron at the active site. My friends working at pharma companies told me, "It'll never work." They said it would be toxic. But they hadn't done the experiments to test that assumption.

Shapiro and Benkovic did the chemistry, and boron-containing compounds turned out to be nontoxic and extremely effective in selectively inhibiting bacterial and fungal pathogens. Suddenly, she says, "we had a new chemical space for drugs."

In 2002, Shapiro and Benkovic started a company, Anacor, to commercialize their discovery. In 2010, Anacor became a publicly traded company, and in 2014, the FDA approved one of their products, tavaborole, marketed as Kerydin. It was, according to Shapiro, the first new antifungal in 50 years. The team further went on to design and gain FDA approval for a new class of boron-containing compound, crisaborole, currently marketed as Eucrisa, that is highly effective for eczema (atopic dermatitis) without any of the side effects of topical steroids. Two years later, Pfizer acquired Anacor for $5.2 billion.

Shapiro has cofounded another company, Boragen, which is focused on developing remedies for fungal infections that devastate crops such as bananas, soybeans, and wheat. She also remains particularly interested in antibiotic resistance—a topic I explore in more detail in chapter 6, highlighting the evidence that some medicines are becoming less effective in counteracting many infectious diseases. This worries Shapiro:

> I want new antibiotics. The trouble is, you make a new antibiotic and doctors put it on the back shelf because they want to save it for something that nothing else is working on. Whereas if they use it routinely, you're going to get resistance in no time. It's a terrible treadmill. My antifungals will ultimately run into the same problems with resistance. I'm trying to work around this by combining drugs, so if you have two drugs in one pill or one spray, the chances of developing resistance to an antibiotic decline enormously.

As with most public health challenges, there are no easy solutions to overcoming antibiotic resistance. But the workaround Shapiro mentions shows why it's a challenge perfectly suited for her, drawing on her deep knowledge of the inner workings of microbial cells coupled with an ability to see solutions where many other scientists only see obstacles.

SHATTERING THE STROKE TREATMENT STOPWATCH

Approximately 750,000 people in the United States experience a stroke every year. Groundbreaking research has recently upended the established wisdom about how quickly stroke victims need to be treated—leading to new guidelines and new opportunities for treatment.

Most strokes result from blood clots going into the brain and disrupting the flow of blood. The effects can be debilitating, including paralysis on one side of the body (and sometimes the entire body), memory loss, vision impairment, speech problems, and even death.

As recently as 1996, there was no effective treatment for strokes, and it wasn't even possible to see a brand-new stroke on any type of brain image. Patients would arrive in hospitals, seeming to be experiencing a massive stroke, and the pictures taken of the brain would be normal. As a result, neurologists couldn't tell where the stroke was, when it started, its magnitude, or whether there had been any irreversible injuries, and this was simply an accepted reality. In medical school, students were taught that there would probably never be an effective treatment for a stroke resulting from a thrombotic occlusion of blood vessels because it causes the brain tissue to die quickly, and thus the brain could not be rescued. The new treatments being tested did not distinguish between one person and another—the exact *opposite* of Precision Health.

The status quo started to change in 1992 when a Stanford radiology professor, Michael Moseley, achieved a major imaging discovery. He identified an

MRI (magnetic resonance imaging) sequence that could see a stroke in real time. This made it possible to see precisely where the brain was injured as well as the size of the stroke. Within a few years, MRI scans were being conducted on every stroke patient at Stanford, and they revealed something astonishing, says Greg Albers, a Stanford neurologist: "Everything we learned in medical school about stroke damage always happening so quickly was totally wrong."

> We would see some patients who would come in, and all of their brain was dead within a few hours. But we saw more patients who would come in many hours later, having been flown in by helicopter, and it looked like they were having a big stroke, and you looked at the new MRI picture, and there was only a tiny amount of damage. But then if you repeated the picture a day later, or two days later, then the big stroke had blossomed. That led us to believe stroke was potentially treatable even for patients who arrived late. While some patients were out of luck because their stroke did grow super-fast, in other people it grew slowly, which meant we could intervene. So we needed an intervention.

It had long been thought that two million neurons died every minute when a patient was having a stroke (the brain contains about 100 billion neurons). If that was true, patients could not be treated successfully at 6 or 12 or 16 hours after a stroke. In 1996, the FDA approved a clot-busting drug, using a three-hour time window. But, as Albers points out, "very few patients were treated because it's so hard to get a stroke patient to a hospital within three hours." (And because nearly one-third of all strokes occur when an individual is sleeping, it was even more difficult to meet the three-hour threshold.) The arbitrary time window did slowly expand, and eventually reached six hours using a mechanical device to physically remove the blood clot from the brain. Even so, countless patients were denied treatment for years. The message from doctors and hospitals was, in so many words, "I'm so sorry it took eight hours for you to get here, but it's too late. You can't be treated."

What these assumptions missed, says Albers, is any analysis of how an individual's brain reacts to a stroke. It was once thought that all brains reacted the same way. The reality is quite different. "Strokes are incredibly heterogeneous," says Albers, "so we need real-time imaging to make the best decision for each individual, and not simply use a stopwatch."

But in the absence of having a way to determine how a patient's stroke is evolving, treatment decisions are highly imprecise, since it's not clear whom to treat. If a patient's brain is dying instantly from a stroke, it doesn't matter if it's treated in 90 minutes, because the brain is already dead. But if a patient's brain is dying very slowly because the other blood vessels are helping, there may be no irreversible injury for 12 to 24 hours.

One of the early keys to more effectively treating a stroke was the development of techniques to pull the blood clot out of the brain. But to ensure that there would still be viable brain tissue to be salvaged by the restoration of blood flow, Albers and his colleagues put a huge amount of effort into the imaging. They focused on trying to determine the eventual size of the stroke if no treatment was given, since a stroke can start small and never grow, while others start small and grow progressively larger.

Then they developed software that could determine how much of the brain had died and how much was salvageable, first using images from an MRI scan and then later from a specialized CT scan. They conducted a trial involving patients who were having strokes but who arrived at the hospital six hours or more after their stroke began. (Six hours was believed to be the outside limit of treating people during a stroke.) The software was used to take a picture of the brain, and if it showed a large amount of salvageable tissue, the patient would be admitted to the trial. The patients were randomized in two similar studies. One was NIH-funded and called DEFUSE 3, and the other was conducted by an industry partner, Stryker, and called DAWN.

In these trials, patients who had substantial amounts of salvageable tissue were randomized into two groups. One group of patients received a thrombectomy, which is a procedure that involves guiding a stent through the circulatory system to the site of the brain clot and then using the stent to extract the clot. The other group of patients received standard medical therapy. The trials revealed that those who received a thrombectomy had much better outcomes than those who didn't. There were improvements among some patients even when their brain clots were removed up to 24 hours after the stroke symptoms had started. In DEFUSE 3, 45 percent treated with the clot removal procedure recovered without a disability. Among those who received standard therapy, only about 17 percent recovered without a disability.

Patients in the study were also followed for 90 days after their strokes. (After this time period, stroke patients typically experience little additional recovery.) At the end of the 90 days, among those who had received standard therapy, 26 percent had died and 16 percent had devastating disability. But among those who had received a thrombectomy, only 14 percent had died, and only 8 percent had severe disability. According to Albers, the DEFUSE 3 and DAWN results represented the largest treatment effect seen in any stroke-treatment trial to date [9].

Spurred by what Albers had discovered, in January 2018 the American Heart Association revised its guidelines on the treatment of strokes, extending the treatment window from 6 to 24 hours [10]. The *New England Journal of Medicine* also published an article coauthored by Albers that spelled out his findings [11]. Walter Koroshetz, MD, director of the National Institute of Neurological Disorders and Stroke, spoke to the significance of the Albers discovery: "These astounding results will have an immediate impact in the clinic and will help us save many lives. I really cannot overstate the size of this effect" [12].

One result of the findings, says Albers, is that the volume of thrombectomy procedures for late-arriving patients is likely to double. One beneficiary of the expanded treatment window is Cindi Dodd, a Salinas, California, graphic designer who shared her story with Stanford Medicine [13]. In April 2017, she experienced a massive ischemic stroke in her sleep. "My husband woke me up at 5 o'clock as planned [she was planning to go in for surgery], and when I started to speak to him, I knew what I was trying to say in my mind, but it had nothing to do with the sounds that were coming out of my mouth," Dodd said. Experiencing paralysis on the left side of her body, she was taken to a local hospital by ambulance. But because the attending physician there did not know when she'd experienced the stroke, she was told that a clot-busting medication could not be administered, and it was too late to undergo a thrombectomy. But an emergency room physician was aware of the DEFUSE 3 trial described above and Dodd's husband agreed to have her participate, which led to her being flown by helicopter to the Stanford Hospital (about 80 miles away, if traveling by car).

The brain imaging software showed that she had a large volume of salvageable brain even though she arrived beyond the six-hour treatment limit that existed at that time. This made it possible for Dodd to have a thrombectomy, and the procedure was successful. Seven days later, she had substantially improved and was discharged from the hospital. A year later, she told Stanford Medicine that she was almost fully recovered, thanks to the thrombectomy, intensive rehab, and personal initiative. "I am literally standing on this Earth as a wife and a mother because of that procedure," she said. "It saved my life" [14].

Resistance to Innovation

The breakthrough achieved by Albers and his colleagues points to the value of challenging established thinking in medicine, particularly when it comes to new treatments or cures, but also the determined resistance that disruptive thinkers can encounter.

When Albers and his team started doing MRI scans on every stroke patient, other doctors said they were imprudent and would ask questions like, "Why do you need that?" "Why are you spending money on MRI scans, when you aren't going to do anything different for the patient?"

Similarly, all the DEFUSE grant requests were originally rejected and needed to be resubmitted because the reviewers were highly skeptical. Even DEFUSE 3—the one that became a major breakthrough in stroke treatment—was criticized in multiple ways, said Albers.

> I was told, "There's going to be nobody home. You're trying to find patients who don't exist by looking in the late window and expecting to find people with salvageable tissue. So, it'll take you forever to do this trial." In fact, the enrollment rate for this trial was twice as fast as any previous thrombectomy study and enrollment was completed in one year.

The resistance was particularly intense at some academic journals. When Albers and his colleagues wrote papers, reviewers were often reluctant to accept them because the results did not fit with their expectations. Sometimes they would publish an accompanying editorial suggesting that imaging findings may not have clinical relevance.

Even with the breakthroughs, and the publication in the *New England Journal of Medicine*, Albers said the controversy has not completely died down. The root of the issue, he says, is non-precision versus the precision argument.

> Many people are invested in treating everybody the same. Their attitude is, "the sooner that we get the clot out, the better it is for the broad population of patients." But in this new world, we have to tailor treatment to the individual, not because the majority of people don't do well if you treat them within a chosen timeframe. That can hold for the population in general, but not necessarily for the patient in front of you [15].

DEVELOPING THE THERAPEUTIC OPPORTUNITIES ASSOCIATED WITH STEM CELLS AND REGENERATIVE MEDICINE

Irv Weissman's scientific career started in the summer of 1956 in the hospital of his hometown—Great Falls, Montana. He was just 16, but a meeting with the hospital's pathologist, Ernst Eichwald, led to an opportunity to work in Eichwald's lab, where he independently started conducting experiments in the area known as immunological tolerance. Those experiments helped spark a deep interest in biomedicine. After earning his bachelor's degree from Montana State University, he enrolled in the Stanford School of Medicine to be part of its five-year program that allowed students up to a half day every day to do scholarly work.

Weissman was hosted by Henry Kaplan, chair of radiology, and made a remarkable number of discoveries during medical school. He demonstrated that the thymus was not simply a gland, but that it produced and emigrated millions of T cells daily that homed to lymphoid organs. He also showed that immunological tolerance could be transferred from a tolerant host to a naïve newborn mouse of the same strain, providing an early, if not the first, demonstration that immune tolerance was not simply a lack of immunoreactive cells. Weissman's research in the intervening years has led him to develop the methods for isolating and lineage-tracing pure populations of lymphoid cells and stem cells, opening the field of modern stem cell biology. He's also led efforts to devise clinical translations in areas such as cancer and regenerative medicine.

His discoveries in the 1980s not only charted the separate locations of T and B lymphocytes in lymphoid organs (and their cohabitation of germinal centers upon antigen activation) but also led to his discovery, isolation, and characterization of homing receptors on both: CD62L for homing to lymph nodes and integrin $\alpha4\beta7$ for gut-associated lymphoid tissues. Antigen-activated lymphocytes replace both of these receptors with $\alpha4\beta1$, thereby enabling these T and B lymphocytes to enter inflamed tissues. Vedoluzimab, an antibody to integrin $\alpha4\beta7$, is currently a therapeutic used in patients with inflammatory bowel disease.

Among his many breakthroughs, in 1988 Weissman became the first person to identify and isolate blood-forming stem cells (hematopoietic stem cells, HSC) in mice [16]. In 1991, he extended this discovery to humans. These breakthroughs unlocked valuable new insights about the immune system. In 2000, Weissman isolated both human fetal brain stem cells and human acute myelogenous leukemia stem cells.

In the mid-1990s, Weissman began investigating bone marrow transplants, which were being done in order to give patients higher doses of chemotherapy. This was becoming a common treatment for women with breast cancer, so Weissman and colleagues at SyStemix and Stanford looked at the cellular composition of mobilized blood to see how many stem cells could be found there. He discovered that if a woman had metastatic breast cancer, her cancer cells were also in the blood and the bone marrow. As he explained in an interview, "The mobilized blood was being removed and frozen, the patient was being treated with a lethal dose of combination chemotherapy, thawing the cells and putting them back in. And when the cells were reinserted, so was the cancer."

He set out to test whether removing all the cancer cells by purifying the stem cells would improve the outcome. He had helped design the trial and was one of the coauthors of a paper published in 2012 by *Biology of Blood and Marrow Transplantation* that reported on a study comparing survival rates over 12 to 14 years among 22 women who received purified stem cells and 74 women whose chemotherapy involved unmanipulated, mobilized peripheral blood [17]. Among the Stanford cohort, most of whom had responded to their last chemotherapy regimen, the women who received the purified stem cells had a median survival of 120 months, and 33 percent of the women were still alive. Among the women receiving the untreated cells, the median time of survival was just 28 months, and only 9 percent were still alive. When the paper was published, another one of the authors, Judith Shizuru, a professor of medicine and of pediatrics at Stanford, said, "Most people in the oncology community feel that this issue is a done deal, that high-dose chemotherapy does not work for patients with breast cancer. But our study suggests that the high-dose therapy strategy can be modified to include the use of cancer-free purified blood stem cells to yield better overall outcomes in women with advanced breast cancer" [18].

In the brain stem cell field, Weissman and colleagues at Stem Cells, Inc., provided preclinical proof-of-principle that these cells could repair by regeneration a congenital lysosomal storage disease and a dysmyelinating disease. Noting that spinal cord–injured immune-deficient mice could overcome paralysis with these human brain stem cells, the studies have been extended to patients in clinical trials.

More recent research by Weissman and his researchers led to the discovery that most cancer cells are enveloped by a protein called CD47, and CD47 transmits "don't eat me" signals to cells known as macrophages, which normally scavenge pathological and dying cells, and also stimulate the immune system. Armed with this knowledge, Weissman developed an antibody, Hu5F9-G4, that counters

CD47 and causes macrophages to "eat" cancer cells [19]. The results from a clinical trial published in 2018 showed that using the antibody in combination with another antibody (rituximab) led half of the 22 patients with relapsed, refractory diffuse large B cell lymphoma (DLBCL) or follicular lymphomas (FL) to experience a clinically significant reduction in their cancers. Indeed, eight of these patients saw their cancer completely eliminated [20].

Harking back to his studies on immunological tolerance, Weissman demonstrated the induction of tolerance in allogeneic hosts with the transplantation of pure HSC from organ donor mice, including tolerance of heart, skin, and islets of Langerhans cells. Because pure HSC lack contaminating T cells, the recipients do not develop graft versus host disease. Transplanting HSC from autoimmune-resistant hosts to mouse strains that are predisposed to the development of auto-immune diabetes (type 1 diabetes) and system lupus erythematosus eliminated the autoimmune parts of the diseases.

To be able to treat patients who would be at serious risk if administered the lethal doses of chemoradiotherapy to eliminate host immune rejection of transplants, as well as to eliminate recipient diseased HSC and blood systems, Weissman initiated antibody conditioning of severe combined immunodeficient mice in 2007, now resulting in a trial with severe combined immunodeficiency (SCID) patients at Stanford. To extend this to non-SCID patients, Weissman et al. have included antibody cocktails that eliminate host immune cells and HSC and have observed their persistent immune tolerance to heart grafts only from the HSC donor [21]. These findings have established methods for the use of purified HSC from donors or pluripotent stem cell lines for regenerative medicine.

Like many innovative scientists, Weissman has encountered significant resistance to his ideas when he's put them forward. He wrote in 2016 that he learned an important lesson from these episodes: "The major barrier to scientific advancement and its translation to medicine are the holders of the conventional wisdom, and these holders may have the power to enforce their own understanding at the levels of journal review, grant review, and, most surprisingly, tenure review" [22]. He added, "I am delighted that Stanford Medical School has decided to reopen the five-to-six-year option, so that many of the leaders we train will have carried out extensive original research as well as learning medicine, which should help discoveries to be translated by those who understand experimental medicine."

Training the future leaders of stem cell biology, immunology, and biomedicine has been a passion of Weissman, and his trainees span the leadership of academia and the biopharma industry. These former trainees greatly value the time spent with Weissman and his ongoing mentorship, gathering to celebrate their mentor at major occasions. Ravi Majeti, former fellow in the Weissman lab and now professor of medicine, chief of the Division of Hematology at Stanford, said, "Training with Irv is an amazing experience due to his brilliant scientific ideas, culture of innovation in his group, and drive to make available all the necessary resources, but more importantly, Irv deeply cares for his trainees and works to ensure their success throughout their careers. Indeed, while his scientific legacy is embodied in his remarkable discoveries, it is equally manifest in the achievements of his trainees."

Weissman has been active outside the lab as well. He was on the founding scientific boards of three companies and was the founder of three companies focused on translating his stem cell discoveries into clinical applications, and recently another to translate the CD47 discoveries. In 2004, he was one of the architects of a statewide ballot initiative in California (Proposition 71) that was approved by 59 percent of the state's voters. The initiative set aside $3 billion in bond funding for support of stem cell research, which has been allocated through the California Institute of Regenerative Medicine. Some of these funds go toward training future scientists, and in a nod to Weissman's early start in science, there are even opportunities for those still in high school.

BRINGING INNOVATION TO IMMUNOLOGY

The quest for medical cures takes many different forms, but one commodity is often present, and has been for decades: mice. There are several reasons why, but most important is that their genetic and biological profiles are similar to those of humans. But curing mice of disease is very different than curing humans, and for a range of immunological and other conditions, mouse-derived conclusions can rarely be applied to humans, according to Mark Davis, the Burt and Marion Avery Family Professor of Immunology and Microbiology at Stanford. "While the mouse has been successful at uncovering basic immunological mechanisms, mice have been lousy models for clinical studies," says Davis, pointing specifically to shortcomings in studies around autoimmunity, cancer immunotherapy, and neurological diseases [23].

Davis happily plays the role of a rebel within immunology and has spent more than a decade trying to get his field to become less "mouse-centric" (as he calls it). He can make this statement with authority because earlier in his career he made many transformative discoveries about immunology from studies in mice, including identification of the first T-cell receptor genes. This work defined the mechanisms that enable T lymphocytes to locate and make a wide variety of responses to foreign entities.

Regarding the limitations of studies in mice, Davis says, "Mice have been 'cured' of many diseases that are thought to model human diseases. And then, with rare exceptions, when these are tried on humans, they don't work." He says there are many reasons for this, such as the evolutionary distance between mice and humans (65 million years) and their very different immune systems, as well as numerous other obvious differences. More fundamentally, says Davis, mice used in research are "artificial organisms living in artificial environments."

> They're something we made up in the laboratory, and they're purely inbred, which we know is harmful in the real world, but it's very convenient for lab experiments because they can all have the same genetic makeup. But

humans have a lot of genetic diversity, and so give a broader variety of immune responses, making it more difficult to isolate variables, but that's real life. And unlike mice, people don't live in cages covered in HEPA [high efficiency particulate air] filters for their entire lives to prevent infections. In the real world, people are outside, continually being exposed to viruses and other micro-organisms, and this is important for how the immune system develops. Or how it fails to develop properly, as the major model to explain allergies in children is that increased hygiene in developed countries has limited kids' exposure to microbes that helps to keep their immune systems in balance. But factors like this don't show up in research that's solely built around mice.

What's the solution? Davis says there's a clear need to collect more disease-specific data from humans.

> That will help with the building of better models, whatever they might be, but at least there will be a much better idea what the diseases are. And those models may lead to conclusions that have nothing to do with the mouse model, in which case researchers will need to go where the data takes them and try to understand the dynamics and the mechanisms that are involved— and attack them directly, rather than being so dependent on a species that just happens to be very convenient to work on.

Davis says he is receiving a better reception than in the past—he has been asked to write reviews in major immunological journals, and he was elected a councilor of the American Association of Immunologists ("probably the first real election I've ever won," he says), which puts him in line to be the association's president. But his goals are not focused on personal recognition. Davis is determined to modernize immunology. He points to the near absence of immunological information in medicine.

> The two main immunological assays that are used in general clinics today are white blood cell counts, which were developed in 1915, and complete blood cell counts, which were developed in 1959. Meanwhile, the field of basic immunology has exploded in the last 60 years, with 15 Nobel Prizes. But that's not reflected in the clinic. That needs to change, and high-quality, actionable human data that shows who is or isn't at risk for a particular disease is a critical springboard to enable that change.

One of those springboards is the Institute for Immunity, Transplantation and Infection at Stanford, where Davis serves as the director. Its focus is enabling researchers to use advanced immunological tools to understand what a healthy immune system looks like and what are the signs of impending illness. Many groups at Stanford have taken advantage of this expertise, particularly with the Institute's unique Human Immune Monitoring Center, with hundreds of projects being carried out to probe the immune system in a wide variety of different diseases.

THE APPROACHING REVOLUTION IN SLEEP RESEARCH

In chapter 1, I catalogued some of the worrying developments in U.S. public health. One simple behavior has the potential to help cure many of these conditions—and even prevent them from arising: sleep. More specifically, sleeping well and enough hours every night. But the United States is, increasingly, a nation marked by sleep deprivation and sleep disorders. Thirty-five percent of the country's adults regularly sleep less than seven hours each night, according to a federal government report published in 2016 [24], and an estimated 50 million to 70 million people in the United States suffer from sleep disorders. The two developments are connected, and while the environment for sleep has become more challenging in recent years, new tools are emerging that enable a better understanding of the biology of sleep— a development that's helping with prediction and prevention of sleep disorders and may eventually improve detection and treatment.

That's according to Emmanuel Mignot, the Craig Reynolds Professor of Sleep Medicine at Stanford. Sleep research has a long and distinguished history at Stanford, beginning with William Dement, emeritus professor of psychiatry and behavior sciences, who was involved in the discovery of rapid eye movement (REM) sleep, a particular stage of sleep in which the body is paralyzed and we dream. Mignot has been studying sleep since 1986. In 2000, he discovered the cause of narcolepsy, which is a disease that leads patients to go so quickly into REM sleep that they experience symptoms of being half awake and half in REM sleep, dreaming awake, or being paralyzed but awake after waking up.

The discovery—the culmination of more than 10 years of research—was enabled by his research into a gene mutation that causes narcolepsy in dogs. (Mignot owned a narcoleptic Schipperke named Bear during much of that period, and today has a narcoleptic Chihuahua named Watson.) This led to the discovery that a total absence of a neurotransmitter called hypocretin or orexin (due to an autoimmune attack of hypocretin cells) causes human narcolepsy—a sleep disorder that affects an estimated four million people globally. New hypnotics and stimulants that modulate hypocretin are being developed today, thanks to this discovery.

Given the nexus between getting enough sleep and staying healthy, it's striking that sleep has only recently started to receive significant attention from medical researchers. There are a few different reasons for this, according to Mignot. One is that many of the most important discoveries are, by medical standards, relatively recent. REM sleep and sleep apnea were only discovered in 1953 and 1965, respectively. The medical and scientific fields have also exhibited skepticism about the very existence of certain sleep disorders. When Mignot attended neurology conferences in the 1990s and talked about narcolepsy affecting hundreds of thousands of people, he was often told variations of "It is impossible,

I have never seen a case" [25]. Another issue, says Mignot, is that sleep researchers don't have a natural home in academic medical centers.

Clinicians and researchers working in sleep medicine come from disparate disciplines. Some are pulmonary medicine physicians because of sleep apnea. Psychiatrists and psychologists often focus on insomnia. Neurologists focus on narcolepsy, restless leg syndrome, and REM sleep behavior disorder (acting out one's dream, a precursor of Parkinson's disease). ENT surgeons can operate on sleep apnea patients to help them breathe. Researchers work in devices, engineering, neurosciences, and genetics. It's very multidisciplinary, and that makes it harder to work within traditional structures of academic medical centers.

But today, research into sleep is undergoing a revolution, thanks in large part to the emergence of better technologies. Mignot notes that the most commonly used tool to measure sleep and diagnose sleep disorders—nocturnal polysomnography (PSG)—is cumbersome and expensive, and does not reflect normal sleep. Multiple electrodes are affixed to the body of patients and they must sleep in a laboratory, on an unfamiliar bed that may be uncomfortable for some people. Once an overnight session has been completed, the results are calculated based on visual inspection and a tally of factors such as depth of sleep (sleep stages), respiratory activity (sleep apnea), and leg movement (restless leg syndrome). The interpretation is very imprecise, according to Mignot. "The process is subject to human errors and depends on the quality of the scorer. It is also non-reproducible in the sense that the same technician will not score the exact same sleep recordings the same way twice" [26].

The PSG has been in use for 50 years, but Mignot says it is in the process of being displaced by something much more modern: machine learning tools. He was the lead author of a 2018 study, published in *Nature Communication,* that showed how these tools are more accurate than humans in scoring PSG and in detecting sleep disorders [27]. He sees them as particularly useful in detecting a disorder such as narcolepsy.

When we started to use machine learning for sleep scoring in narcoleptic patients, we discovered that very often the program had trouble distinguishing wake and REM (dreaming) sleep, giving equal probability to both, almost as if the patient was in between these stages. We then developed a new algorithm based on this to diagnose narcolepsy. It's an example of how machine learning can replicate what normal humans do (scoring sleep stages on a PSG), but also do better by providing more information that enables a narcolepsy diagnosis. It is cheaper and simpler than the current standard for diagnosing narcolepsy, which involves studying patients when they nap during the day. Here we can just go through a night PSG and automatically output if someone has narcolepsy.

The use of machine learning is just one way in which the field of sleep research is going to be transformed, says Mignot, pointing to the development of smaller, less obtrusive devices to measure sleep signals.

In my lifetime, people will no longer go through a traditional in-laboratory PSG sleep study, unless they have very unusual problems. Instead, they will go home, have a small electrode attached to their forehead, a tiny microphone close to their throat, and a monitor on their legs. It will all be wireless, and the data that's generated will be automatically uploaded and scored by machine learning—making it possible to know if someone has a sleep disorder and how severe it is. All of this information can be processed weekly or monthly, and the individual will be notified if something starts to look wrong. We may also be able to predict the development of psychiatric disorders and neurological problems before they show up in daily life. Sleep could be monitored as a brain health check to see if something starts to go wrong and develop preventative at-home therapies.

Using sleep monitoring as a tool of prediction and prevention can hopefully translate to people sleeping better—and longer. That could have far-reaching ripple effects, for the simple reason that "sleep is really important to everything," says Mignot. He cites multiple health hazards associated with impaired sleep patterns. "If you have sleep apnea," he says, "your risk of stroke goes through the roof." Sleep disorders also contribute to metabolic conditions, such as diabetes and obesity, as well as psychiatric ones, such as depression and anxiety, and they feed on each other in a vicious circle: when people are depressed, they start to sleep poorly, which exacerbates depression.

But amid hope for greater progress in prediction and prevention, cures remain elusive—those with sleep apnea need to make do with an unwieldy device that delivers pressurized air to the back of the throat. The shortage of therapies is partly a product of something basic: there is still much more to learn about sleep. As Mignot points out, while there has been an explosion in clinical approaches to sleep, it's "an oversized clinical field with relatively little basic science" [28]. Even the molecular mechanisms of why we feel sleepy when we don't sleep enough are not well understood.

THE PROGRESS UNDERWAY IN PREDICTING, PREVENTING, AND CURING ALLERGIES

Allergies are among the most common medical conditions in the United States, and their incidence has been rising. But more precise diagnostic tools are emerging to predict their onset, and we're learning that early interventions with infants can help them ward off allergies throughout childhood and perhaps for the rest of their lives. Kari Nadeau, director of the Sean N. Parker Center for Allergy and Asthma Research at Stanford University and Naddisy Foundation Professor of Medicine and Pediatrics at Stanford, has been at the forefront of efforts to inject the Precision Health tenets of predict, prevent, and cure into allergy and asthma care.

Approximately 26 million adults are believed to suffer from a food allergy, according to a 2019 article coauthored by Nadeau and published in the *Journal of the American Medical Association* [29]. About 5.6 million children also suffer from such allergies [30]. From 1997 to 2011, there was a 50 percent increase in the incidence of food allergies among children [31].

Allergies can stem from a wide variety of factors. One culprit is the poor state of the current diets around the world, as being overweight or obese wreaks havoc with the dysfunctional immune system, which can increase vulnerability to one type of allergy, asthma. Lack of dietary diversity early in infants, increases in skin dryness, decreases in vitamin D levels, and lack of good microbes in the gut are some of the reasons why allergies are on the rise. Another culprit is climate change. Nadeau points out that "pollens are being emitted about two to four times longer in a year than they were in the past, and when coupled with pH change in the air (our air is getting more acidic because of the CO_2 emissions), it means that on any given day, there can be tenfold as much pollen in the air because the chemistry of the pollen from the plants is now different."

Allergies can also be triggered when misinformation drives unhealthy behavioral changes. Nadeau says the incidence of allergies mushroomed around 2000—a product of ill-advised recommendations by the American Academy of Pediatrics and other entities throughout the world not to give infants milk, peanuts, shrimp, and other products until they turned two or three. "But then a major study was done," says Nadeau, "and it showed precisely the opposite—so we think that diversifying the diet early is important because the gut naturally tolerizes itself to items that you eat." She points out that some of the lowest food allergy rates in the world are in countries like Norway and Austria, where the guidelines were seldom followed.

In addition to dietary patterns, more is being learned about what works and what doesn't when it comes to preventing allergies in children. This includes ensuring that they have sufficient levels of vitamin D and even exposing them to "more dirt." "We now know that among children who lived in a home with a dog during their first year of life, allergies and asthma are reduced by a factor of five," says Nadeau. "There is something about having a dog and exposing all of its outside microbiota to the infant. While we can't go back to our old lifestyles of living on the farm, it's clear that our bodies were likely meant to evolve with other animals, with a good skin barrier, and with a diverse diet."

Even with increased emphasis on prevention, there will still be a need for diagnostic tools, which today are "subpar and not precise," says Nadeau. She points out how little progress there has been in this area until recently. "We've been relying on skin prick tests for about a century and they haven't changed much. Nor are they particularly good at actually diagnosing allergies or asthma." Blood tests are also used to detect allergies, but they only search for a single antibody, IgE, out of many other features of the immune system involved in allergy.

Nadeau's lab has been developing a more comprehensive blood test. Instead of looking at only the IgE levels, the test also is designed to look at all the cells and molecules involved in an allergic response. They incubate two drops of blood with about 96 different allergens (cat, insect, food, drug, etc.) in order to detect an allergic reaction. This saves individuals from having to be exposed to these allergens via a skin prick test—and, says Nadeau, "it might allow us to predict allergies before they start and allow us to follow allergies and their severity if they have already started."

Research conducted at Stanford's Sean Parker Center for Allergy and Asthma Research has led to patented technology, and Stanford has been involved with the launch of three companies focused on allergies—one for prevention, one for care, and one for therapy. Stanford has also conducted clinical trials that involve gene therapy to eliminate food allergies.

Nadeau is excited by the flurry of activity happening in allergy and asthma research, pointing to a large increase in NIH funding to study fatal allergies and more than a dozen new companies developing drugs to combat allergies and asthma. Ten years ago, says Nadeau, there weren't many companies doing drug development in severe allergies and asthma. "It's been incredible to be in this field for the last decade and to see how much progress has been made."

Nadeau's research is helping to drive that progress. So is her entrepreneurial spirit. She's the cofounder of a company called Before Brands, which is focused on preventing the onset of allergies in children. The company's product, SpoonfulOne, can be served to infants, starting from liquids that can be mixed with other foods to puffs that can be consumed once an infant has transitioned to solids. The products contain all the food groups that cause more than 90 percent of food allergies. "With precise portions," says Nadeau, "it takes repeated dietary exposure over time to safely allow a baby's immune system to grow up accustomed to a diverse range of foods. Exposure to the product helps train the child's digestive system to accept food as food, rather than as an allergen."

Nadeau says she wanted to start a company focused on an infant food supplement for a simple reason: "The vast majority of allergies can be prevented, and the earlier we introduce preventive measures with infants, the greater the likelihood that we'll succeed in inhibiting the allergens and reduce the need for medical therapies." And while there will always be exogenous factors contributing to allergies and asthma (like climate change), it's clear that the future holds much greater precision when it comes to diagnosis and treatment.

THE PROGRESS TOWARD PREDICTING, PREVENTING, AND CURING MENTAL ILLNESS

Mental illnesses pose one of the biggest challenges to public health. They afflict an estimated 44.7 million adults in the United States (close to 20 percent of the total number of adults), according to the National Institute of Mental Health, a federal government agency [32]. Globally, it's estimated that the most common such illness—depression—affects 323 million people globally. Those large numbers mask one of the heartbreaking realities about the U.S. medical system: it's very poorly equipped to diagnose and treat mental illness. Also, there is considerable imprecision in the treatment of depression and other mental health conditions. As Stanford's Leanne Williams explains,

> While there are many effective treatments for depression, guessing who will respond to which treatment is all too often a shot in the dark. Depression is a catch-all diagnosis that lumps together patients experiencing a wide range of symptoms with different underlying brain dysfunction [33].

Williams is a professor of psychiatry and behavioral science as well as director of Stanford's Center for Precision Mental Health and Wellness, which launched in April 2018. She sees an urgent need for a greater understanding of how malfunctioning brain circuitry causes specific symptoms in each patient, and how to guide treatments that correct these underlying malfunctions.

The U.S. medical system has been poorly equipped to diagnose and treat mental illness. But even without that misguided framework, there hasn't been a sufficiently deep understanding of the brain to predict, prevent, or cure mental illness with much accuracy. That's beginning to change, though. "The breakthroughs have really escalated in just the last five years," says Williams, "to the point that we have enough understanding of the human brain in action to develop a model giving us a biological frame for how to diagnose mental diseases."

Williams attributes some of this progress to the Human Connectome Project, a National Institutes of Health undertaking that's roughly equivalent to the Human Genome Project. The Connectome Project has been focused on mapping the detailed, defined structure and functions of the human brain. The project has led to advanced sequences of brain images that are enabling much greater precision related to temporal and spatial resolution. The result, says Williams, "has been a whole new set of maps of what is wiring an actual brain. We have a deeper understanding of how the brain communicates—we can see the literal cables, blood flow changes in activation, and the functional and structural connections between regions."

As a result of this deeper understanding, we can accelerate our discovery and translation in at least three directions. We can elucidate the progression of brain changes across different stages or phases of illness, between people with different mental illnesses, and across subtypes within an illness. We can also predict which treatments may be best suited to each illness and subtype, and the mechanisms by which the treatment works. In addition, we can use structural and functional connectivity measures to understand risk factors and develop novel approaches for early detection, intervention, and ultimately prevention.

New technologies have also helped unlock new information about the brain. One of them is called *transcranial magnetic stimulation*. It is an FDA-approved noninvasive approach to stimulating brain networks and returning them to a healthy state. It involves attaching an electromagnetic coil to the scalp and stimulating those nerve cells associated with depression.

Williams has been at the forefront of using another breakthrough technology, known as *multi-band imaging*, with functional MRI. Rather than providing a single image of the brain, which has been the standard for many years, the functional MRI, optimized for spatial and temporal precision with the multi-band technology, enables multiple snapshots of the brain (as many as 400) over five minutes and tracks how it is communicating. The functional MRI also illuminates different types of depression (known as *biotypes*), which show faulty neural networks. "It gives us a way to look at how the brain is functioning in real time, and that gives us a way to understand healthy regulation of the emotions and thought because we can literally see what the brain is doing second by second. Armed with this information, we can measure and quantify what happens when that healthy regulation of emotions and thoughts breaks down."

Big data, blended with computational horsepower, is also enabling new insights. Each of the functional MRI's precise multi-band images generates about 50 gigabytes of data, and Williams typically works with thousands of images. She says that 10 years ago, it would take her and colleagues five months to quantify all the data and reach conclusions. Today, she says, her team is road-testing the system for processing and quantifying the same volume of images in five hours.

Williams and her colleagues have drawn on these developments when conducting the first translational trials backed by neuroscience. They have the largest data sets in the world, and they have characterized eight biotypes for different types of depression. Subtyping precision is informing which therapies to offer for depression. In the current system, it is necessary to try one treatment, wait for two to three months to see if it works, and then try another if it does not. Typically, only one-third of people recover after the first treatment they try. Clinicians, patients, and families alike all want tools that will help get the right treatment, the first time, for many more people. In her translational trials, Williams assessed patients with functional MRI and other neuroscience measures, including genetics, before they received treatment with commonly used antidepressants. She found that, with knowledge of faulty neural networks, the accuracy of predicting who would respond well to treatment could be increased to over 70 percent.

As Williams and her colleagues work toward developing better predictive powers, the translational trials backed by neuroscience have also revealed a breakthrough using genomic information to predict how individuals are likely to respond to specific therapies. "If you are prescribed an antidepressant, but we know you have a gene that is very slow in shifting the chemical across the blood-brain barrier, then we can prescribe a higher dose of that antidepressant. We can also uncover subgroups of people who might benefit—because of their genes—from starting on a less common antidepressant, rather than going through trial-and-error with more common antidepressants. Genes turn out to be very relevant to saying not only what medication is relevant but what dose and how to minimize side effects."

> We are continually refining the biotypes to consider personal variations—using genetics, life experience, social and clinical information. No two brains are the same. One brain might respond to certain medications and therapies,

but another might need an entirely new form of treatment. By precisely identifying the type of short circuit in the brain, we can design customized treatments and, ultimately, preventions to target that specific short circuit, for the right person at the right time.

In 2017, Williams completed a study, known as RAD ("Research on Anxiety and Depression"), that was the first of its kind to take a large cohort of people with different levels of depression and anxiety. Using advanced, precise imaging, she mapped how their brains were functioning, with an emphasis on serving as an early-detection system. She also took detailed measures of their symptom experiences and daily coping. The RAD study built on a decade-long effort to accumulate standardized information about depression and anxiety. With this pool of data, she identified different types of anxiety and depression that are replicated across samples. These subtypes correlate with the activation of different brain networks and relate to different aspects of daily functioning.

She says the next step is to fuse the genetic information and the brain imaging "because we know from fundamental neural science that genes influence how brain circuits develop and function. Your genes might make you more prone to stress, for example." The goal, she says, is to understand how the brain imaging map relates to the genomic map. "That space needs a lot of attention, because the combination will be really powerful—just as it has been for cancer medicine."

The progress in developing precise cures is leading to a renewed focus on predicting which individuals may eventually develop a mental disease. Williams says that once there's been more progress in developing a new diagnostic system, based on the identification of specific conditions, it will be possible to focus on the predictors of those conditions. "What are the early signs of that happening before the illness develops? It is very hard to assess prediction or to raise any question until you know what the actual consequence is."

Williams and her colleagues look at first-degree sons and daughters of parents who have had depression. "They are healthy, but they have a familial predisposition to depression. We can use imaging to track how their brain is functioning, and then look at what's changing that could be an early sign of risk, even in the absence of any symptoms." She draws a parallel to women getting mammograms on a regular basis to see if a risk factor is emerging. "Something like that could be done with brain scans. If you know you have some genetic risk, regular scans will give you a sense of whether that genetic risk is getting expressed."

But even amid extensive medical progress, challenges remain. Predictive and preventive tools focused on mental health are far less developed than they are for other conditions. There is nothing equivalent to the Apple Watch that has been used in a study to detect atrial fibrillation (described further in chapter 5). Even if there were, its utility might be limited. "The research linked to the Apple Watch was anchored in our understanding of how the heart functions and the signals we need to track in real time," says Williams. "Today, while brain sensors are being developed, we have a very incomplete understanding of how the brain functions.

We're often relying on subjective symptoms, and if we use those subjective symptoms as our standards, that means the sensors are going to be tied to something suboptimal and an incomplete picture of the underlying process."

There is one other significant barrier: the long-standing stigma associated with mental conditions. Williams recounts how she meets with very smart, and very high-performing, people from Silicon Valley's technology companies. "They feel like if they're diagnosed with depression, that it's a sign of character weakness. Or that they've somehow 'failed.' They're often uncomfortable even discussing it. They believe they should be able to cope and push through."

What's encouraging, however, is an erosion in that stigma. "The precise measurement of mental health that's now possible is making things more tangible and really giving people a way to talk about depression without feeling stigmatized," says Williams. She often describes one's mental health as being akin to one's blood pressure. "It varies across everyone. And each person's mental health will fluctuate." She says that she talks about how the circuits in a person's brain go into an extreme state and take over the ability to feel anything, which is what constitutes one form of depression. "When people I meet with can see an actual picture of it happening, they are much more understanding and want to know how treatments could bring their brain back into the healthy range. It's just a different way for them to talk about it so that they don't think their depression is their fault."

The changing perception about depression is emblematic of the progress we're seeing across the mental health landscape. Much of that progress is reflected in the precision that's become infused into efforts to predict, prevent, and cure mental illness. That progress is long overdue and will benefit millions of people in the United States and throughout the world.

Disrupting Mental Health Diagnoses

Amit Etkin, a professor of psychiatry and behavioral sciences at Stanford, is determined to bring greater precision to mental health—with a focus on developing treatments that are uniquely tailored to each individual. To achieve this, he wants to upend many long-established practices in the mental health field. He's generating valuable new insights, particularly as his research leverages the potential of machine learning.

Etkin's approach starts from the premise that psychiatric diagnoses are riddled with shortcomings. He sees them as highly imprecise—based on arbitrary checklists of symptoms that may not reflect the challenges being faced by an individual. He also says that these diagnoses do not describe biology very well. In other words, brain imaging does not reveal the kinds of differences you would expect between diagnoses if they described biologically distinct entities. Likewise, Etkin has found that perhaps the strongest signal that emerges with brain imaging when comparing diagnoses is a set of abnormalities that every psychiatric diagnosis shares relative to healthy individuals. "Psychiatric diagnoses may have misled us more than they've helped us in terms of understanding what's actually wrong with the brain and how to treat it."

The focus of mental health treatment, says Etkin, should shift from diagnosis to developing a deep understanding of each individual's brain and then making judgments or predictions based on that understanding. Etkin calls this a "circuits first" approach. As he explained to *Scientific American,*

> We understand behavior is essentially underpinned by brain circuits. That is, there are circuits in the brain that determine certain types of behaviors and certain types of thoughts and feelings. That's probably the most useful way of organizing brain function. If you can start characterizing circuit disruptions for compensatory symptoms at an individual subject level and then link that to how you can provide interventions, then you can get away completely from diagnoses and can intervene with brain function in a directed way [34].

Etkin has been particularly focused on antidepressants—seeing them as a symbol of how the mental health field has poorly served its patients. He points to the work of Irving Kirsch, who in 2008 published a paper that was based on the first large-scale meta-analysis of clinical data on antidepressants submitted to the FDA. Kirsch concluded that antidepressants were only slightly more effective than placebos—and not clinically significant enough to have patients use them [35].

But Etkin thinks it's misguided to worry about whether antidepressants are effective treatments for depression. "The hand-wringing should really be about whether depression even works as a diagnosis." The real focus, he says, should be on identifying whose brain is most amenable to the actions of an antidepressant, since the antidepressant is going to work differently in different people. Once that amenability has been pinpointed, "you can actually use the medication to define the patient, as opposed to using the patient to define the medication."

Etkin has also been part of the largest study on record seeking to understand how baseline brain function predicts clinical outcome with an antidepressant versus placebo. His group was the first to use machine learning, building on a novel method developed in his lab, to find a brain signature that distinguishes between who will respond to the antidepressant specifically, and not to placebo. Doing so identifies people not only who will see a clear benefit of the antidepressant— expecting a response rate that is double that with placebo—but also whose outcome with an antidepressant will be worse than with a placebo. The latter group of people would be those for whom the medication does not work, and all they experience is the medication's side effects. Indeed, the very fact that response to medication could be distinguished from that to placebo using baseline brain data and machine learning suggests that the drug may act in specific and potent ways, but that since it is given to a broad and unselected patient population, its impact is diluted by mixing responders and nonresponders. In other words, it does seem that the medication can better define the patient than his or her diagnosis.

According to Etkin, the study "sets the stage for a much more rigorous and effective approach to precision medication in psychiatry by just knowing what you are doing with brain data." He argues that there are multiple meaningful ways to objectively anchor such studies, including a wide variety of interventions, each of which will push our understanding of both psychiatric illnesses and their treatment further in a clinically useful direction. With brain data more easily accessible, Etkin says, clinics could conduct low-cost tests of electrical activity in the brain (known as EEG tests). This brings access to the brain—the organ at the heart of mental illness—directly into the point-of-care clinically. As EEG technology improves, driven in part by clinical applications of EEG, Etkin also foresees these becoming take-home tests using even lower-cost devices.

The machine learning was preceded by what Etkin identifies as another highly significant development: "We've moved from using brain imaging as a way of characterizing groups ... to characterizing individuals" [36]. He is also particularly enthusiastic about marrying tools like EEG to a form of neuro-modulation called *transcranial magnetic stimulation* (TMS). As a form of non-invasive brain stimulation, TMS is useful for understanding how brain activity can be shaped through repetitive stimulation. Indeed, first-generation TMS has already been developed for the treatment of depression. However, since TMS makes it possible to turn brain circuits on and off, using a focal magnetic field, its ultimate full potential has yet to be realized. "Using brain imaging, we can see the effects on the brain while it's being stimulated, and using that combination we've started to identify regions that act like those brain circuit switches. This allows us to manipulate brain circuits in a targeted manner" [37]. That targeted approach offers much more precision than the standard form of treatment for depression: a pill.

> There's been this assumption that medications are either preferred or maybe the best way to go about treating things, and that comes a bit from the history of psychiatry but also from the rest of medicine. I'm not sure that a pill is necessarily going to be the best approach for psychiatry. Washing the brain in a drug that affects many parts of the brain, and also affects many parts of the body, is a pretty crude and nonspecific way to affect a very discrete part of the brain. In contrast, as our neurostimulation approaches have proved, we can have a lot more specificity for our target [38].

Etkin is enthused by the progress that's been achieved in just the past few years. But for that progress to continue, he says, "we need to come up with a different way of understanding mental illness—a way that involves the brain, a way that involves new flexible therapeutics, and really take advantage of the revolutions in brain science that have yet to permeate psychiatry" [39].

Transforming Mental Health Treatment through Measurement

Paul Dagum is another innovator in the world of mental health. He's the founder and CEO of Mindstrong, a company founded in 2014 and dedicated to reorienting the treatment of mental illness, with an emphasis on using digital tools in two ways: to improve the diagnosis of mental illnesses and to help treatment become less reactive and more preemptive.

As with many innovators, Dagum's background is a few steps removed from the field he's looking to transform. He earned a medical degree from Stanford in 1994 and later published widely on the intersection of computer science and medicine. He's credited with achieving breakthroughs in several areas, such as quantifying the pathophysiological mechanism of mitral valve disease. But frustrated by the inability to have health and medical innovations make their way into the clinic, he left the practice of medicine in 2000, and for about the next 15 years he worked at several successful technology companies. (One company he cofounded, Rapt, was later acquired by Microsoft.) He has published more than 75 peer-reviewed articles and book chapters, encompassing both medicine and computer science, and he's been awarded more than 25 patents, in areas from algorithms used with big data to digital measures of the central nervous system.

While he was a senior executive at a cybersecurity company from 2009 through 2013, he and his colleagues discovered that they could synthesize all the information generated by individuals' online activity and use it to create a *digital fingerprint*. He wanted to learn more, and he knew that the societal burden of mental health and neurodegenerative disorders was worsening at an alarming rate.

> We still had no major clinical way to measure brain health, whether it was neurodegeneration and/or mental health outside of the laboratory. I was very intrigued by the possibilities connected to the digital fingerprint we had discovered. It wasn't simply idiosyncratic but that there was some component of that fingerprint that was a systematic measure of cognitive ability or disability in the moment or in that day. That's what intrigued me, and that's what I set out to investigate.

In 2013, he and some of his former Stanford colleagues launched two Institutional Review Board–approved clinical studies in the Bay Area. The studies involved an app they created that would sit on a smartphone and capture every touch-screen interaction that individuals had with their phones, to reconstruct the digital fingerprint—also known as a *digital phenotype*. One hundred and fifty participants were consented and enrolled in the studies, and each of them received a four-hour cognitive assessment from a neuropsychologist. Over the next year, the app collected data from each participant's activity, monitoring routine actions during normal day-to-day use of their smartphone—all of which was expected to help provide insights into the individual's mental state.

The primary finding of the study was startling: the conclusions reached by studying the data captured by the app paralleled the conclusions reached by the neuropsychologist. The digital fingerprint, in other words, wasn't just an idiosyncratic timestamp. As Dagum explains,

> We were very excited to learn that we could take passive data from how individuals use their phones, such as the touch-screen patterns of interaction, and the temporal variability within those patterns, and that we could apply specific

algorithms and mathematical transformations to predict the neuropsychologist's test scores. When we further looked at the daily data for the full year, it taught us that when people are being tested in the laboratory, they're in a very controlled environment. The neuropsychologist is trained to get the best measure out of the people they're testing. But the test is not emotionally challenging or provoking the patient in any way. By contrast, when people are out in the real world, their emotional state affects their ability to think and perform. That's what we're trying to measure, in a passive and ecological way. Because when patients step out of that laboratory and they are in the real world, they can be dealing with a variety of possible conditions: job stress, family stress, substance use disorder, medication for mental health issues, lack of sleep, etc. These conditions can vary from day to day, and so we were measuring those variations—not just providing a single snapshot from a meeting with a neuropsychologist. Those measurements became very powerful. And that was what propelled us to the next phase of the company.

Mindstrong explored information in areas such as websites visited, time spent on specific apps, and volume of emails and text messages being sent and received. But they discovered, says Dagum, that behavioral data is idiosyncratic, situational, and not very predictive, given that changes in behavior have poor specificity and are not a clinical measurement. Instead, they focused on neural circuit function that can be measured by a neuropsychologist using very simple tests that gauge reaction time to certain complex information.

Mindstrong's discovery occurred in 2014 when it focused on individuals' phone activity—the tapping, scrolling, etc.—and used that to measure ecological cognitive function, such as cognitive control, to determine whether there's more volatility than usual, which can be a worrying sign. Some individuals, says Dagum, never had great cognitive control on the population norm, but they were within a narrow band around their baseline. "Those are the things that we're measuring. We get at a very quantifiable neuroscientific level of measurement."

Today, the app is available to people under care for a serious mental illness or other significant behavioral health disorders. (As of December 2018, Mindstrong also had a contract with 15 counties throughout California, with its app available to patients in those counties.) Once it has been installed on a user's phone, it records the activity described above, synthesizes this activity into data, and then uses the data to create five daily clinical biomarkers: cognitive control, processing speed, memory, executive function, and emotional valence. The clinical biomarkers generated go to both the Mindstrong health care team and the user. Machine learning is used to analyze the data, and if it ever starts to look worrying, Mindstrong receives an automated alert—as does the user. A Mindstrong health adviser makes contact, via a text message, and starts with some open-ended questions along the lines of "Hey, is everything OK?" The communication then becomes more structured and inquisitive. If the adviser believes everything is OK, the communication stops. But if the user shows decline or is in denial, Mindstrong continues to engage.

Sometimes the engagement is all that's needed. Other times, the situation escalates to higher levels of care, which can include recommendations for therapy or motivational interviewing. It can also escalate to adjusting medications. The intent, says Dagum, is for the interventions to happen early. "We want to predict and preempt versus what we have today, which is diagnose and treat when you receive a call from the emergency department."

What Mindstrong offers, says Dagum, is the ability to measure people, via a smartphone, and see how they're functioning.

> We think of it as digital phenotyping. It is clinical biomarkers constructed from a user's digital data patterns without the need to use personal information such as content. It gives us insight on whether they're having troubles, whether they're having stress, whether they're depressed, and whether they're getting better. Having this window into our users provides an ability to start to understand signatures of illness, and the ability to create predictors of disease and deliver early interventions.

All the work being undertaken by Dagum and his colleagues, who include Tom Insel, the former director of the National Institute of Mental Health, is focused on filling a void. The second-rate system for treating people with mental health illnesses is, says Dagum, a product of the fact that there has been no clinical measurement in mental health.

> Look at every other discipline in health care. With diabetes there is fasting blood glucose and HgA1C. With cardiac care, there is an echocardiogram, an EKG. All very objective measures of the physiology and the pathology. And these become your targets. And then all your treatments and your therapies are around restoring normal physiology and function. But in mental health, we have nothing. We rely on patient-reported symptoms and family reporting. Even with something as severe as schizophrenia, the assessment is based on unmeasurable symptoms such as auditory hallucinations. Yet they are the basis of how a patient will be diagnosed and treated for life with medications. What's clear is that as humans, when we don't understand something, we create superstition, fear, and stigma. And we don't understand mental health, perhaps because we haven't had good clinical measurements that can help shed more light on these disorders.

ADVANCING EARLY DETECTION AND TREATMENT OF AUTISM

One of the most striking medical developments of the past few decades has been the dramatic increase in the incidence of autism—rising from 1 in 150 among children born in 1992 to 1 in 59 among those born in 2006, according to the Centers for Disease Prevention and Control [40]. While the precise factors behind the increase remain unclear, there is pioneering work underway that leverages new technologies to improve early detection and treatment.

Autism is a developmental disorder that's typically diagnosed in children. As with many of the conditions described in this book, early intervention is one of the keys to minimizing autism's effects. In the United States, the average age of autism diagnosis, which is four times more common in boys than in girls, is 4.5 years. At that age, children are still accessible to behavioral therapy, points out Dennis Wall, an associate professor of pediatrics, psychiatry, and biomedical data sciences at Stanford's School of Medicine. "Interventions at four-and-a-half can be impactful, but it's at the outer edge. If you can intervene earlier and you detect and diagnose definitively at two-and-a-half or three years, and begin running behavioral programming, that's much more effective."

Indeed, numerous studies have shown that the earlier autism is detected, and the earlier the children diagnosed with it receive therapeutic services, the greater the likelihood that they will overcome autism-related challenges. One study of 48 children, published in the journal *Pediatrics,* showed that those who were randomly assigned to a group receiving a comprehensive developmental behavioral intervention for two years, starting with children between 18 and 30 months of age, experienced an IQ gain of more than 17 points. A separate group of the children, who received interventions from community providers, saw an IQ gain of seven points [41].

But one of the obstacles to progress is a shortage of personnel. Wall points out that for every 10,000 children at risk for a diagnosis of autism, there are only about five developmental pediatricians. As a result, parents often face long delays before their child can receive a diagnostic evaluation—up to 18 months in many parts of the United States. That evaluation is critical, as it's typically required for parents to be reimbursed for their child to receive one-on-one therapy. But here, too, there is a shortage of behavioral technicians who are trained to deliver this therapy, which translates to more delays for children who need care.

Given the critical importance of early intervention, these delays mean lost opportunities to improve and can be highly detrimental to a child's cognitive and social development. The staffing challenges are only mounting, given the growth in the number of children diagnosed with autism.

"With autism, therapy is preventative," says Wall. "Kids actually get better. And if you detect the phenotype [the actual physical characteristics] before it stabilizes and intervene with behavioral programming, you can reverse it or even 'prevent' it. But there aren't enough clinical practitioners to meet the demand." The solution, he says, is to reinvent detection, diagnosis, and intervention.

Wall has contributed to that reinvention by starting a company called Cognoa. It uses an artificial intelligence platform, which in October 2018 was recognized by the FDA as a "breakthrough" medical device for autism, to assist primary care pediatricians with diagnosis and treatment of autism and other behavioral conditions. "The platform empowers pediatricians to effectively and efficiently render decisions during the brief time they have allotted for each child," says Wall. That means reducing the waiting time for a diagnostic evaluation by a specialist.

Cognoa also seeks to empower parents. The company offers an app that includes a series of multiple-choice questions, which parents can answer to help Cognoa better understand their child's development. Questions include "Has your child had any developmental challenges so far?" and "Does your child imitate your actions?" Parents can also upload videos showing their child's everyday behaviors, and they are given guidance on activities they can undertake to help with their child's development.

While the app is not a substitute for diagnosis by a clinician, parent-directed methods of treatment can help overcome the lengthy delays that result from having too few clinicians in the field. As Wall and a coauthor have pointed out, "The earlier and faster that parents are able to move to the therapeutic starting line, the sooner they can begin to engage in activities that equip them and their child with invaluable skills to thrive" [42].

Convincing potential investors that parents would share data about their children was an early challenge for Cognoa, as the company's CEO, Brent Vaughn, explained in 2018.

> One of the … questions that came up quite early, even from early potential investors and clinicians, was can you actually get parents to give you the information on which you could base a clinical diagnostic decision? Can you get them to do this reproducibly without a clinician being in a room? … So we certainly had to address that.
>
> I remember sitting down with one venture capitalist who looked at me and said, you know what—you're never going to find 5,000 parents that are going to do this. And that are going to be able to do this reproducibly. … Within a couple of years, we were up over a quarter of a million parents that had actually done it—and we learned a lot about how to reproducibly collect information on which you can build a clinical diagnosis but collecting it outside of the clinical setting. Parents providing us information in their living room in the evening. So that was certainly one major step for us. And in doing that, we showed that the unmet need was much, much bigger than we originally had estimated [43].

Cognoa's reliance on artificial intelligence is one of the ways its approach to autism breaks with long-established practices in the world of autism research and therapy. That has generated resistance from others in the field. "I think it's partly a clash of cultures," says Wall. "We're coming in from data science computational approaches, and bioinformatics, so we have a very different perspective from others. We look at things differently in general and set up our research studies differently as well."

The other issue, for some, was his decision to launch Cognoa as a for-profit entity (it has raised more than $50 million in venture capital funding). "I think there's this general concern about commercialization being tantamount to greed and exploitation," says Wall. "But the reality is if you don't commercialize, you can't complete the clinical evaluation studies and build a product that will serve the hundreds of thousands of people who need it."

Cognoa's projects have included securely capturing videos as well as developing videos for viewing by children diagnosed with autism. Both are labor-intensive and capital-intensive, says Wall, and difficult to implement outside of a for-profit company.

> You can't just say, "We believe we can see autism in short home videos" and run a machine and a classifier and publish papers on that. We have to build a mechanism that enables families to upload video in a way that's seamless, that's secure, robust, and fault tolerant. And that takes a significant amount of capital.

While it's too early to reach any definitive conclusions about the effectiveness of Cognoa's methods, the early evidence is encouraging. A paper published in *Autism Research* in May 2018, and another published in the *Journal of the American Medical Informatics Association* a few months later, reported on the results of a study involving 230 children, with four long-standing autism screening measures compared with Cognoa's screening tools. The authors concluded that Cognoa's tools were more effective in distinguishing between children with and without autism [44].

The Unlikely Role of Google Glass in Treating Autism

Wall also pursues autism research through the Wall Lab at Stanford. Perhaps the most noteworthy research has involved a device called Google Glass, which in a pilot study was shown to be effective in treating autism.

In 2014, Google began selling the device, which is a head-mounted display worn like eyeglasses. The person wearing it can control what appears on the display with voice commands or by swiping a touchpad on the side of the frame. The device can also be used to take pictures and record video.

Not long after Google Glass's release, it attracted the attention of a Stanford computer science student from Germany named Catalin Voss. He wondered if the device could benefit his cousin, who has autism. Voss was working under an emeritus professor of computer science, Terry Winograd, who is also the founder of the field of human-computer interaction. Their work led them to Carl Feinstein, a professor of psychiatry and behavioral sciences at Stanford, who started the autism center at Lucile Packard Children's Hospital Stanford. He, in turn, referred them to Wall, who had been exploring the use of video as a diagnostic tool. At the time, Wall was still worried about the therapy bottleneck once children were diagnosed with autism, and so he was searching for home-based options. Once Voss came to him, recalls Wall, "I knew it was exactly what we needed."

They started working with Winograd and Feinstein, as well as a postdoctoral scholar, Nick Haber. Seeing the potential of Google Glass, they began hiring people and building the technology that would enable each Google Glass to be adapted for use by children and for processing the information needed to make it effective as a therapeutic tool.

Children diagnosed with autism are typically taught to recognize emotions of others through rote memorization, using flashcards. That approach is effective, but it consumes significant time. There are also limits on the variations of human faces that can be captured on flashcards. This was important. As Wall explains,

> Children have to figure out how to interpret different facial emotions. They eventually do, through socialization, but children with autism struggle with this. They focus on things that are totally not social, and so they miss opportunities to learn organically the variation of human faces.

The Google Glass project put forward an entirely new approach. Wall and his colleagues built a smartphone app, which is underpinned by AI-trained tools that draw on hundreds of thousands of photos of faces showing the eight different facial expressions children need to learn: happiness, sadness, anger, disgust, surprise, fear, non-emotive, and contempt. The app is linked to the Google Glass, and the child wearing the device receives real-time guidance regarding the facial expressions of others.

The app developed by Wall and his colleagues also allows the development of games for the kids to play, as well as giving them the ability to record video and enable playback that labels different emotions. This allows parents to review with their child moments when an emotion was recognized or when one was missed. These features have made the device into more of a holistic therapeutic intervention, says Wall, as well as a data capture system for each child, delivering actionable guidance and more precise therapy. The data element is critical, he says.

> Traditionally, data has not been captured. There is on-the-spot care, and it can be effective in that one moment, but all of the information that's important about that interaction, and what's effective about that care, is lost. In this system, there is immediate data feedback, and through machine learning that data is used to build better models for treatment.

The early evidence about the effectiveness of Google Glass is encouraging. A pilot study by Wall and some of his Stanford colleagues showed that children with autism improved their social skills by using the app that's paired with Google Glass [45]. (Some of the kids in the study said that when wearing the device, they felt like they had superpowers, such as the ability to read minds, so it became known as "Superpower Glass.") In the study, which was published in August 2018, 14 families tested the Superpower Glass setup at home for an average of 10 weeks each. Each family had a child between the ages of 3 and 17 with a clinically confirmed autism diagnosis.

The families used the therapy for at least three 20-minute sessions per week. The mean score of the children on the SRS-2, a questionnaire completed by parents to evaluate children's social skills, decreased by 7.38 points during the study, indicating less severe symptoms of autism. None of the participants' autism symptoms worsened (based on SRS-2 scores), and 6 of the 14 participants had their level of autism reclassified—four from "severe" to "moderate," one from "moderate" to "mild," and one from "mild" to "normal."

Although the study had a small sample size and no control arm, it nonetheless suggests the potential of an innovative technology to help remedy a challenging condition—and help overcome the staffing bottlenecks that currently delay diagnoses and treatments. "While the factors contributing to autism are extraordinarily complex," says Wall, "it's now becoming clear that diagnosis and treatment can happen much faster, and with much more precision, than in the past. That's going to go a long way toward helping kids overcome the condition and help them thrive in everyday life."

THE BENEFIT OF BIG SCIENCE / BIG PHARMA COOPERATION

There is tremendous complexity and cost associated with drug discoveries. The most recent research from the Tufts Center for Drug Development, based on 106 new drugs from 10 different pharmaceutical companies, showed the average cost of a new drug to be nearly $2.6 billion (and nearly $2.9 billion when post-approval R&D costs are incorporated) [46]. While there's no guarantee of success until this lengthy and expensive process is completed, pharmaceutical companies often play a critical role in translating research into new therapies. The development of one medicine in particular shows how these companies can leverage their resources and scientific knowledge to great effect.

Cervical cancer is the second-leading cause of cancer death among women in the world (500,000 women are diagnosed with it annually). Research by a German virologist, Harald zur Hausen, revealed that cervical cancer is caused by human papillomaviruses (a discovery that led to his being awarded a Nobel Prize in 2008). He first published this research in 1976, but three decades passed before a vaccine to protect against the virus was approved by the FDA.

Merck, a U.S. pharmaceutical company, set out to develop a cancer vaccine by preventing the infection that causes the cells to become cancerous. The company drew on the talents of people throughout the company, but particularly teams of chemical engineers and bio-process engineers. The work before them was anything but simple, points out Peter Kim, who was Merck's head of research and development when the vaccine was being developed.

> Over a number of years, they figured out how to ferment the yeast in large fermenters to get better-quality product. And then they figured out how to take the particles that were isolated from the yeast, disassemble them, and then get them to refold and reassemble with correct disulfide bonds. And all along, they were doing analytical analyses and electron microscopy analyses to see which steps were going in the right directions and which were not.
>
> They also had to figure out how to formulate the vaccine product together with adjuvants, which help to stimulate the immune response. This took years of work by hundreds of people to end up with preparations of virus-like particles that were stable for many months or years at room temperature. When

you took electron microscopy pictures of the product, it was shown to be highly ordered and homogenous.

Kim, who today is the Virginia and D. K. Ludwig Professor of Biochemistry at Stanford, says he emphasizes this part of the process because it often gets glossed over when talking about drug development. "The story often jumps from basic science to the clinical science, but there's actually a lot of engineering in the middle that has to take place."

Once the vaccine was developed, clinical trials involving more than 10,000 women showed it to be extremely effective in protecting against two of the types of HPV, type 16 and type 18, which together account for about 70 percent of cervical cancers. In June 2006, the FDA approved the vaccine, which Merck marketed as Gardasil. Subsequently, components were added to protect against additional types of HPV, so the vaccine now covers viruses that are the cause of about 90 percent of cervical cancers.

Fundamental to the progress, says Kim, was having the resources needed to see the project through to its completion.

> It wouldn't have been possible to do something like this without having big teams of people with all sorts of different expertise—basic scientists, biochemists, biologists, statisticians, clinicians, bio-process engineers, and chemical engineers. Big teams were also needed to work together in the same direction. If you don't work with teams, you're not going to get anything done. That's not always appreciated or understood by people who haven't worked in this industry.

Basic science lays at the foundation of this work, says Kim, "but if you want to translate a discovery into a vaccine, it requires people who work on things that would be considered mundane by some who work in basic science." Without those people doing that work, he says, "you don't get new drugs."

MAKING BABIES WITH MODERN TECHNOLOGY

One of the 20th century's most meaningful medical innovations was in vitro fertilization (IVF), which refers to the process of combining an egg and sperm in a laboratory and then transferring the embryo to a woman's uterus. In July 1978, the first baby was born that had been conceived through IVF. (This was the so-called test tube baby, even though the procedure did not involve test tubes.) Since then, IVF and other assisted reproductive technologies have led to the births of more than eight million babies worldwide, and more than one million in the United States.

The science and technology underpinning IVF have become progressively more advanced over the past four decades, and that's contributed to a dramatic increase in success rates, though there are still significant variations based on the age of the mother. For women under the age of 35, nearly 40 percent of IVF cycles lead to having a baby. For women over 40, the success rate is less than 12 percent.

Barry Behr, a professor of obstetrics and gynecology (reproductive endocrinology and infertility) at Stanford Medicine, is one of the pioneers in the IVF field, as well as a clinical and scientific leader in research about human reproduction. More than 20 years ago, he developed a special recipe for a nutrient-rich culture medium to keep artificially fertilized embryos growing in the lab for a few extra days, allowing for extra development. This was a critical breakthrough, as it helped address one of the many challenges with IVF: determining which embryos have the highest likelihood of viability. In the early years of IVF, explains Behr,

> we could only grow embryos up to the stage of the day-two or day-three stage. That early in their development, our ability to discriminate between viable and nonviable was very poor—they all looked the same. It was kind of like the three-mile mark during a marathon race—everyone is mostly packed together.
>
> We knew that a high percentage of these embryos created were not able to make a baby, but we had no way to tell which ones. So we would put in six and hope for one good one. Sometimes there was a good one, sometimes there wasn't, and sometimes there were more good ones than we expected. And that's when you saw the sextuplets and quadruplets, which really gave IVF a black eye.

Behr's work helped reduce the incidence of these multiple pregnancies. But viability was still largely determined by specialists viewing embryos under a microscope. About a decade later, Behr codeveloped a process that involved a form of time-lapse imaging whereby snapshots of an embryo are taken every five minutes during the first 48 hours of cell division. Behr and his colleagues developed an algorithm that generates an assessment of the embryo's viability, looking at factors such as how rapidly the cells are dividing and the size it achieves, compared with a benchmark embryo. This is known as Early Embryo Viability Assessment, and in 2014 it became the first FDA-approved tool to help fertility specialists with their decision-making.

There's been another major benefit to keeping the embryos alive in a culture for five or six days—it enables what Behr refers to "embryo interrogation." It's possible, he says, to minimize some of the randomness in fetal development and, in the process, help reduce the incidence of fetal abnormalities. "Today we can eliminate any single gene disorder from a family's gene pool through embryo selection," says Behr. This includes a range of conditions, including spinal muscular atrophy, Tay-Sachs disease, and muscular dystrophy.

Today, says Behr, about 65 percent of his patients involved with fertility procedures have their embryos genetically screened. If one or both parents are a carrier for a particularly harmful condition, such as those listed above, they are given the option of two forms of pre-implantation genetic testing. One is pre-implant genetic screening, which involves identifying embryos with the correct number of chromosomes. The other is pre-implantation genetic diagnosis, which involves identifying a single gene that can trigger the conditions described above. In this process, a few cells are removed from embryos, and the DNA is analyzed for genetic abnormalities. The embryo(s) without any abnormalities are then placed in the mother's uterus. Behr is aware of the moral dilemmas that can arise from genetic screening, but he sees it contributing to the health and vitality of future generations.

Some Ethical Principles That Should Guide Decisions about Starting a Life

As Behr alludes to, moral dilemmas can arise when doctors are engaged in medical procedures that involve decisions about when life begins and how embryos are treated. David Magnus, director of the Stanford Center for Biomedical Ethics, highlights the principles that need to guide medical research and clinical care.

> In carrying out precision health research, the research will need to conform to the three core ethical principles identified in the Belmont Report. The first principle is respect for research participants. This includes the duty to treat people as autonomous agents, and to protect those with diminished autonomy. The second principle is beneficence, which includes the duty to "do no harm" and also the duty to maximize benefit and minimize harms as much as possible. The third is justice, the duty to create a fair way of allocating the benefits and burdens of research. These principles form the basis of our oversight and evaluation of the ethics of research on human subjects.
>
> Some have attempted to apply refined versions of these principles to the ethics of clinical care (as opposed to research), often supplemented with principles related to veracity (the obligation to tell patients the truth) or fidelity (the duty to maintain trust in the patient/physician relationship). The challenge with applying these principles to precision health or precision medicine (as opposed to precision health research) is that they derive their force from the dyadic patient-physician relationship. But the reality of modern medicine is that a patient's relationship is with a health system and a team. Many decisions are made that constrain the range of physician choices, and for the benefits of precision medicine to be realized, there will likely need to be further limitations. The principles of precision health have yet to be fully developed.

The Creation of "Savior Siblings" to Save Lives

Another innovative practice undertaken by Behr is something called *savior siblings*. As he describes it, "this is essentially creating a genetic match for someone whose health is failing." That "genetic match" is the creation of another human being. As Behr explains,

> Consider a child who has a blood disease that can be treated with a bone marrow transplant. The chance of finding someone in the general population with a precise match is approximately one-in-64,000. But the odds of finding a match from one's parents is about one in eight. In situations like these, some parents who still have the ability to bear children can go through IVF and genetic screening to find one embryo that is a tissue match for the sick child. That embryo is then transferred to the mother, and if a pregnancy ensues, the

blood from the umbilical cord is used for the bone marrow transplant—and saves the life of the sick child.

This is another area where Behr recognizes the ethical dilemmas around this practice—some of which are explored in a 2009 movie starring Cameron Diaz called *My Sister's Keeper*. When he first learned of it, he was adamantly opposed, believing that it was not an appropriate reason to bring a child into the world. But his objections have relaxed as he's seen how having the option can be life-changing for families, and in recent years he's helped about five families to deliver a savior sibling.

An IVF Success Story

IVF enables pregnancies under conditions that in the recent past would have been considered impossible. Every success story is life-changing for the parents. One mother who was trying to get pregnant, amid very challenging circumstances, came to Stanford for assistance. She shared the details of her story with Stanford Fertility and Reproductive Health Services, which later published an article about it on its website. That article follows.

Shortly after starting a new job in 2007 as a legal specialist in a technology company, Denise Wong, who was 27 at the time, was diagnosed with breast cancer. The treatment that would save her life—a lumpectomy, four rounds of chemotherapy, 30 days of radiation and five years of tamoxifen—would also decrease her chances of ever being able to conceive a baby.

"At that point, I wasn't thinking about becoming a mother," Wong remembers. "But to have the choice stripped away was probably the hardest part." Over the next 10 years, Wong says, she stayed in remission and life got back to normal.

In 2016, Adolfo Polanco, the boyfriend who had been at her side throughout her cancer diagnosis, treatment and recovery, became her husband. And they began to imagine what had once seemed out of the question: starting a family.

"We always knew it wasn't going to be high probability," says Wong. "But we did try for several months after we got married, and it clearly wasn't working. That's when we talked about going to Stanford."

With each month that passed—each cycle releasing one of the limited number of eggs Denise, like all women, was born with—Wong knew that her chances were diminishing. She needed to act quickly.

Wong and Polanco reached out to several fertility treatment centers. Stanford Fertility and Reproductive Health Services was the first to respond. It proved to be a fortunate match since the Stanford team was one of the first to have a fertility program for cancer patients and survivors. On top of that, the program takes care of patients that other centers might deem too risky or unlikely to conceive.

"Stanford prides itself on taking the most unusual and challenging cases," says Steven Nakajima, MD, director of the Stanford IVF Outreach Program. With

the most advanced technology and approaches, he adds, the team is on the cutting-edge of reproductive sciences.

"*A lot of times, people will come to us because they've already been to three or four other clinicians who won't take their case, either because of their weight or because they have too many medical risk factors," he explains. "We don't have arbitrary cut-off points where we say we won't take care of someone because we're afraid it will decrease our pregnancy rates. Our group really embraces the fact that we try to give everyone a chance."*

Nakajima says that while Wong's case wasn't unusual medically, her chances of conceiving were very low. Her ovarian reserve test—also known as an ovarian assessment report, or OAR—showed that although she was just 36 years old, she had the ovarian function of someone closer to 42. "In a reproductive sense, this is very depressed function," states Nakajima. A test of Wong's anti-Mullerian hormone (AMH)—another indicator of a woman's remaining egg supply—also came back low at 0.48 nanograms per milliliter.

"*Dr. Nakajima said that my chances of having a baby naturally were about 8 percent or less per month," says Wong. "With intra-uterine insemination (IUI), about 10 percent. The success rate if we went through IVF would be slightly higher but still low, about 15 percent. So, the thinking was, why not jump to the most aggressive path?" Wong's insurance company—which, unlike most, covered her fertility treatments—disagreed. They wanted her to begin with less aggressive approaches. But her doctors knew this would cost her precious time, so they appealed the insurance company's decision on her behalf and received the approval she needed.*

"*Because of her diminished ovarian reserve, we didn't know how much longer she'd continue to ovulate or have good-quality eggs," explains Nakajima. "So, we did ... a special kind of IVF cycle to prevent her from having a too-high estrogen level that might reactivate her breast cancer."*

Wong was supplied with multiple medications, and had to learn, with her husband, how to do injections at home. She also came to the clinic for twice-weekly blood draws. "IVF is not fun," Wong confesses. "You're going through a personal struggle while also trying to manage things logistically. The good news is the nurses are fantastic and help you with scheduling."

The following month, Wong underwent her egg-retrieval procedure. "The nurses were so warm and sweet," remembers Wong. "So were all the techs and doctors. It was a very warm experience for something so clinical."

After the egg retrieval, five eggs were identified and two showed signs of fertilization the next day. Of those two zygotes, one embryo was viable on day five. Nakajima decided to biopsy it to ensure it was chromosomally normal, which it was. "Some people would not have biopsied the embryo because of the fact that it might harm the embryo," says Nakajima. "But in this case, it was more important for her to know." They froze Wong's single embryo in case she wanted to try again. Ultimately, understanding that a second IVF cycle might increase her risk of breast cancer recurrence, she chose to implant their one frozen embryo.

"You have to understand how emotionally trying this is for her," remarks Nakajima. "She has this one chance as a breast cancer survivor who probably can't make many more eggs in the future. It's her one chance, and she's willing to go through the embryo transfer procedure."

On May 19, 2017, Nakajima and his team thawed Wong's single embryo and placed it in her uterus. "You're holding your breath," says Wong. "You always have to be cautiously optimistic because you know there are so many obstacles along the way and so many challenges that you have to be prepared for anything to go wrong."

Four weeks passed, and Wong missed her next period. Her pregnancy was confirmed, but she was hesitant to celebrate knowing that most miscarriages happen in the first trimester. "Once we got past the first trimester, then we fully exhaled," she discloses. "You have these pictures from the ultrasounds showing the progress your baby is making every couple of weeks, and that's when it starts to feel more real. I wouldn't say we celebrated. We exhaled."

Soon, Nakajima marked another major milestone for Wong and Polanco by graduating them from fertility treatment. "He said there's no reason for you guys to see us anymore because you're pregnant and your chances of holding on to this baby are the same as everyone else's."

When she was 37 weeks pregnant, Wong sent Dr. Nakajima a photo of herself to update him on her progress. "I was really touched by it," shares Nakajima. "I thought, I can't get over this. It's really something. We knew we weren't going to have a lot of chances to make this work, but the fact that she had this one embryo that made it through—it was just the perfect storm for her."

On February 11, 2018, Maxwell Polanco was born at Good Samaritan Hospital in San Jose. When Wong's labor wasn't progressing, her doctors opted for a C-section. It was a fortunate choice because Maxwell's umbilical cord had knotted and wrapped around his neck. They were able to carefully unwrap it, protecting his fragile chances at the final moment, and deliver a healthy baby boy.

"When I first saw him, he just seemed like a little miracle, like a one-in-a-million baby," says Wong. "He gave three loud cries when he came out of the womb, and then he quieted down and started sucking his fingers. He was born 6 pounds, 7.7 ounces and 19 inches long. He looks like both his mother and father, we think. He's gaining weight fast. Yeah, he's perfect" [47].

ADVANCING SCIENCE THROUGH CITIZEN SCIENTISTS

One of the most intriguing developments in science today is the emergence of so-called citizen scientists. It's a catch-all term for individuals who may not have formal academic training in scientific disciplines but who nonetheless pursue research, and sometimes achieve breakthroughs that have eluded credentialed scientists. The example I am most familiar with is a project called Eterna, and it involves research related to ribonucleic acids (RNA). It is led by Rhiju Das, a computational biochemist at Stanford's School of Medicine, and it draws on the insights of people from throughout the world.

RNA is important because all biological processes in human beings are encoded by RNA molecules. RNA genomes are present in several pathogens, such as influenza, HIV, the Zika virus, and a panoply of other pandemic infectious agents. There is also an RNA dimension to neurological diseases, and one of the leading mysteries in medicine right now, says Das, is the etiology of neurological disease and why are there so many RNAs that seem to be involved. RNAs' actions within a virus's genome have also been a mystery, and that has delayed the development of therapeutics that could attack viruses at the RNA level.

The work that became Eterna started in 2009 when Das was researching the idea of using RNA molecules as new kinds of drugs and encountering problems related to RNA engineering that he couldn't solve, supercomputers couldn't solve, and Nobel laureate scientists couldn't solve. Out of desperation, he turned to the internet, soliciting solutions to these problems from people who could play a video game that involved sequences of RNA molecules. The objective was to develop hypotheses about RNA engineering and to design experiments that would test these hypotheses. Within months of the project being launched, a community of the video gamers solved problems that had gone unsolved by computer algorithms that were themselves based on 30 years of hard-core RNA biochemistry and computational biology. Das's reaction to the players' outperforming computers? "One of the really shocking moments of my life" [48].

The Eterna community has continued expanding since that initial work, and more than 150,000 people have been involved with the project. A 2019 reference paper coauthored by Das explains how the system works.

> After playing starter puzzles and gaining entry to Eterna's "Lab," players virtually design RNA sequences on-screen. Their designs are synthesized and experimentally analyzed. These data are returned directly to players, providing feedback of whether their submissions fold into the predicted structures [49].

The paper also describes the outcomes from this work: "Eterna players outperformed existing computational prediction algorithms in novel secondary structure prediction algorithms, and the heuristic rules discovered by players were turned into a predictive algorithm 'EteRNAbot,' which also outperformed all prior existing algorithms" [50].

The Eterna project has led to several breakthroughs, with some players even publishing articles about their discoveries for academic publications. One such article, which had two Eterna players as its lead authors, appeared in the *Journal of Molecular Biology* [51]. Another one described how the author coded an algorithm for automated RNA design—a design that, according to Das, "dramatically outperforms deep learning methods that were being developed simultaneously by professional scientists."

One of the most noteworthy undertakings has involved building on the work of Stanford's Purvesh Khatri, a professor of medicine and biomedical data science, who has discovered a three-gene signature from blood that could predict the onset of tuberculosis in a person six months before it becomes infectious. (About one-fourth of the world's population is infected with bacteria that cause tuberculosis—a condition that leads to 1.7 million deaths annually.) But the signature depends on measuring three RNA molecules—and there is no molecule in existence that can act like a molecular calculator, nor is there any technology that can create a molecule that can carry out the calculation.

That's where Eterna came in. Khatri came to Das and asked if he could help. Das talked to his team and realized that they could set up a puzzle that might elicit an RNA molecule that could calculate the needed RNA signature. That signature would, in turn, enable the creation of the first-ever paper-based TB test, which would be much more cost-effective than current tests, and help expand access in poor areas.

Within a few months of the puzzle being launched, Eterna had received 30,000 potential solutions. Das then worked with some of his Stanford colleagues to develop a throughput experimental method that would enable them to test all 30,000 molecules. Those tests led to about 100 solutions that look like they will work in a test tube. (Several of the solutions came from someone who lives in Switzerland and who had no prior connection to science, other than being a former computer hacker.) In the fall of 2018, Das was testing whether these molecules could be used for a paper-based test.

If this TB project succeeds, says Das, and it becomes a point-of-care diagnostic, "it will be the first example I'm aware of where a new form of medicine has arisen from data that is publicly available or donated by the public. And it will have the potential to benefit hundreds of thousands—if not millions—of people."

So who are the players? Das describes them as people who

> don't have a connection to science but they love science and they particularly love the idea of confronting ideas that we have about Nature and subjecting those ideas to actual lab experiments. I'm someone who loves getting experimental feedback, even if I'm wrong. And what's been really interesting about dedicated Eterna players is they seem to get the same rush from experiments that I do, despite not having trained as academic scientists.

Das points out that the players' lack of formal training may afford them perspectives that are shut off to those with such training. "I get ideas from Eterna players that I don't see from folks in my lab," he says. One of the players, whose online name is Wateronthemoon, has explained why this might be. "The difference between us and scientists (and there are scientists among us), is we have no idea what should work so we try everything. We're more creative" [52]. Das emphasizes that the players are not mere savants.

> A lot of them have read the scientific literature on RNA folding and RNA medicine. One of them occasionally corrects me on which RNA bases can

form which kind of non-canonical base pairs of RNA structure. And he can do that because he's read the literature. I think the top players truly are scientists—just not academic ones.

The Eterna work comes at a time when RNA is assuming a more prominent place on the medical landscape, says Das. "While it's been promising for a long time, there hasn't been deep basic science understanding of RNA until recently." But now, he says, "there's an explosion of activity," pointing to therapeutics that target RNA and drugs that are made of RNA. (The treatment for spinal muscular atrophy, which I describe in chapter 7, was made possible by expanded understanding of how RNA functions.) And CRISPR Cas9—the gene-editing mechanism I describe in chapter 7—is guided by RNA.

The ultimate objective, says Das, is to be able to create RNA that can be transcribed into cells and deactivate a virus. While he sees steady progress, he thinks it will be several years before this goal is met. What's likely to happen sooner, he says, is making RNA that will have an impact in medical clinics, and the OpenTB project is emblematic of the progress.

> This process of taking public data, and the invention of molecules by the public, is a new route to medicine. Even in this day and age of being pretty advanced technologically, there's a potential for 100x the number of people who are in academic research or pharmaceutical research to be engaged with taking on extremely difficult challenges, like the invention of the actual molecules. Having so many more people engaged has the potential to bring forth new insights that contribute to breakthrough discoveries.

The Profile of a Citizen Scientist

Andrew Kaechele is one of the standout citizen-scientists who are active in Eterna. His unconventional background is a reminder of what can be achieved when hidden talents are allowed to flourish.

Kaechele grew up outside Pittsburgh but never finished high school. When he was 18, he joined the Army, where he held a variety of positions, including crew chief on a twin-engine aircraft. After being discharged, he spent nearly two decades as a commercial fishing boat captain in the Gulf of Mexico.

In 2012, he saw an episode of the PBS show *Nova* that was devoted to Eterna. That led him to start playing the games found on the Eterna website. His interest grew over time, and he became more involved, particularly with the OpenTB project. One recent undertaking entailed developing about 100 designs that calculate the OpenTB signature in vitro, with the RNA synthesized and tested. All of Kaechele's solutions were robust, says Das, noting that "Andrew proposes novel design strategies that don't exist in the literature."

> An example involves a paper TB test, where we would want a molecular calculator to be triggered to turn a line on the paper red when a patient appears to have active tuberculosis. And we want to have other calculators that cause

the red line to disappear when there's active tuberculosis. But all the solutions failed for the ones that make the line go from absent to red. Andrew went on to develop new strategies with molecules that could be adapted to both turn on and turn off when the patient has active TB. And they're the same basic molecules, but then he's developed a new strategy to essentially toggle them to go in either direction. It's an exciting idea I've never seen before.

Kaechele says he devoted about 10 hours a day, for six days, to coming up with the solution. Asked about the origins of his ideas, he replies, "To be sure, I have my own perspective on things. And it's not totally a bad thing not to be a trained scientist. This is not my job—it's more of a hobby, something that I enjoy doing, with some free time when I have it."

In December 2018, Kaechele earned an associate's degree in social work from Butler County Community College in western Pennsylvania, and he'd enrolled in Slippery Rock University. Even with his extensive knowledge of RNA design, he was planning to study social work but stay involved with Eterna— ensuring that he will remain a citizen scientist.

DEVELOPING NEW THERAPEUTICS AND REPURPOSING EXISTING DRUGS

Biomedical research involves a never-ending quest to better understand the intricacies of the human body. As knowledge advances, so too do the opportunities to translate discoveries into new therapies that can help treat (or prevent) illness and disease. But even when breakthrough science occurs at the bench, it doesn't always translate to the bedside. Bridging this gap is the focus of a program at Stanford called SPARK, which was founded by Daria Mochly-Rosen, the George D. Smith Professor in Translational Medicine in the Department of Chemical and Systems Biology at Stanford.

The idea for SPARK originated with Mochly-Rosen observing, over many years, a range of discoveries that were never commercialized.

> There is an inherent risk that early-stage programs will fail during development, no matter how promising the science. Such nascent programs are unlikely to attract interest from industry until they have reached significant milestones, and very little funding is available from the NIH, foundations, or private enterprise for this critical transition.

Kevin Grimes can speak to the challenges of drug development. Currently a professor of chemical and systems biology at Stanford, and codirector of SPARK, he has also worked as a health care consultant and at biopharmaceutical companies.

> During my time in industry, I saw some really promising therapeutic technologies that no one would develop, merely because the appropriate patents were not filed. Drug companies require a period of market exclusivity in order to

obtain an adequate return on their investment. If you're looking at investing hundreds of millions to a few billion dollars, which is the average cost to develop a new therapeutic, and there's no patent position you can hold, what investors are going to put their money there? Drug companies have a fiduciary responsibility to investors to maximize profit, for better or worse. They're not going to invest in the development of a therapy if the generic companies can come right in and do a copycat drug.

Mochly-Rosen had firsthand experience with the phenomenon. She is a protein chemist, and in 2000, her laboratory discovered that a particular peptide inhibitor could be administered following a heart attack and reduce the size of dead tissue by 70 percent in lab animals. This discovery might, in turn, mean dramatically reducing the likelihood of heart failure or death in people suffering from heart attacks. Academic journals published articles on the topic, but there was no interest from pharmaceutical companies.

That would have been the end of the story, but Mochly-Rosen started talking to representatives of the pharmaceutical companies. They recognized the significance of her discovery but didn't see a way to translate it into a drug. "They basically told me to go away," she recalls. Instead, she worked with one of her former students to look for funding, figuring that the two of them were smart enough to succeed. They met with venture capitalists, but there was no interest. (She says she was rejected about 50 times.) "Raising money takes a lot of stamina, determination, and humility," she says. "You can't have any ego, because it would quickly break. And academics like me are not accustomed to being told 'no.'"

But she kept talking to anybody who would listen. "I had a picture of a heart with the drug and one without the drug, showing a big difference in infarct size and I would just show it to people." A chance encounter with her neighbor—they were both taking out the trash—led him to draft her business plan. Her persistence paid off. In 2003, she succeeded in raising $27 million from venture investors.

She took a one-year leave of absence from Stanford and hired several Stanford students. "I assumed that because we were all smart, we could figure out what we needed to do." In fact, she recalls, "we were all totally clueless about what needed to be done."

> There is a huge body of knowledge that we are never taught in academia. The business part is actually the easiest. The hard part is the intricate process of drug development. We in academia have an attitude that this is not intellectually challenging. So, we have kind of disregard for that. But it's extremely intellectually challenging. It's also unintuitive. There are so many ways to fail—many more than there are to succeed. And it's not like academia, where failure is fundamental to research and can be written up in a paper as a success story. The measures are just completely different.

When Mochly-Rosen returned to Stanford, she wanted to help bridge what she described as a "vast chasm" between industry and academia. She concluded that the best way to do that would be to put representatives of both sides in a room together on a regular basis. "This would help people start to respect each other and potentially continue to learn from each other." The initiative started with five volunteers from industry (a venture capitalist and a regulatory science expert in addition to clinicians and basic scientists). There were also clinicians and basic researchers involved. They all signed confidentiality agreements and they were not paid. "I simply asked them to help us select the right projects," recalls Mochly-Rosen, "and teach us what we needed to know."

That was in 2006. Since then, SPARK has evolved into a multidimensional program, and Mochly-Rosen serves as its director. There are graduate-level courses focused on the drug development process, but the major activity relates to the SPARK Scholars, who must apply to the program, which is open to Stanford professors, clinicians, postdoctoral scholars, and graduate students. The selection criteria for the SPARK Scholars are based on three factors:

- Does the proposed therapeutic address an unmet medical need (preferably an important one)?
- Does it involve a novel approach?
- Is there a reasonable chance that the project will advance to an industry partnership or to a clinical trial at Stanford?

More than two-thirds of the people on the selection committee are senior executives from the Bay Area biotech industry, including health care investors, officers of companies, and scientists who have deep disciplinary experience in areas such as medicinal chemistry, regulatory science, and the design and execution of clinical trials. The rest of the committee is composed of academics who have firsthand experience translating their discoveries into new drugs. The committee receives about 60 proposals each year, and 10 to 12 are typically accepted.

The accepted proposals receive modest funding for product development—typically lasting two years. The greater value typically comes from the mentoring provided by industry experts. About 100 such mentors are involved with SPARK. They have expertise across the drug development spectrum, in areas such as assay development, clinical trial design, intellectual property law, funding, regulatory requirements, and university compliance. "It's important to have multiple advisers," says Mochly-Rosen, "because there is no one path to success, but one bad piece of advice can derail the best project."

At weekly meetings held on the Stanford campus, 30 to 40 of the industry advisers are typically present. The meetings alternate between instruction on the process of drug development and getting updates on individual SPARK projects. A key element of the meetings, says Mochly-Rosen, should be disagreements. For example, one adviser will recommend moving quickly into a mouse study with an early version of the drug to show a proof of concept, another will say that studies in mice are useless until the drug has been optimized, and a third will recommend further validation of the target before moving to a proof of concept in mice.

Seeking consensus, she says, "means that you don't take risks." Although pharma companies take the long way to characterize the pharmacological characteristics of a compound and would consider beginning an early proof-of-concept study in mice a risky shortcut, Mochly-Rosen hopes that SPARK fellows will choose this riskier option. Risks can also be inherent in the particular type of drug target; inhibiting a protein-protein interaction or correcting a genetic mutation in an enzyme by small molecules are considered very risky projects by industry. SPARK welcomes these types of projects, as they move into "white space"—there is no competition, and if they are successful, the impact will be substantial.

The ultimate goal of the projects started each year is to advance them through the applied science of drug development and de-risk them to the point where one of two things can happen. One desired outcome is to hand the project over to a commercial partner, who sees the promise and is willing to make the investment for further development. The other outcome may involve projects that do not appear to be commercially attractive but are nonetheless good for patients. In those cases, the objective is to take the projects into the clinic at Stanford or find public-private partnerships or other not-for-profit ways of supporting the development. In many of these latter cases, successful clinical studies at Stanford result in a licensing agreement; an investor or a company sees the value in the program and finds a way to make it commercially viable.

In addition to educating academics about the processes involved in the dis-covery of new drugs, SPARK has been remarkably successful in identifying new clinical applications for already-approved drugs. As Grimes explains,

> Developing a new drug is costly, time-consuming and risky. Repurposing a drug that has already been shown to be safe in humans for a new clinical indi-cation reduces the up-front costs of developing the molecule and reduces the risk that the drug will have unintended side effects. We largely focus on deter-mining whether the existing drug is effective for the disease of interest. Nearly one-third of SPARK projects take this approach. To our surprise, a significant number of these projects are licensed to commercial partners because we create new drug formulations, routes of administration, or other patentable approaches. Repurposing projects are particularly attractive because they are less expensive and advance effective treatments to patients more rapidly.

One example of drug repurposing involves sildenafil (Viagra). Pfizer origi-nally developed sildenafil as a potential treatment for hypertension and for angina caused by coronary artery disease. During clinical trials, the drug was not particu-larly effective for these conditions, but patients reported that it was helpful for male patients with sexual dysfunction. This led to the creation of an entirely new market for erectile dysfunction drugs. Sildenafil, when given at higher doses, was later determined to be beneficial in the treatment of pulmonary arterial hypertension.

Alfred Lane, emeritus professor of dermatology at Stanford, identified another repurposing opportunity for this drug. He was taking care of children with lymphatic malformations (very rare disorders that result in benign growths of lymphatic tissue that can, because of size and location, cause serious detriments to health). One of these children was receiving sildenafil as treatment for pulmonary arterial hypertension, a condition for which sildenafil has also been shown to provide benefit. Lane noted that the lymphatic malformations in this child dramatically diminished in size. He approached Grimes about designing a clinical trial to evaluate the utility of sildenafil in the treatment of these children with lymphatic malformations. Grimes describes the findings:

> Dr. Lane secured approval from the FDA and Stanford's ethics committee to conduct a small clinical study. Pfizer generously donated the drug. After 20 weeks of treatment, there was a significant shrinkage in six of the seven children in the study. Under a special program to support treatments for rare diseases, the FDA is now financially supporting a larger corroboratory study. Based on the initial academic publication, physicians around the world have started treating afflicted children with the drug.

SPARK has also had considerable success in accelerating progress toward being able to translate discoveries into new therapies. Within two years of completing the program, approximately half of all SPARK projects move into industry startups or existing companies, and/or enter clinical studies. This compares with an industry standard of about 5 percent. More than half of SPARK projects address child and maternal health, global health, and orphan diseases.

There are about 60 SPARK-inspired programs spread across every continent but Antarctica. The program's popularity underscores that drug development is a challenge throughout the world—and that there's a great need to streamline the process of training people in how to do development.

SPARK's success in facilitating discovery, clinical application, and iteration is critical at a moment when the drug development and approval process has not kept pace with the rapid technological progress. As much as the program has already accomplished, there is much more that can be done to promote the development of new therapies that can improve lives throughout the world.

ACCELERATING INNOVATION IN HEALTH TECHNOLOGY

Historically, physicians have been the leading source of ideas for new medical technologies, and engineers have been tasked with translating mature ideas into actual products. The leaders of the Stanford Byers Center for Biodesign wanted to adjust that sequence and enable physicians and engineers to work together as a team of equals, focused on addressing unmet medical needs—and doing so in an interdisciplinary way.

In 2001, the center launched an innovation fellowship for young physicians who have completed their residency and engineers who have earned a master's degree or PhD. Since then, 12 fellows have been selected each year. They are brought together into teams of four—typically two engineers and two physicians—for 10 months. The center, which administers the fellowship, looks for people who may have tried to pursue their own medical technology ideas but haven't been able to make them work. Upon coming to Stanford, the fellows are assigned to a clinical area—typically one in which they have no formal training. "They're just more creative that way," says Paul Yock, who founded the center in 2001. "They have less constraints in the way they think about the issues."

For two months, fellows are given wide access to clinics and hospitals— observing doctors, talking to nurses, interviewing patients, and even spending time with them in their home environments, to get a better understanding of what can be done better. The center leadership tells the teams, in so many words, "Don't come back until you've seen at least 200 clinical needs that, if there was a good technology, would be interesting to solve."

Why 200? "Our young inventors can fall in love too easily with clinical needs," says Yock. "Because getting new technology to patients often takes ten years and tens of millions of dollars, you want to be really careful about what you choose. That's why we purposely overpopulate the bucket of needs that they're considering, and then we force those needs to compete. That makes each team choose the two or three of those 200 that they think will be truly important to solve." Once fellows have identified the top two or three needs, they are asked to propose two or three new approaches to each of those needs. Those solutions then compete to produce a single best concept to move forward into prototyping and testing.

Fellows consult about 150 experts, and as part of that process, they explore several issues that could be obstacles, such as the patent landscape, the reimbursement pathway, and the likelihood of regulatory approval. When they winnow their list down to one idea, the focus turns to how the product will ultimately be developed to benefit patients. For example, will it be licensed? Or will a company be launched to support it?

It's a very thorough process—and sometimes the last step is a decision by the team *not* to pursue the idea. "We actually love that," says Yock, "because these young innovators need to know how to do that in their career later on."

But many ideas have turned out to be worth pursuing. Since the innovation fellowship started in 2001, the trainees have founded 50 companies—48 of which are still operating. They have raised more than $740 million in startup funds, and the inventions have reached more than 1.5 million patients.

One of those companies is iRhythm. Its founders, who were innovation fellows in 2005–06, wanted to improve diagnosis of heart arrhythmias. Typically, a diagnosis depended on the arrhythmia happening while a patient was meeting with a doctor. Some people would wear a device, known as a Holter monitor, that had multiple electrodes attached to the skin for 24 to 48 hours. But the electrodes were cumbersome, the unit was not water-resistant, and the time period was too short to detect intermittent arrhythmias. The Holter also needed to be retrieved from the hospital, and returned there, for doctors to access the data it collected. The fellows saw a clear need for a single-use product that was comfortable and that could generate a flow of data over one to two weeks—and enable a prompt diagnosis. It also needed to be affordable for payers.

The fellows developed a user-friendly heart monitor, known as the Zio Patch. The three-inch patch is applied to the chest via an adhesive and can be worn for up to 14 days, offering uninterrupted cardiac monitoring. The patient then mails the Zio Patch to a service center, where the data is downloaded, with a diagnosis to follow. It's more convenient for patients and doctors, and it saves money by reducing the number of referrals.

In 2009, the FDA approved the Zio Patch for use, and it has proven very popular. Hundreds of thousands of people have used it, and in October 2016 iRhythm became a publicly traded company. The company's founder, Uday Kumar, has said that the Center for Biodesign's approach was critical to the success of the Zio Patch. Although he's since left iRhythm, he said that "I've used the process [taught at the center] to launch multiple companies, and I'm even more confident that it's the most effective way to do health technology innovation" [53].

The effectiveness of the Biodesign process has also been tested in different global settings. The Stanford-India Biodesign program has trained a generation of in-country fellows who have developed new technologies that are serving resource-constrained patient populations. Joint training programs have also been established in Singapore and Japan (cultures that are not traditionally known for innovation or risk-taking). The Biodesign fellows in both countries have had considerable success in inventing new health technologies, several of which are now entering clinical care. Trainees from the global programs understand that the key to successful inventing in any cultural context is a disciplined focus on researching the needs in that specific setting. As the Biodesign faculty leaders like to emphasize: "A well-characterized need is the DNA of a great invention."

HOW DATA CAN IMPROVE MEDICAL EDUCATION AND HELP MEASURE PHYSICIAN PERFORMANCE

How should medical students be taught? And how should the skills of doctors be quantified? Those are critically important questions that don't always have easy answers. But Carla Pugh, a professor of surgery at Stanford, has provided valuable new insights in both areas. She has been a pioneer in developing advanced engineering technologies that generate data that can be used to bring precision to medical education and to assessments of how effectively physicians perform a variety of procedures.

Pugh has an extremely rare set of credentials—she has a medical degree and a PhD in education. (She was the first surgeon in the United States to have both credentials.) She decided to pursue the education degree after finding one element of her medical school education unsatisfactory.

> I was a visual learner, and there are pros and cons to that. In anatomy, I had a photographic memory. I could see things in 3-D. But the positive side was also the negative side: I wanted my books to be in 3-D and they weren't. I would spend a lot of time in the library looking at every picture of the folding and rotation of the heart tube. It was a pivotal moment of frustration—until I was able to draw the picture in series. Textbooks would show one or two portions of the heart tube and expect you to be able to grasp it. That was very frustrating for me. So I would check out books that we weren't assigned, and I would dive deep to find those images.

She had similar experiences once she started as a surgery resident, which led her to want to help develop better textbooks, better ways of training, and better ways of visualization in preparation for anatomy or surgery.

While pursuing her doctorate, she learned about sensor technology—which generates data based on motion and force—and she recognized that it could be used to help teach surgical procedures. She used that technology to develop a simulator (a realistic imitation of a patient), which led to a patent and then her own company, Medical Teaching Systems (MTS). "I was on a mission to find out how we can use technology to drastically change the face of medical education and surgical education." The first MTS product is used in more than 200 medical and nursing schools. Students can utilize the devices to simulate experience in the clinic, and instructors can use the data that's generated to measure students' performance.

Pugh has been particularly focused on haptics, which is the art and science of touch. It means knowing how to touch something, knowing how it is supposed to feel, and being able to discern the difference between what's normal and what's abnormal. It's a critical skill for physicians—and surgeons in particular. But as Pugh has pointed out,

> The tricky thing about haptics is we don't have a sure-fire way of teaching it and we don't have a way of measuring it. Therefore, we don't have a way of ensuring competency. How are doctors supposed to learn? How do you master a body of knowledge when some of the most important things you're supposed to know can't be taught in a lecture, can't be read in a book, and sometimes can't be experienced in an emergency situation when things are so moving so quickly [54]?

This is part of her larger complaint with how doctors are trained:

> Doctors go through years and years of training to become top-notch elite professionals, but when you look at our training, it pales in comparison to other professionals. Athletes, for example, have access to instant replays, video reviews, and years and years' worth of performance data and metrics that help them to understand exactly what it is they need to do to master their craft. The best we have in the medical field is the tried-and-true board examination, but this is a pencil-and-paper test. A test of cognitive and declarative knowledge. We don't have a test for hands-on skills and we desperately need one [55].

In 2016, Pugh founded another company, called 10 Newtons. It is focused on cultivating the measure, analysis, and understanding of the process of touch, with an emphasis on data analytics and data visualization. Instead of building simulators for teaching (like medical teaching systems), the goal is to build sensor-enabled systems that allow for mass data collection and characterization of mastery learning curves.

Ten Newtons has developed more than 15 sensor-enabled training tools, and many of them can also be used for patient care. They're being utilized along with video and motion-tracking technologies, which has enabled "data acquisition methods ... to capture hands-on clinical performance at every point of contact" [56]. And that has generated a comprehensive database that yields new insights about medical decision-making and clinical performance in areas such as breast health, laparoscopy, pelvic exams, and intubation. A critical factor in the data and training tools is an additional focus on decision-making and team communication during procedures. While most motion research has focused on technical skills metrics, Pugh and her team have noted that lack of motion (idle time) within a complex motion signal indirectly represents procedural planning and intraoperative judgment. To facilitate an in-depth assessment of performance, her team also collects audio-visual data along with the sensor data. Their goal is to fully realize "the quantified physician"—using wearables to track personalized performance data. This approach enables a broader focus than technical skills alone.

Although Pugh was expressly warned by others in the medical profession not to study physicians' hands-on skills—because of the wide variety of approaches—she and her team have repeatedly found that the sensor data reveal a striking number of similarities when the desired procedural outcomes are achieved. This is especially true for the clinical breast examination.

She and her colleagues conducted a study revealing that experienced physicians who missed a breast lesion all had one element in common—failure to apply the needed amount of pressure when conducting the clinical breast exam to properly locate a mass. The study, which was the basis of an article that Pugh coauthored in the *New England Journal of Medicine* in 2015, showed that in a simulated environment, if examiners apply less than 10 Newtons of force—equivalent to a light-to-medium back massage—they are seven times more likely to miss a breast lesion. "Since variations in force cannot be reliably measured by means of human observation," wrote Pugh and her coauthors, "our findings underscore the potential for sensor technology to add value to existing, observation-based assessments of clinical performance" [57].

Pugh has developed a simulator called BEST (Breast Exam Sensory Training) Touch that measures the pressure being applied to a lifelike model. The model has a sensor on the bottom of the ribcage, and it delivers real-time feedback on the amount of pressure being exerted. There is also a lesion on each breast, which the user is instructed to find. She points out, "Within 10 minutes max, 5 minutes for most people who didn't get it right in the beginning, they're able to figure out, 'Wow, OK. I didn't know that that's how I was supposed to do it'" [58].

Getting the medical profession to improve performance measurement is ultimately going to depend on technology, says Pugh. "There is a lot of great technology out there. Sensors, motion tracking, wearables, physiologic monitors, you name it. Most of this technology is not built with medical training in mind, or human performance measurement. All that means to me is that there are incredible opportunities to repurpose currently available technologies and expand their use." She also believes that once doctors have access to instant replays and video reviews of their performances—something that's largely unavailable to them, for legal reasons—"then we'll really be able to take education and assessment to the next level. That's the final frontier" [59].

DEVELOPING NEW AND BETTER DIAGNOSTIC TOOLS

For all the progress that's been achieved in medicine, there are still areas where treatment options have changed very little over the past 20 years. Consider the diagnosis of infections. Physicians are routinely forced to make decisions about how to treat an infection before it's been diagnosed—a practice that is virtually unheard of elsewhere in medicine. It's a problem that Adam de la Zerda is trying to solve. An assistant professor of structural biology at Stanford, he is also the founder of a company called Click Diagnostics that is seeking to accelerate the time needed to diagnose infectious diseases.

De la Zerda has a personal connection to the issue. One evening, when his daughter, Noa, was about 18 months old, she arrived home from a playdate and a few hours later started signaling that she had a stomachache. She eventually vomited, but the pain continued. De la Zerda called a nurse, and after reporting the symptoms, he and his wife were told to bring Noa to the emergency room. A team of doctors and nurses was assembled when they arrived, and they took chest X-rays and a swab from Noa's nose. She was hooked up to an oxygen monitor, and while the X-rays did not show any foreign objects in her lungs—there was a fear that she may have inhaled part of a toy during the playdate—there was still uncertainty about what was causing her pain. When her oxygen levels began to decline, the doctors recommended a procedure under anesthesia to check to see if she had a foreign body in her airway. De la Zerda and his wife opted against that step, but the doctors came back to them many more times over the next 24 hours and made the same recommendation.

Eventually, the lab results came back from the nose swab—and it turned out Noa had a very common condition called respiratory syncytial virus. At that point, recalls de la Zerda, the environment at the hospital changed.

> Everybody calmed down. No longer did they tell us that we're bad parents for not letting them operate on our child and look into her lungs. They even started talking about releasing her back home, with just us monitoring the

symptoms. But if we had only known when she just checked into the emergency room that she had the virus, this entire episode would have been very, very different.

Click Diagnostics seeks to prevent episodes like this by enabling much faster diagnoses of infectious disease. The company focuses on a tool called Polymerase Chain Reaction (PCR), which is the gold standard for diagnosing infections. (Its inventor, Kary Mullis, received the Nobel Prize in Chemistry in 1993.) PCR is typically used in connection with a very large instrument—about the size of a small sofa—that's found in medical labs. While PCR tools are very accurate at diagnosing infections, they depend on having a tissue sample, which is sent to a lab for tests, and the lab then contacts the doctor to provide the results. The machines that run PCR can cost over $100,000, take hours to run, and require specialized trained personnel to operate.

De la Zerda wants to make PCR tools much more accessible. "We want to empower anybody—from health professionals to individual patients—anywhere to run PCR diagnostics to look for any infection and know that they're getting good and accurate answers, whoever they are." And he wants to achieve that by transforming a very large, slow-moving instrument into a small handheld device that generates diagnoses in less than 30 minutes. If he succeeds, diagnosis of infectious diseases would be transformed. Having the PCR result available while the patient was still in the physician's office could help reduce unnecessary antibiotic prescriptions, as physicians would have a definitive diagnosis indicating viral versus bacterial infection for common upper-respiratory infections. Moreover, such a small, inexpensive, rapid, and accurate test for infections could transform the way patients take ownership of their health, by empowering them to test themselves or their loved ones for common infections in the privacy of their own home.

As that work continues, de la Zerda's research at Stanford has a similar diagnostic objective, which is to gain a more rapid understanding of whether therapies like chemotherapy are successfully treating cancer in individual patients. To achieve this, he is focused on bringing greater precision to medical imaging. Approximately 25 trillion cells reside in the human body, and they are in constant communication with one another, with proteins and other signaling molecules being sent back and forth as messages. His goal is to make it possible to listen in real time to the ongoing communication that's going on—one billion cells at the same time.

Today, it's possible only to get a snapshot of how cells communicate with each other, and that severely limits our understanding of cells, says de la Zerda.

We know individual "words" that are being said by the cells, but we've never heard an actual conversation. And that means we're lacking context. We don't know anything about how the cells had been communicating or how they will respond. And the analysis misses the billion other cells that are communicating with each other. It's a very incomplete picture.

Monitoring communication will also make it possible to see how cells are responding to treatments like chemotherapy. "Today, it typically takes us two to three months to see if somebody's responding to chemo. Those are two, three months where a patient is going through really nasty treatments without even knowing if the treatments are effective or not. If they're not responding, we'll know to stop the treatment right away."

Technology is fundamental to meeting this challenge. Achieving a complete picture depends on looking into tissue and being able to see billions of cells simultaneously, in three-dimensional models. Today, the most powerful tools make it possible only to capture images that represent thousands of cells. De la Zerda is working to bridge this gap so that cell communications can be captured in much greater detail. Once this capability is developed, there are many different applications. In addition to therapies being analyzed for their effectiveness, tumors will be detected much earlier. More generally, seeing and monitoring cell communications will enhance our fundamental understanding of cancer biology, which will lead to more innovative and more precise guidelines for cancer treatment.

LEVERAGING INTERDISCIPLINARY INNOVATION TO ADVANCE GLOBAL HEALTH

The flurry of activity and innovation at Stanford and in Silicon Valley can unleash opportunities to improve the well-being of people in developing countries. While most of these countries have achieved significant progress in recent decades, they are also home to many of the world's most pressing health challenges. Medical breakthroughs can (and should) benefit people in these countries, but there is still tremendous value in efforts that are entirely devoted to improving well-being worldwide.

That's the focus of Michele Barry, who is director of the Center for Innovation in Global Health at Stanford, senior associate dean at the School of Medicine, and the Drs. Ben and Jess Shensen Professor of Medicine. The center seeks to leverage its connection to Stanford by making grants primarily for interdisciplinary projects that benefit the developing world. More specifically, applicants are encouraged to demonstrate that their projects will involve at least two of Stanford's graduate schools, in addition to the School of Medicine. "I don't think you can precisely attack problems of global health without thinking about larger components than just the disease," says Barry. "There are many social, cultural, and business aspects to a global health problem that one needs to incorporate to be able to precisely cure it or predict it. That's why we look to projects crossing multiple disciplines."

The center has funded some remarkably innovative and successful initiatives. One of them was a "mini-lab" to authenticate counterfeit medications and permit small-scale providers in Africa to manage safe pharmaceuticals and inventories. Another project funded low cost, point-of-care audiometry to identify and prevent hearing loss caused by tuberculosis medication. An incredibly successful center-funded project led to the development of a $20 foot brace that serves children born with clubfoot, a condition that affects 1 out of every 750 newborns worldwide. Known as Miracle Feet, it is now used annually by about 5,000 children in 21 developing countries—and it has won multiple awards for its creative and accessible design. "It's super easy to put on and take off," said the mother of a child born in Brazil with clubfoot. "It's quite different. In my opinion, it's better than the other brace" [60].

The center also enables Stanford clinicians to work in communities that have limited resources to meet health challenges. Each year, more than 50 Stanford physicians are sent to low-resource settings that are in long-term relationships with Stanford—avoiding parachute-in missions. "I don't think you can be a really good doctor, taking care of immigrants, unless you really understand their approach to health, how they treat themselves, and how they define 'health,'" says Barry. Residents and faculty see patients and pursue research, in developing countries and/or on American Indian reservations bringing back a more precise understanding of cross-cultural health concerns.

A cardiology fellow at Stanford, Andrew Chang has worked in Rwanda and treated patients at a hospital in the capital city, Kigali. He's also spent time in Uganda studying women with rheumatic heart disease. The experiences gave him an important insight: "Practicing medicine overseas makes you realize that, in many ways, people are all the same," he told *Stanford Medicine*. "It's the same base emotions. Fear, regret, anger, sadness—these things are universal. When someone starts crying, you hold their hand" [61].

Another area of emphasis is what Barry calls "planetary health," saying that "one cannot achieve human health if one doesn't look around and see what's going on with your planet. Planetary health is more than just the climate's impact on health. It's also about the impact humans have had on the natural systems of Earth, such as its biodiversity, animals, water infrastructure, and air."

Emblematic of that focus is support the center has given to a program in Borneo called Health in Harmony. The habitat around one of the island's last orangutan parks, Gunung Palung National Park, was being decimated by logging. A program funded by the center offered a local village's residents low-cost health care in exchange for an end to logging. The effect has been transformative. Logging has declined by 88 percent, child mortality and disease have plunged, the overall health of the community has improved, and more than half of the residents who had been employed in logging are now in farming.

Barry is also working to cultivate a new generation of women leaders in global health, as women occupy less than 25 percent of leadership positions in the sector despite being responsible for the majority of health care provided. Empowering women and girls has been shown to impact health—and "placing them in leadership health positions is key," says Barry.

One part of this effort involves the launch of new training opportunities throughout the world, with a goal of reaching up to 3,000 mid- and senior-career women over the next decade, through fellowships of about one year, complemented by real-world practice plans that can contribute to better help and more inclusive leadership, as well as mentorship, peer support, and residential experiences. "It's not just about giving women leadership skills," says Barry. "I also want to try to be catalytic in changing the environment that they work in as well."

BRINGING TRANSPARENCY TO DRUG PRICING

One of the internet's great benefits has been enabling the emergence of platforms, like Amazon, that deliver transparency about the prices companies charge for products that are similar, if not identical. Alas, this transparency has been slow to penetrate the health care industry, where prices for products and services can vary widely, based on a constellation of factors. But one company—GoodRx—has succeeded in collecting prices and discounts for thousands of drugs, with all the information published on its regularly updated website.

The company's origin can be traced back to 2010, when its founder, Doug Hirsch, made a routine visit to a pharmacy to fill a prescription. The pharmacist told him the price was $450. He decided to visit another pharmacy, where the price was $250. At a third pharmacy, the price was $350. When Hirsch balked, the pharmacist offered to negotiate. "That opened my eyes," says Hirsch, "because I just assumed that the person with the white coat and the computer had a fixed price list. And I had no idea there was a variability in drug pricing."

Hirsch had a background in technology—he had previously been a senior executive at Yahoo and Facebook—and so he approached a friend, Trevor Bezdek, who had founded a technology firm that served health care companies. They decided to explore further, and although they had no experience with health insurance or pharmacies, they wondered if it might be possible to organize a comprehensive database of drug prices. They discovered that 14 states had laws that required a website to publish the prices of common prescription drugs. "But half the websites were down," recalls Hirsch, "and the other half were just totally wrong."

Hirsch and Bezdek started trying to manually collect the cash prices for different drugs—a process that taught them that there were several ways for consumers to pay far less than the posted price. That launched them on a seven-year odyssey to organize drug pricing, understand the variability of drug pricing, and provide consumers with the information that would enable them to choose from a variety of pricing options.

The way it works is simple. Users enter their zip code and the medication they're looking for. In return, GoodRx provides a list of prices in their area, for comparison shopping. There is no charge to use the service, and it doesn't require users to provide any personal information—not even an email address. As of the summer of 2018, about eight million people were using the service each month. The company has called itself "the Expedia of prescription drugs."

Pharmacies were initially suspicious of GoodRx, but they've become very supportive. Hirsch explains why:

> Imagine if you're a pharmacist, and you're asked to fill a prescription. You get the bottle. You put the sticker on it. You measure out the pills. And then the consumer doesn't show up. Or the customer shows up but can't afford to fill the prescription and walks away, which happens 200 million times a year. Pharmacies have realized that GoodRx helps consumers who otherwise wouldn't have filled their prescriptions. And that's helped make our relationships with pharmacies really strong.

There's another benefit—helping people find the lowest price for the pharmaceuticals increases the likelihood that they will buy them and use them. Patients' non-adherence to their recommended treatments has been estimated to cost the U.S. health care system up to $289 billion annually, while also causing approximately 125,000 deaths [62].

Like many innovators, Hirsch and Bezdek initially met resistance when seeking feedback on their idea. Everyone from pharmaceutical sales executives to a medical school dean (not me!) told them they were wasting their time. What these people overlooked, says Hirsch, was that 90 percent of prescriptions today are for generic drugs, which can have significant price variation. "People told us we were playing in the wrong swimming pool," says Hirsch, "but we realized the swimming pool we were in was actually huge."

DOING THE "IMPOSSIBLE": USING PLANTS TO PRODUCE "MEAT"

Pat Brown has an audacious goal: eliminating the use of animals in the food system and causing the animal-based food industry to fade away. How does he plan to achieve that? By creating food that replicates meat, fish, and dairy products and having consumers decide that they prefer these versions to the ones that are made using animals. "We are not interested in coexistence with the incumbent industry," he says. "We want to completely take their market away by fair competition of the marketplace with better products, and to do it by 2035."

Brown is the founder and CEO of Impossible Foods—a company based in Redwood City, California, that has attracted $750 million in funding (as of May 2019) since its founding in 2011. Its investors include Bill Gates and the venture capital arm of Google. The company's product is the Impossible Burger, which is designed to look and taste like animal meat, despite being made without any animal products. As of April 2019, the Impossible Burger was available in more than 5,000 restaurants in the United States, Hong Kong, Singapore, and Macau—these restaurants include chains such as Carl's Jr., White Castle, and Burger King—with plans to have it sold in grocery stores as well.

Brown's background does not suggest someone who would start a food company. He was trained as a molecular biologist and joined the faculty of

Stanford's School of Medicine in 1988. His initial research focused on how the AIDS virus replicates, but he transitioned to developing tools for using the genome sequences to systematically study how genes work and how they specify the properties of cells. He applied that knowledge to understanding, classifying, and diagnosing cancers and to understanding basic physiology. "The last thing I ever imagined myself doing was founding a company," he says. "I also had essentially zero interest in food. I never really gave it much thought, and if you had asked me, I would have said, 'Food as a topic of research is as boring as it gets.'"

But like many successful entrepreneurs, Brown had a contrarian streak—and an appetite for challenging established industries. Earlier in his career, he confronted what he calls "the grossly antisocial dysfunctionality of the scientific publishing system." Angered by the practice of scientific publishers charging for access to their articles, he helped launch a public repository of scientific literature called PubMed Central. He also founded the world's first successful open-access publisher, the Public Library of Science (PLOS).

While on a sabbatical from Stanford in 2009, Brown gave himself a bold assignment: identify the most important problem in the world that he could help solve. He quickly settled on trying to combat the environmental impact associated with using animals for food. While he'd been a strict vegetarian for a decade, he was never an evangelist about it. "I didn't feel like it was my job to tell anyone else what to do." But that changed when he concluded that the existing system "was the thing most likely to push us into a complete environmental catastrophe. I decided it was not just a personal choice—it was something I have to figure out in order to change the world. And nobody was seriously trying to solve it, so I felt like 'OK, I'll do that.'"

In 2010, he initiated a workshop under the auspices of the National Academy of Sciences and the National Academy of Medicine (he's a member of both). The event brought together several experts in public health, nutrition, the environment, and economics, and Brown asked them to focus on the impact of transitioning away from animals in the food production system. While the workshop was productive, Brown realized that simply issuing a report on the topic was going to have little or no influence on what he wanted to change: people eating animal-based products.

He also thought it would be futile to try to get people to stop eating meat. He sees meat consumption as a "cultural habit" that's complemented by an intrinsic attraction to the chemical profile of heme, which is the molecule that's responsible for the unique flavors and aromas of meat and fish. "Some of the odorants produced by heme-catalyzed reactions have a striking effect on the behavior of carnivorous animals, which suggests they have a really strong drive for it." He concluded that

> the only way to address the issue was to do something akin to what I did with
> the Public Library of Science, which was to beat the incumbent industry at
> their own game by competing in the marketplace and taking their business

away from them. And the way to do that was to find a way to satisfy the demand for meat that doesn't involve using animals to produce these foods.

Brown approached three of the multiple venture capital firms operating near Stanford with what he says was a "very amateurish pitch," focused on how to compete with the animal-based food industry. One of his final slides highlighted that it's a $1.5 trillion industry based on technology that hasn't fundamentally improved for thousands of years. "All three firms were ready to invest. I just picked one and went with it."

Brown's primary focus is environmental protection. He says that eliminating the animal-based meat industry is "the only way we avert—and hopefully reverse—an ongoing environmental catastrophe that's due to the use of animals to develop food." This process of food production is, he says, "increasingly recognized by environmentalists around the world as the most destructive technology on Earth." According to the company, animal agriculture takes up nearly 50 percent of the earth's land, consumes 25 percent of all freshwater, generates 15 percent of all greenhouse gas emissions, and "destroys our ecosystems" [63]. In 2019, a sustainability firm hired by Impossible Foods compared the environmental impact of buying an Impossible Burger with buying a burger made from a cow. The analysis showed that an Impossible Burger involved 87 percent less water use, 96 percent less land use, 89 percent fewer greenhouse gas emissions, and a 92 percent reduction in aquatic pollutants [64].

Better health will ultimately be realized from the environmental improvements associated with ending animal-based food production, says Brown, and will dwarf the public health benefits of people not consuming meat- and dairy-based products. But he projects that public health will improve as people transition to products like those produced by Impossible Foods.

> We only release products that we believe, based on the best available evidence, are better for the consumer than what they replace. [The quarter-pound Impossible Burger has 0 mg cholesterol, 14 grams of total fat, and 240 calories in a quarter-pound patty, while the equivalent patty from a cow has 80 mg cholesterol, 23 grams of total fat and 290 calories.] In terms of global health and nutrition, there are nearly one billion people whose health and growth and development are impaired by inadequate protein intake, and there are nearly two billion people globally who have clinically significant iron deficiency. The product we're developing is an excellent source of both protein and iron.

Impossible Foods is one of the biggest actors in a space that's undergone considerable growth in recent years—and that growth is likely to continue. As CB Insights points out in a January 2019 report titled "Our Meatless Future," "We can expect to see more experimentation across the globe on alternative protein sources" [65]. It's too early to tell how successful these companies will be, but the experience of the past decade shows how hidebound industries can be challenged by upstart companies delivering a traditional product or service in a new way. That's something the animal-based food product industry can't afford to ignore.

MINIMIZING MISTAKES IN MEDICAL RESEARCH

In any given year, more than five million articles are published in scientific journals. The volume is so high that supercomputers are now used to synthesize the conclusions contained in these journals, to help ensure that medical researchers are always drawing on the most up-to-date information. That sounds like an innovative way to help improve treatment and care of patients, but it does raise a fundamental question: Are the published conclusions accurate?

"I think there are errors in every single scientific study," says John Ioannidis, a professor of medicine at Stanford, and codirector of the Meta-Research Innovation Center, which focuses on strengthening the research enterprise to improve the quality of scientific studies in biomedicine and beyond. He has been at the forefront of highlighting factual mistakes in scientific publishing. In 2005, he wrote a celebrated paper titled, "Why Most Published Research Findings Are False" [66]. (It has been the most-accessed article in the history of the Public Library of Science.) He points to a range of factors contributing to errors in research:

> You have the basic drive to come up with something that looks unusual—and the more unusual something looks, the less likely it is to be correct. The burden of evidence to prove that something is really unusual, and that no one has seen before, is pretty high. Another issue is the reward system, which does not reward people for finding non-significant results—not for "failing." And there is a misconception that finding non-significant results is failure. Very often, non-significant results are very informative. They're telling us that, "Here's a very large block that you can exclude," or, "By excluding this, you know that the answer is going to be there." So negative results can be extremely informative—far more informative than some of the "positive" results. A third issue is limited funds. There are lots of very smart people trying to do research, and each one of them, on average, gets a very thin slice of funding. If you're in an environment where studies are small, this means that you're underpowered, which means that a lot of interesting things to be discovered will not be discovered. Worse, in an environment of small studies, when something is discovered, it has a higher chance of being entirely wrong or grossly exaggerated.

Ioannidis doesn't see fraud as a common driver of the research errors, but rather problems with handling complex data that require a high level of expertise from everyone involved in the research. As an example, he points to a 2013 study, published in the *New England Journal of Medicine,* on the benefits of the so-called Mediterranean Diet [67]. The study received considerable attention, but in June 2018 the lead authors retracted it, after they discovered that approximately 14 percent of the people who participated in the study had not been randomly assigned to the two different diet groups (Mediterranean and low-fat) [68]. According to Ioannidis,

There were 241 authors and collaborators in the author masthead. Apparently not all of them had full expertise about how to run an important trial. And there were probably hundreds of other people who were collecting data at all of the sites where the study was happening. Some sites just violated very basic, elementary rules about how to randomize people.

There are a few basic principles that should guide research, he says. One is collaboration with other researchers, which can translate to larger sample sizes and more oversight. He also points to the importance of replication—"If you see something happening again and again, it's more likely to be accurate." Another point of emphasis is protection from bias, which can be challenging. "I was involved with a study that identified 235 different biases," says Ioannidis [69]. "So researchers have to think ahead of time about which of these 235 biases might be influential in the study they're conducting and then figure out a way to preemptively eliminate them or at least try to limit their influence."

Most important of all may be transparency—and data sharing in particular. Ioannidis says that while most biomedical researchers do not share their data, "there's clearly been progress." In a random sample of 441 biomedical research papers published from 2000 to 2014, the raw data was not made available for any of them [70]. A more recent random sample of research papers published in 2015–17 showed that the raw data was available for almost 20 percent of them [71].

INNOVATION GONE WRONG: THOUGHTS ON THERANOS

In many industries, it's generally understood that an innovative product will go through many failures before it gets traction in the marketplace. That's accepted, since a consequence of these failures is often some consumer inconvenience, but not much more. It's a very different environment for innovations related to health and health care. While trial and error is part of any product development, once a product is being used in the marketplace, failures can have a profound impact on the users—illness, injury, and even death.

In Silicon Valley, the search is always underway for innovations that could be the "next big thing." The optimism comes from many different factors, not the least of which is that Silicon Valley *has* given rise to products and companies that have been, at different times, actual versions of the next big thing: Google, Facebook, and Netflix are a few recent examples, and earlier ones include Hewlett-Packard, Cisco, Intel, and Apple.

It was out of this environment that one particularly celebrated Silicon Valley startup emerged: Theranos. Founded in 2004, it promised to revolutionize health care through a simple blood test. With a young, female founding CEO, Elizabeth

Holmes, and a board of directors composed of many notable figures, the company attracted widespread publicity and significant capital.

As we now know, Theranos could never back up its bold claims. According to news reports, it went to extraordinary lengths to misrepresent itself to regulators, investors, scientists, and—most important—patients. That deception could not be sustained, and the Securities and Exchange Commission announced in March 2018 that it was charging the company, Holmes, and another senior executive with having engaged in an "elaborate, years-long fraud"; it said Theranos "deceived investors into believing that its key product—a portable blood analyzer—could conduct comprehensive blood tests from finger drops of blood" [72]. (Holmes later paid a $500,000 fine and agreed not to serve in a leadership position at a publicly traded company for 10 years.) Holmes also faced criminal charges, having been indicted on two counts of conspiracy to commit wire fraud and nine counts of wire fraud. In September 2018, the company informed its shareholders that it intended to cease operating.

Much of what is known about Theranos comes from the legwork of an enterprising *Wall Street Journal* reporter, John Carreyrou. His book, *Bad Blood: Secrets and Lies in a Silicon Valley Startup*, which was released in May 2018, makes for gripping reading. But the first article questioning Theranos was written by Stanford's John Ioannidis. Published in the *Journal of the American Medical Association* in February 2015, the article pointed out that Theranos had made several bold claims but had never subjected them to the peer-review process that is a staple of biomedical literature [73]. Following the article's publication, the general counsel of Theranos contacted Ioannidis and suggested he meet with Holmes, Theranos's founder, with the idea that the two of them could collaborate on a paper. But the company lost interest when Ioannidis replied that any paper he might be associated with would require the company to be willing to publish its data.

Ioannidis's initial skepticism has been validated, and when interviewed for this book, in the aftermath of Theranos being brought to its knees, he commented on the company's shortcomings:

> Retrospectively, what was wrong with Theranos? I think the major problem was an absence of transparency. They were not making any of their data available. Nor were they making any of their science available, not even an advertisement in a scientific journal. It's impossible in 2018 to accept biomedical research where the researcher says, in effect, "I have a secret. I'm not going to tell you." We need to see how it works. If it's a laptop and someone says, "Well, this is a better laptop. The battery lasts five hours more than others," it's very easy to see. You just open it and you wait until it dies. But for Theranos and for health in general, if you say that this is going to be good for your health, we cannot wait 80 years for someone to die, and you don't need just one person to die. You need a population to be followed. So, we need transparency, and transparency was not something that Theranos was after. It was completely the opposite.

Another point of interest for many in Silicon Valley's technology community was the composition of the Theranos board. Holmes had attracted several high-profile individuals. This included many distinguished leaders with highly successful careers in government and business, but there was a near-absence of anyone with a science background.

Linda Avey of Precise.ly had some of the same concerns about governance. But her skepticism about Theranos also grew out of her initial experience with one of the company's blood testing clinics at a Walgreens in Palo Alto. She and a professional acquaintance asked the clinic technician some very basic questions, such as how many tests could be run based on a single blood prick. "The guy got a little bit uncomfortable," recalls Avey, "and then he just said, 'Well, that hasn't been worked out yet.' The whole thing just struck me as so odd. That was my first indication that something wasn't right."

The Theranos episode has prompted soul-searching about the culture in Silicon Valley and how the company was able to attract so much attention and money when its products were never backed by peer-reviewed science. Ioannidis says the company's practices should be viewed as emblematic of a larger trend—not of cheating and fraud, but of deficits in sound research practices and scientific rigor.

> Once a colossus like Theranos crumbles, everybody who was dissatisfied with the company—particularly former employees—will say that cheating was rampant. But I do worry about that narrative because it creates the impression that problems that arise in science are due to fraud and psychopaths and sociopaths. I don't think that that's true. In general, when things go wrong, we don't have sociopaths and psychopaths and fraud. We have people who struggle. They may put in an amazing number of hours and an amazing amount of effort, and then they get it wrong. I think that that's human, and especially nowadays with science being so complex and so convoluted, it's very easy to get it wrong. I think that if you take today's unicorns [privately held companies with valuations exceeding $1 billion], there may be many like Theranos. They're not engaged in fraud, but they have other major problems. Some of that is unavoidable. We cannot expect everything will turn out and everything will work all the time. But we can work on improving our success rates by improving how well we apply the scientific method to do, evaluate, share, and communicate research.

* * *

The Theranos episode aside, it's difficult to exaggerate the importance of innovation when it comes to human health. While the individual examples of innovation are too numerous to mention, their cumulative effects have transformed everyday life. One way of measuring this is to consider a simple indicator. At the start of the 20th century, life expectancy in the United States was just 47 years [74]. Disease and famine alone could kill millions of people. Today, with a plethora of innovations having contributed to advancements in detecting, preventing, and treating disease, U.S. life expectancy is 78.6 years (though as I noted in chapter 1, this has slightly declined in recent years) [75]. There have been similar—if not greater—gains in other countries throughout the world.

We take many of these advancements for granted, but it's important to remember that there was nothing inevitable about them. In many instances, the progress has been—and will continue to be—a product of men and women working together (often in academic medical centers) to challenge established ideas and conventions. Many of the individuals featured in this chapter have challenged—or are challenging—those ideas and conventions, and in doing so they are helping to lay the groundwork for breakthroughs that contribute to an improvement in human health, while helping to advance the Precision Health vision, across the United States and throughout the world.

As we contemplate the many different developments underway today, we shouldn't lose sight of what helps make many of them possible: an understanding of basic science, as well as the quest to continue unraveling the mysteries of human biology. That is the subject of the next chapter.

FUNDAMENTAL, DISCOVERY-FOCUSED RESEARCH: THE FOUNDATION OF BIOMEDICAL BREAKTHROUGHS

In the previous chapter, I discussed some of the keys to innovation, such as diversity, combination, collaboration, and chance. Each of those could apply to innovation regardless of the industry, but there's another key to innovation that is of critical importance in the world of biomedicine: discovery-focused, fundamental research, sometimes referred to as *basic science*. The goal of fundamental research in biomedicine is to increase our knowledge and understanding of living organisms and the biological systems that are essential for life.

The importance of fundamental research cannot be overstated. Every breakthrough in the diagnosis and treatment of disease is based upon our knowledge of fundamental biomedical principles and concepts. Without fundamental research, there would be no translational medicine because there would be nothing to translate. The Nobel Prize–winning chemist Sir George Porter observed that there are two kinds of research—that which is applied and that which is not yet applied. Many of us whose scholarship has led directly to an improvement in the care of patients can clearly trace our contributions to advances in the knowledge of fundamental biological mechanisms and processes. My discovery of superior canal dehiscence syndrome was directly related to the work that I and others had done to understand how the inner ear balance system controls movements of the eyes.

I include this chapter here because our ability to innovate in the prediction, prevention, and cure components of Precision Health will be dependent on continued insights that advance our knowledge about how biological systems work. There's a natural inclination to focus nearly all our energies on what seem like (and often are) pressing needs. That could be treating sick patients. Or it could be pursuing therapies, based on existing knowledge, that will make it

Discovering Precision Health: Predict, Prevent, and Cure to Advance Health and Well-Being,
First Edition. Lloyd Minor and Matthew Rees.
© 2020 John Wiley & Sons Ltd. Published 2020 by John Wiley & Sons Ltd.

possible to treat those afflicted with disease. These pursuits, and others like them, have inestimable value. But we can't lose sight of the fact that ongoing progress in these areas rests on continuing to unravel the mysteries of how the human body functions.

The real value of discovery often comes into focus during times of crisis. It was in that environment that a distinguished engineer named Vannevar Bush offered a compelling explanation of basic science, in 1945. He was serving as director of the U.S. government's Office of Scientific Research and Development. He had been in this role throughout World War II, which gave him an acute appreciation for the value of open-ended inquiry. "Basic research," he pointed out, "is performed without thought of practical ends."

> It results in general knowledge and understanding of nature and its laws. The general knowledge provides the means of answering a large number of important practical problems, though it may not give a complete specific answer to any one of them. The function of applied research is to provide such complete answers. The scientist doing basic research may not be at all interested in the practical applications of his work, yet the further progress of industrial development would eventually stagnate if basic research were long neglected [1].

Bush's words have only become more relevant over time. Knowledge of basic science continues to underpin and enable virtually all medical breakthroughs, and expanding that knowledge will play a vital role in advancing our ability to predict, prevent, and cure disease precisely. There has never been a better time than now to pursue discovery-focused research in biomedical science. As described in chapter 1, multiple fields of science and technology are now focused on problems and questions in biomedicine. In this chapter, I will highlight the enduring value of basic science, as well as several biomedical pioneers who are grounded in basic science and whose breakthroughs have dramatically increased our understanding of human biology.

It's not my goal here to provide a comprehensive overview of discovery-focused, fundamental research in biomedicine. Rather, I hope that the brief overviews of discoveries and the remarkable people who have made them will be informative and inspiring.

THE MANY DIFFERENT REASONS FOR RESEARCH

Research serves many different purposes. A useful shorthand description introduced by the late Donald E. Stokes, who served as dean of the Woodrow Wilson School at Princeton, featured three categories (or, as Stokes labeled them, "quadrants"). The first, named for the Nobel Prize–winning Danish physicist Niels Bohr, was described by Stokes as including "basic research that is guided solely by the quest for understanding without thought of practical use."

The second quadrant, named for the American inventor Thomas Edison, "includes research that is guided solely by applied goals without seeking a more general understanding of the phenomena of a scientific field." The third quadrant, named for French biologist Louis Pasteur, features "basic research that seeks to extend the frontiers of understanding but is also inspired by considerations of use" [2].

Given the academic affiliations of the individuals featured in this chapter, their research falls into the Bohr and Pasteur quadrants. I have also included descriptions of people whose research is focused on developing technologies that will help them and others make fundamental discoveries. The common denominator is a foundation of basic science, as the next two examples demonstrate.

A BREAKTHROUGH ENABLED BY BASIC SCIENCE

Suzanne Pfeffer is the Emma Pfeiffer Merner Professor in the Medical Sciences and professor of biochemistry at Stanford. Her research is helping to unlock insights about Parkinson's disease—a chronic, degenerative neurological disorder that affects about 1 percent of all people over the age of 60 and 5 percent of people over the age of 85 [3]. The progress she's achieved showcases how a long-term investment in basic science can pay dividends.

For the vast majority of people with Parkinson's disease, the cause is not well understood. In about 10 percent of cases, however, it is inherited, with the affected individual carrying mutations, typically involving one of two different proteins. One of those proteins is known as a kinase, which is an enzyme that modifies other proteins by adding phosphates to them.

For the past 30 years, Pfeffer has been studying a set of small enzymes called Rabs. She calls them "master regulators," given that they direct traffic between membranes. In 2015, two biochemists in Europe contacted her about their research into Parkinson's disease. They had discovered that Rabs are the main target of the kinase that's involved with inherited Parkinson's. Pfeffer and the biochemists are now collaborating, with researchers in Pfeffer's lab drawing on their knowledge of membrane traffic to better understand the molecular basis of Parkinson's. What made it possible, she says, "is our 30 years of basic research."

> Understanding how Rabs function has greatly jumpstarted our ability to discover exactly what goes wrong when they are modified by the disease-associated kinase. Identification of the molecular targets helps us know exactly where to look for defects in the brain, and it is already helping drug companies monitor the effectiveness of candidate drugs being tested to help patients with Parkinson's disease.

This progress, says Pfeffer, "attests to how investment in basic science can advance our understanding of disease—and do so with a remarkable level of precision."

MEDICAL RESEARCH AND UNEXPECTED DISCOVERIES

For scientists exploring molecular structures, Parkinson's disease, or just about anything else, it's useful to remember a fundamental principle of research: it is an unpredictable process, it cannot be rigidly structured, and at times it can seem haphazard. When scientists are looking for one thing, they often find something else. "Discoveries can't be planned," says Pfeffer.

> There's serendipity involved. And luck. You never know where that next breakthrough is going to come from. There are many, many examples of things in the clinic today that were discovered by accident. It was because people were just following their nose and following their gut feeling about what we needed to understand. It's paid off time and time again.

Roger Kornberg, the Mrs. George A. Winzer Professor in Medicine and a professor of structural biology at Stanford, points out that four of the most important discoveries underpinning modern medicine—X-rays, antibiotics, genetic engineering, and noninvasive imaging—did not result from attempts to solve a specific medical problem. "They resulted from the pursuit of knowledge for its own sake, the pursuit of basic science."

> People often fail to understand that the pursuit of knowledge is the source of discovery. You can't predict where solutions are going to come from because discovery cannot be anticipated. That's the definition of the word. These discoveries, and many others, all came about in that way. And that's the way discoveries will happen in the future.

Consider the accidental discovery of antibiotics. In September 1928, a scientist, Alexander Fleming, returned from a summer vacation and discovered that a mold called *Penicillium notatum* had contaminated his Petri dishes. But the mold had stopped the growth of bacteria—a finding that led to penicillin becoming one of the most valuable weapons to combat infectious diseases throughout the world. "When I woke up just after dawn on September 28, 1928," Fleming wrote later, "I certainly didn't plan to revolutionize all medicine by discovering the world's first antibiotic, or bacteria killer. But I guess that was exactly what I did" [4].

A more recent example of an accidental discovery that led to the creation of an entirely new scientific and medical field involves the revolutionary gene-editing tool, CRISPR. In 1993, a doctoral student named Francisco Mojica was examining bacteria taken from a marsh in Spain when he noticed a pattern of repeating DNA, with spaces between them—something he later characterized as "very unexpected and very amazing—and very peculiar" [5]. A decade of research followed, with Mojica trying to better understand what he had discovered. While others have subsequently built on the foundation he helped establish, he's said that his primary motivation has always been knowledge for knowledge's sake—not technological applications. "I have to confess that [technological applications are] not my goal. I just want to know" [6].

That desire for knowledge has been (and still is) a character trait among the world's most distinguished scientists. Not surprisingly, it's also a trait found among a group of Stanford professors whose work has greatly expanded our understanding of the inner workings of the human body. Profiles of a few of these individuals and their discoveries follow.

DISCOVERIES IN MOLECULAR BIOLOGY THAT ENABLED GENES TO BE CLONED

Paul Berg established himself as a pioneering scientist in 1953, when he was just 27. A biochemist at Washington University in St. Louis, he was, in the words of one science writer, "already conspicuously surefooted, fast, and precise" [7]. He challenged two senior scientists—one of whom was about to win a Nobel Prize—on an issue that had been lingering in biochemistry for years: how do mammalian cells make a molecule called acetyl CoA that is involved in the production of long chain fatty acids? The scientists had advanced a theory, which Berg investigated. Within a few months he'd discovered that their theory was completely wrong, owing to impurities in the preparation of the enzymes they had used. That research also led him to the discovery of a new kind of compound: acyladenylates. As he described it, "ATP could react with a variety of fatty acids and other compounds containing carboxyl groups in a specific way, thereby generating an activated acyl function which could then undergo a second reaction to produce a variety of compounds" [8].

It was an important discovery: that compound has become fundamental in the production of many different biochemical metabolites, and years later Berg would say that he took more pride in this discovery than any other in his career: "It was original research, the results weren't predictable, and it transpired when I was really just starting out as a scientist" [9].

In the course of that work, Berg discovered a large group of enzymes that participate in protein synthesis. The role of these enzymes is to activate the amino acids prior to their assembly into proteins. He was the first person to purify several of these enzymes from bacteria and from yeast that came from one of St. Louis's many breweries [10]. Each of these enzymes attaches one amino acid to the "tail" of an RNA molecule (tRNA), and each amino acid–tRNA is used in the process of protein chain assembly.

In 1959, Berg came to Stanford to help establish a department of biochemistry. His focus was gene function, but, as he points out, "the general paradigm for how genes work and the nature of genes was already established. We knew what a gene was. We knew largely what the structure of a gene was. We knew how it was transcribed into RNA." But all of this had been learned using bacteria and the viruses that infect them. What Berg wanted to know was if the way bacteria expresses its genes was also the case for the more complex eukaryotic and human cells. He realized that he had to change the focus of his research to accomplish this goal. His work with *E. coli* on the enzymes involved in protein synthesis shifted to exploring the nature of the genetic system in eukaryotes. "It was a big question to answer," he recalled years later.

In the years that followed, Berg's research led to numerous advances, which explored using the SV40 tumor virus and its DNA as a means of introducing new genes into mammalian cells. With that intent, he and his colleagues developed a method of joining together two different DNAs in vitro—an innovation that led to the emergence of recombinant DNA technology and resulted in Berg's being awarded the Nobel Prize for Chemistry in 1980.

Recombinant DNA marked the start of a new era in genetics. It had "pushed genetics from the realm of science into the realm of technology," writes Siddhartha Mukherjee in *The Gene: An Intimate History*. "Genes were not abstractions anymore. They could be liberated from genomes of organisms where they had been trapped for millennia. Genes were no longer just the subjects of study, but the instruments of study" [11].

Indeed, recombinant DNA assumed the most prominent place in biotechnology, medicine, and research. It has contributed to advances in the use of insulin, human growth hormone, blood clotting, hepatitis B, and HIV. The technology was a key enabler for cloning DNA—a breakthrough resting on a foundation of basic scientific research. As Berg has pointed out,

> Cloning became the disruptor of genetics. It enabled the isolation of human genes, or any genes, and propagating them to the point where large quantities could be obtained for analysis. From there, researchers could begin to make mutations in any of these genes that were cloned to study their properties. This breakthrough made possible all the advances in genetics that followed. The genome project could not have been done without being able to clone individual pieces of DNA, sequence those, and then develop algorithms that assemble them into the correct order. The discovery of oncogenes came about through recombinant DNA. Almost everything in genetics today stems from the basic technology of joining disparate DNA molecules together that enable scientists to devise new experiments and answer questions that could not be asked before that development. It didn't disrupt the science. It changed the paradigm of how we think about molecular biology.

THE BIRTH OF BIOTECHNOLOGY: CLONING GENES TO PRODUCE PROTEIN

Biotechnology has been one of the most dynamic industries of the past 40 years, and it has helped to deliver a range of therapies that have contributed to improvements in human health and well-being. But it's sometimes forgotten that the industry's creation rests on a foundation of a scientific discovery pioneered by two researchers working at academic medical centers.

The discovery came in the early 1970s, when Stanley Cohen was a professor of genetics and medicine at Stanford (a position he still holds today, as well as being the Kwoh-Ting Li Professor in the School of Medicine). Herbert Boyer was a professor of biochemistry at the University of California, San Francisco. Cohen's research was heavily focused on plasmids (circular double stranded DNA molecules), and in 1972 he and two colleagues pioneered an approach to removing plasmid DNA from bacterial cells, and then cloning single molecules of plasmid DNA by reimplanting each into a bacterium. The practice helped illuminate plasmid structure and antibiotic resistance [12]. Around the same time, Boyer's lab made a similarly important discovery. As the science historian Sally Smith Hughes describes it,

> A graduate student had isolated a restriction enzyme (the soon to be widely employed EcoRI) that cut DNA predictably at a specific position in the molecule.... Especially exciting was the finding ... that EcoRI did not cut evenly through the double strands of the DNA molecule. Instead, it made a staggered cut, creating two single projecting DNA strands. Each single strand was able to bond with a complementary DNA strand, as one Velcro strip unites with another [13].

She points out that the use of "sticky ends" to join DNA fragments had existed for about a decade, but the process was quite laborious. That changed with the enzyme discovered in Boyer's lab, as it "offered a substantial leap in ease and efficiency in splicing together DNA pieces to form recombinant molecules" [14].

Cohen and Boyer did not know each other, but in November 1972 they both traveled to Hawaii to attend a conference focused on plasmid biology (Cohen was one of the conference organizers and invited Boyer). Cohen spoke about being able to implant plasmid DNA into *E. coli*. Boyer discussed his work with EcoRI.

In an episode that is now part of science history, Cohen and Boyer took a walk together after a day of the conference proceedings. Along with a few colleagues, they ended up in a Korean-owned kosher delicatessen near Waikiki Beach. Over sandwiches and beer, Cohen and Boyer talked about their work and realized that fusing their findings could be the basis of genetic engineering. They envisioned a way for individual genes to be produced in amounts sufficient for them to be isolated and studied. EcoRI would be used to slice DNA into multiple fragments. The genes carried by a DNA fragment could then be propagated and cloned by joining the fragment to a plasmid and introducing the combination into *E. coli*. Potentially, this strategy also would enable proteins made by human cells to be manufactured in bacteria. The experiments that followed over the next year resulted in the cloning of DNA molecules.

The discoveries by Cohen, Boyer, and their colleagues laid the foundation for the birth of the biotechnology and enabled the development of medical treatments and vaccines that have contributed to advances in human welfare. The ability to clone genes also helped bring a new level of precision to the diagnosis of disease.

While the commercial opportunities that arose from the Cohen-Boyer methods are often emphasized, such as the founding of Genentech (which Boyer cofounded), it's useful to remember that the simple and powerful approach was made possible by basic science that built on the pioneering work of others in fields such as molecular biology and biochemistry. As Cohen has written,

> Our DNA cloning experiments resulted from the pursuit of fundamental biological questions rather than goals that most observers might regard as practical or "translational." I was investigating mechanisms underlying the ability of plasmids to acquire genes conferring antibiotic resistance and to exist separately from bacterial chromosomes; Herb Boyer was studying enzymes that restrict and destroy foreign DNA. The PNAS [Proceedings of the National Academy of Sciences] publications resulting from these pursuits generated considerable scientific excitement—and work aimed at repeating and extending the findings was undertaken almost immediately by other researchers [15].

A 1995 interview of Cohen by Hughes drives home Cohen's emphasis on basic science.

HUGHES: It was not your idea to develop what later became recombinant DNA technology.

COHEN: That's correct.

HUGHES: What you were trying to do was to pursue your science, and for your science you needed this particular method.

COHEN: Right.

HUGHES: Is that the order of priority?

COHEN: Yes.

HUGHES: I think we now look back and tend to see the technology as being the dominant thing, where in actuality it was the science.

COHEN: I think that's an important point, Sally, and that was also probably true for at least some of the other people that were working [in the field] as well. In my case, the technology was developed out of necessity so that we could study antibiotic resistance plasmids [16].

DISCOVERY OF A NOVEL MECHANISM RESPONSIBLE FOR REGULATION OF GENE EXPRESSION

There are approximately 20,000 genes in each human's genome. The process by which a gene is expressed in a cell involves copying DNA to messenger RNA, which is known as transcription. Andrew Fire, Craig Mello, and their colleagues investigated the regulation of gene expression in nematode worms—a process summarized by the Nobel Committee:

> Injecting mRNA molecules encoding a muscle protein led to no changes in the behaviour of the worms. The genetic code in mRNA is described as being the "sense" sequence, and injecting "antisense" RNA, which can pair with the mRNA, also had no effect. But when Fire and Mello injected sense and anti-sense RNA together, they observed that the worms displayed peculiar, twitching movements. Similar movements were seen in worms that completely lacked a functioning gene for the muscle protein. What had happened?
>
> When sense and antisense RNA molecules meet, they bind to each other and form double-stranded RNA. Could it be that such a double-stranded RNA molecule silences the gene carrying the same code as this particular RNA? Fire and Mello tested this hypothesis by injecting double-stranded RNA molecules containing the genetic codes for several other worm proteins. In every experiment, injection of double-stranded RNA carrying a genetic code led to silencing of the gene containing that particular code. The protein encoded by that gene was no longer formed.
>
> After a series of simple but elegant experiments, Fire and Mello deduced that double-stranded RNA can silence genes, that this RNA interference is specific for the gene whose code matches that of the injected RNA molecule, and that RNA interference can spread between cells and even be inherited. It was enough to inject tiny amounts of double-stranded RNA to achieve an effect, and Fire and Mello therefore proposed that RNA interference (now commonly abbreviated to RNAi) is a catalytic process [17].

The discovery, which *Nature* published in 1998 [18], led to pivotal changes in our understanding of gene regulation. As the Nobel summary noted, it "revealed a natural mechanism for controlling the flow of genetic information." And as a geneticist with Britain's prestigious Medical Research Council told the BBC at the time of the Nobel Prize announcement, "It is very unusual for a piece of work to completely revolutionize the whole way we think about biological processes and regulation, but this has opened up a whole new field in biology" [19].

The scientific accomplishments of Fire, now the George D. Smith Professor in Molecular and Genetic Medicine at Stanford and a professor of pathology and of genetics, have created new lines of inquiry for researchers and opened the door for new RNA therapeutics. In 2018, the FDA approved the first therapy that's directly based on RNA interference. The FDA commissioner at the time, Scott Gottlieb, MD, hailed the approval as "part of a broader wave of advances that allow us to treat disease by actually targeting the root cause, enabling us to arrest or reverse a condition, rather than only being able to slow its progression or treat its symptoms."

ELUCIDATION OF THE STRUCTURE OF COMPLEX PROTEINS

Roger Kornberg is a scientist's scientist. His father, Arthur, was a professor of biochemistry at Stanford and won the Nobel Prize in Physiology or Medicine in 1959. As a high school student, Roger worked in the lab of Paul Berg, the Nobel

Prize winner whose work is described above. After earning a PhD from Stanford in chemical physics, Roger Kornberg pursued an issue of extraordinary significance: advancing understanding of the structure of the enzyme that converts DNA into messenger RNA. It involved more than 20 years of research, but the effort paid off: He became the first scientist to discover the enzyme's three-dimensional image. The breakthrough was fundamental to his being awarded the Nobel Prize in Chemistry in 2006. The designation also made it the sixth time a father and son had won Nobel Prizes, along with one mother/father and daughter (Marie Curie/Pierre Curie and Irène Joliot-Curie).

Roger Kornberg's discoveries were rooted in basic research, and they prove how investing in research can pay substantial dividends. Without RNA polymerase, all the DNA contained in the human genome would be useless. Understanding how RNA polymerase directs transcription helps explain how the process sometimes goes awry, leading to birth defects, cancer, and other diseases.

Kornberg remains dedicated to research. Having discovered the enzyme and its structure, he also discovered the molecular computer that underlies the regulation of the process and the selective expression of the right genes at the right place at the right time. He and his colleagues continue to study the components of that machinery to this day. It's of particular interest, he says, "because almost every one of the components of that molecular computer, which guides the activity of the RNA polymerase, is now known in one or another mutant form to predispose to cancer. Not surprisingly, perhaps, but nevertheless remarkably, these are all candidates or potential targets for therapy in the future."

Brian Kobilka is another pioneer in elucidating the structure of proteins. Kobilka, the Helene Irwin Fagan Chair in Cardiology at Stanford and a professor of molecular and cellular physiology, won a Nobel Prize in Chemistry in 2012. His research showcased not only the value of basic scientific research but also the power of perseverance.

Advancing our understanding of a family of proteins called G protein-coupled receptors (GPCRs) was (and still is) the focus of Kobilka's research. GPCRs are responsible for most of the responses to hormones and neurotransmitters in the body. They're also responsible for vision and the sense of smell. No less important, a significant portion of the drugs on the market today—perhaps as many as 30 percent—derive their effectiveness from how they interact with GPCRs.

Kobilka became interested in GPCRs as a postdoctoral fellow, and when he started a lab at Stanford, one of his goals was to develop a better understanding of their structures. At the time, crystallography was the only way to do this. He began by trying to work out the procedures for making enough GPCRs to start crystallography trials. Eventually, he was able to conduct the trials, but a major breakthrough did not come for 17 years.

Kobilka and his colleagues ultimately succeeded in getting the first inactive state structure of a receptor for adrenaline. A few years later, in 2011, they obtained a structure of the receptor activating its intracellular protein, called the G protein. These were major breakthroughs. As Kobilka would later write, they "provided unprecedented insights into GPCR signaling at the molecular level" [20]. There were also potentially significant clinical applications. Understanding the receptor's structure, which is the target for many drugs, can contribute to the development of more precise therapies.

Asked about how people viewed his research while it was underway, he says, "Most people think that 17 years was a long time to continue working on the same problem." And he concedes that had he known how difficult it would be to learn the structure of the receptor from crystallography, "I might not have done it." But his single-minded devotion, coupled with what he has described as his "irrational optimism," kept him going. "When something didn't work, you'd be a little down; then at the end of the day at home, you'll think, 'Oh, maybe this will work.' You always think something is going to work" [21].

FOUNDING THE FIELD OF COMPUTATIONAL STRUCTURAL BIOLOGY

Michael Levitt, the Robert W. and Vivian K. Cahill Professor in Cancer Research at Stanford and a professor of structural biology and of computer science (by courtesy), is widely recognized as the founder of a field known as computational structural biology. He was a pioneer in the use of computers to analyze and predict the shapes of important biological molecules. His work opened the door for research into computational analysis of changes in the structure of proteins. In 2013, he and two others (Martin Karplus and Arieh Warshel) were awarded the Nobel Prize in Chemistry, in recognition of the work they did to develop "methods that combined quantum and classical mechanics to calculate the courses of chemical reactions using computers" [22].

Levitt recalls that when he was 14, he was amazed that computers could play chess. Later, he became fascinated by the fact that, as he describes it,

> all of biology and life is built up from tiny little machines called proteins that have very precise structures—a bit like a watch that has a very precise structure. Proteins have moving parts, and these moving parts are not made of metal but of amino acids. You have a protein machine doing everything in our bodies—whether they're enzymes or structural proteins or receptors or messengers. It still boggles my mind. If somebody wrote a science-fiction story saying this is how life works, it would seem ridiculous.

Levitt merged his two interests in ways that drastically expanded scientific understanding. One of his early breakthroughs, in 1967, was working with Warshel to develop the first computer program that could perform energy-minimization calculations for small molecules as well as entire protein structures. This helped lay the foundation for more important discoveries. As the School of Medicine explained on the occasion of the Nobel Prize announcement, "The computer-simulation and molecular modeling techniques pioneered by Levitt reproduce the structural, thermodynamic and dynamic properties of a macromolecule in as accurate a way as possible, profoundly expanding the range of protein structures that can be discerned and unlocking the door to studying these proteins' function" [23].

Levitt's discoveries are also a clear example of the value of basic theoretical research to practical medicine. They greatly benefited the field of pharmacology, which is the study of how drugs interact with living organisms, and they've contributed to the antibody humanization that is fundamental to anti-cancer drugs such as Avastin and Herceptin.

Today, Levitt and Roger Kornberg are affiliated with a company, InterX, that is trying to make quantum mechanical treatments of large molecules less expensive. One goal, says Levitt, is to "treat the whole drug molecule quantum mechanically and then use some of the distinct properties of quantum mechanics to design drugs that will bind more tightly to proteins or to nucleic acids. So instead of just thinking about the drugs as being little constructs of billiard balls, we now think of the drugs as actually containing electrons, protons, and neutrons. And this allows us to produce better-designed drugs."

UNRAVELING HOW NEURONS COMMUNICATE WITH ONE ANOTHER

In 2013, Thomas Südhof, the Avram Goldstein Professor in the School of Medicine at Stanford and a professor of molecular and cellular physiology, won the Nobel Prize in Physiology or Medicine in recognition of his discoveries related to how neurons in the brain communicate with each other. But his scientific training came in an area very different from the research that won him the Nobel. As a young scientist, he worked in the laboratory of Michael Brown and Joseph Goldstein at the University of Texas Southwestern Medical School. They were internal medicine doctors, who had extensive scientific training, and they explored the question of how cholesterol and blood are regulated. When Südhof was a postdoctoral fellow in their lab, they discovered mechanisms that are involved in this regulation. Brown and Goldstein won a Nobel Prize for their discovery, and their work laid the foundation for statins, which have been one of the most important drugs to come on the market in the past 50 years. "One of the things I learned from them," recalls Südhof, "was the importance of fundamental research in approaching a medical question."

He also learned from them the importance of tackling problems that not only advance our understanding of human biology but have practical implications as well. That led him, once he had concluded his training in their lab, to work on something entirely different.

> I decided that the brain was unknown. I was a little too optimistic about how much we would understand over the years, but I thought that maybe by focusing on the brain, I could make a contribution that would differ from those of previous contributions. So in 1986 I decided to work on the problem of how cells in the brain communicate with each other.

Südhof's work, which was exploring a fundamental question in neuroscience, occupied him for much of the next 20 to 25 years. He was particularly focused on the synapse, which is where neurotransmitters convey information from one neuron to another. Several of his discoveries greatly advanced our understanding of synaptic transmissions—a significant achievement, given that these transmissions are central to everything that happens in the brain. As with much of the best work in science, though, he had no magical "aha" moment but rather an accumulation of knowledge that steadily built on itself. As he has explained,

> In my career, no single major discovery changed the field all at once. Instead, our work progressed in incremental steps over two decades. I think this is a general property of scientific progress in understanding how something works—a single experiment rarely explains a major question, but usually a body of work is required [24].

Today, he is particularly interested in learning and memory because, he says, "it is something we can measure reliably in animals, and because it is one of the earliest impairments we see with Alzheimer's disease." And even amid his many achievements (he also won the Lasker Prize in 2013), he remains convinced of the value of basic science: "Disciplines like neuroanatomy or biochemistry cannot claim to understand functions or provide cures, but they form the basis for everything we do."

ILLUMINATING OUR UNDERSTANDING OF THE BRAIN

The brain is one of the least-understood organs in the human body—as well as the most complex, with about 100 billion nerve cells that compute with highly precise electrical signals and an array of biochemical messengers. These factors begin to explain why there's been only modest progress in developing therapies for neurological conditions, from Alzheimer's to mental illness. It's also meant that the therapies that do exist tend to be imprecise, one-size-fits-all solutions. Stanford's Karl Deisseroth, the D. H. Chen Professor of Bioengineering, and of psychiatry and behavioral sciences, has labored to remedy this state of affairs. In the process, he has dramatically expanded our understanding of brain functions—as well as dysfunctions, and how to treat them in a more precise way.

Deisseroth attended medical school at Stanford, but he did not develop a deep interest in mental illness until making a required psychiatry rotation. He encountered a patient with schizoaffective disorder—a condition that typically involves hallucinations, delusion, depression, and manic behavior. The experience with the patient, who was able to lucidly depict his alternate reality, "changed the whole fabric of my life," says Deisseroth. "After that, I knew I wanted to do psychiatry." He started an adult psychiatry residency at Stanford—hungry for knowledge about the functioning of the brain. "It was the unknown that grabbed me," he told a reporter for the *New Yorker*, which published a profile of him in 2015. "I knew how far we were from a glimmer of understanding."

> A cardiologist can explain a damaged heart muscle to a patient. With depression, you cannot say what it really is. People can give drugs of different kinds, put electrodes in and stimulate different parts of the brain and see changed behavior—but there is no tissue-level understanding [25].

Deisseroth's fascination with the brain led him to want to shed more light on it—literally. Early in his career, he used electrodes to stimulate individual cells and then recorded the effect. That inspired him to seek a tool that would have the same response time as electricity, but with greater specificity. He found that light was the most effective tool.

> There's no light in the brain, so the cells don't normally respond to it. But if you could make the cells even a little bit responsive to light, that would give immense leverage. Maybe the cells could be specifically turned on or off with light because the cells that aren't being modified aren't going to be affected.

This was the foundation of a discipline Deisseroth created called optogenetics. It involves using light to control genetically defined elements of the neuronal circuitry. He began experimenting with it in 2004, and he encountered significant skepticism from science colleagues that his vision would ever be realized. Five years later, optogenetics was a reality—and it's been transformative. One of Deisseroth's colleagues, Rob Malenka, has said that optogenetics "revolutionized neuroscience," making it possible for neuroscientists "to manipulate neural activity in a rigorous and sophisticated way and in a manner that was unimaginable 15–20 years ago" [26].

Optogenetics provides the primary benefit that cells can be manipulated, with a level of precision that was once unthinkable, and in ways that influence behavior. Says Deisseroth, "Now we have ways of playing in hundreds of individual cell-sized spots of light, so we can function like a conductor of an orchestra and play very complex patterns and see behaviors in animals."

In the past decade, thousands of discoveries using optogenetics have been published, and even clinical trials guided by optogenetics have been launched. They involve using insights that reveal what's actually causal in a symptom—insights that have been largely absent from neuroscience and psychiatry. "We know what matters because we can turn things up or down and see the symptom change," says Deisseroth. "That's been exciting, and it could guide any kind of therapy." Indeed, optogenetics has already been used to inform treatments for a range of conditions, including substance abuse and depression.

In a particularly recent example, optogenetics has helped provide new insights about drug addiction. Optogenetics experiments using rats addicted to cocaine involved stimulating prefrontal regions of the brain, which caused the rats to stop seeking cocaine. Today, this causal insight is being applied, via transcranial magnetic stimulation, for a noninvasive, safe, clinically approved method.

Once the key elements of optogenetics had been finalized, Deisseroth set out to plug some of the gaps.

> We didn't know enough about the neurons we were controlling. While we knew where they were, and we knew a little bit about them, such as a few genetic features, we didn't know the wiring pattern of the cells that we were controlling by light. Nor did we know in great detail what kind of cells they were.

That led him to an idea: to marry optogenetics with a way of getting a deep understanding of the molecular identity and wiring of those same cells. He's written that the goal was "making the intact, mature, mammalian brain transparent—while still allowing detailed labeling of diverse molecules within" [27].

Earlier in his career, Deisseroth had explored working with hydrogels, which are gelatin-like 3-D polymers that retain water, and that can be transparent and allow the exchange of small molecules like nutrients and cellular labels. After developing optogenetics, he wondered about its utility for his next challenge. One approach would have been to build a gel and then seed cells on the gel to try to build a tissue. But Deisseroth wanted to start with a mouse brain that been subjected to optogenetics and then transform that brain into a gel.

His idea was to create a very robust gel-tissue hybrid where all the interesting biomolecules—the proteins and nucleic acids—would be locked into place onto a gel that he would build everywhere within the tissue—all at once. Next, he would remove any components that were a distraction, such as lipids, and preserve only the important features. This became what is now known as hydrogel tissue chemistry (HTC), initially known by the first form of HTC called CLARITY [28].

According to Deisseroth, this procedure has created "a way to see into the intact brain—and to both determine the trajectories and define the molecular properties of individual connecting fibers that weave through the brain's intricate inner workings." The effect has been to enable the equivalent of a fully annotated circuit map of a computer. "Instead of knowing a little bit about the pieces," says Deisseroth, "now we know just about everything about the pieces. And not just in a static, dry way—we also know their dynamics and their importance in behavior."

A theme running through Deisseroth's research has been trying to bring greater precision to neuroscience. He describes the problem he wants to remedy in the context of what has been a popular form of treatment for depression: transcranial magnetic stimulation (TMS).

> The population effects from TMS were tiny. There was nothing patient-specific about it because there was no understanding of how to make it patient-specific. The TMS coil would be put over the dorsolateral prefrontal cortex. But where precisely? The protocols called for putting the coil 5 cm anterior to the part that causes a twitch in the thumb—for every person regardless of their head size or brain size. It's a miracle that anything was reasonably consistent at all.

Today, a form of imaging known as *diffusion tractography* is used to look at a person's brain. The imaging can identify whether that person has a tract of axons from one brain-surface spot that links to deeper areas such as the nucleus accumbens, which is involved with reward processing. In Deisseroth's optogenetics experiments, it's possible to very precisely adjust up or down the activity of neurons that contribute to a specific tract across the brain, providing causal knowledge regarding symptoms for a given tract. Deisseroth and his colleagues are now exploring strategies to target specific known causal tracts based on the positioning and trajectory of these tracts in individual patients.

PUSHING PHYSICS—AND OTHER DISCIPLINES—TO NEW FRONTIERS

Steven Chu's remarkable career has spanned multiple disciplines and leadership positions—some of the highlights include serving as professor of physics at Stanford, director of the Lawrence Berkeley National Laboratory, and U.S. Secretary of Energy. In 1997, he was a recipient of the Nobel Prize in Physics. Today, he's the William R. Kennan, Jr., Professor of Physics and professor of molecular and cellular physiology at Stanford.

His life's work has contributed to advances in our understanding of many different areas, including atomic physics, polymer physics, biophysics, biology, bio-imaging, and energy technologies. Like Steve Quake, who did his undergraduate honors thesis with Chu and returned to his lab as a postdoc, Chu has used his exceptional background in physics to approach biomedical problems from different perspectives and vantage points.

Early in his career, Chu was interested in how to hold on to atoms with light. However, the feeble forces required him to first develop methods using lasers to cool atoms—a counterintuitive idea, since directing light at the atoms would be expected to raise their temperature, not lower it. But Chu and his colleagues at Bell Laboratories showed that lasers dramatically reduce the speed at which atoms move—from 4,000 kilometers per hour to just centimeters per second. Or, as Chu puts it, "from the speed of supersonic jet planes to scurrying cockroaches."

This so-called optical molasses allowed Chu to hold on to atoms with a single focused laser beam in 1986. When the Nobel Committee awarded their prize to Chu, they singled out the work he and others had done on "development of methods to cool and trap atoms with laser light." Chu went on to show how laser cooling and trapping greatly improved atomic clocks and other ultra-precise physics measurements. Also in 1986, Arthur Ashkin and Chu demonstrated that optical tweezers could be used to trap micron-sized particles in water, and a year later Ashkin showed that individual bacteria and viruses could be held by optical tweezers.

After arriving at Stanford in 1987, Chu used the laser trap to hold on to a single molecule of DNA. The tweezers used to manipulate individual DNA molecules also enabled the measurement of forces exerted by a myosin molecule on a molecular actin filament, the molecular system responsible for muscle contraction. As he explains it, "Together with Stanford Professor Jim Spudich, as well as Bob Simmons and Jeff Finer, we used two optical tweezers introduced into an optical microscope to grab the plastic handles glued to the ends of the molecule." His use of the tweezers to study individual DNA molecules marked a breakthrough. Another advance was his demonstration that fluorescence resonance energy transfer (FRET) can be used to measure the dynamics of individual biomolecules tethered to a microscope slide.

Optical tweezers and single molecule FRET have changed biological research. By focusing on single molecular systems function, says Chu, "you're beginning to see things you simply could not see with bulk experiments." (Chu is working with Stanford's Brian Kobilka in single molecule FRET to unravel the dynamics of receptor molecules.) Today, the tweezers are used by many biologists, given the potential to realize much greater precision. For example, Steven Block in Stanford's Biology Department can resolve how RNA polymerase transcribes DNA into messenger RNA with the precision of a single nucleotide at speeds that occurs in cells. The value of optical tweezers received a powerful validation in 2018 when Arthur Ashkin was awarded the Nobel Prize in Physics for introducing them to biology.

Chu, while continuing to push the frontiers of single molecule optical imaging, is now developing new methods in ultrasound imaging. For example, he and his postdoc are creating an imaging method where two different ultrasound frequencies are used to create a signal vibrating at the difference frequency. They have shown that this so-called non-linear difference frequency ultrasound generates images that more clearly reveal tumors linked to glioblastoma. The hope is that this difference frequency imaging can be used in conjunction with current methods to deliver more precise diagnoses.

Chu believes it's going to be possible to generate high-quality images of features smaller than a millimeter, 20 centimeters deep. He says, "Ultrasound is the cheapest imaging modality, and the images will be much better than conventional X-rays. They may rival MRIs, but the machine is priced at about $150,000, not $8 million." It would be a "very big deal," he says, to be able to quickly image patients with no radiation exposure in minutes and at low expense. "It could really transform clinical diagnostics."

EXPANDING OUR UNDERSTANDING OF THE BRAIN'S DEVELOPMENT—AND COUNTERING ITS DECLINE

Carla Shatz, the Sapp Family Provostial Professor at Stanford and a professor of biology and of neurobiology, is fascinated by the process of how brains change through learning and experience. Her research—spanning more than 40 years—has greatly expanded our understanding of brain development, particularly before birth.

When Shatz was 19, her grandmother had a stroke, which left the right side of her body completely paralyzed. The absence of any treatments at the time was a catalyst for Shatz wanting to become a neuroscientist. She also wanted to understand other aspects of the brain.

> I was captivated by how the brain wires itself during development, and particularly how it is, and why it is, that the child's brain seems like such an amazing sponge, which makes it so easy for children to learn languages and other things whereas it's so difficult for adults—particularly me—to learn French without an accent.

Shatz realized that if it was possible to understand the underlying cellular and molecular mechanisms that regulate the early "sponge" periods of brain development, then it might be possible to reactivate them in adulthood to assist with the recovery from stroke, or to counteract the cognitive decline of normal aging or even the pathology of Alzheimer's disease.

She conducted her research against the backdrop of a striking feature of the way in which the adult visual system is organized from eye to brain: input from the left and right eyes is segregated across the surface of the brain. The developing brain lacks this organization entirely. She has contributed greatly to our understanding of how this precise binocular architecture emerges during development. She showed, for example, that neural activity was essential for this process, and her research ruled out the idea that brain circuitry was hard-wired by guidance molecules.

Shatz's first major discovery, in the early 1980s, involved exploring the interaction between the eyes and the brain during fetal development. She discovered that the adult set of connections from eye to brain were not present early on and that the adult connections need to be "tuned up" during development. Given that the baby's brain is not just a smaller version of the adult brain—it has a set of dynamic circuits that change with learning and use—she wanted to understand the underlying molecular mechanisms that drive this tuning-up process. More specifically, she wanted to know if the systems being used in the brain were activated even before eyesight—and before birth.

> My colleagues and I had a thought that maybe this tuning process starts earlier because it would be genetically extremely expensive to have to mark molecularly every single connection in the brain. We thought if that process is happening, then there should be ways of blocking this tuning and preventing the adult pattern of connections from forming.

Their experiments revealed the need for the early tuning process, which then set Shatz down another path: how did the tuning process work? They knew that cells send electrical signals in order to communicate across long distances. So they set out to monitor those signals early in development, figuring that perhaps they could understand something about the logic of brain tuning and sculpting of the circuits. They were able to use what were then new techniques for studying the neural activity and the signaling of many nerve cells at once. They recorded and monitored the activity of 50–100 neurons at the same time.

The research led to the discovery in 1991 that even before birth, the eye is sending coherent test signals to the brain, and those test signals are used to check the circuits between the eye and the brain. Incorrect connections are removed. If that signaling is blocked, those incorrect connections are preserved, and the adult-like pattern of circuits fails to form. This discovery has important takeaways for how drug abuse, which alters nerve signaling, may affect the developing fetal brain.

This breakthrough also opened new avenues for inquiry. For example, how does the signaling, which is a chemical and electrical process, cause the remodeling of the connections to happen? Similarly, why do some connections get eliminated and other ones get preserved? And what are the molecules and mechanisms involved in that remodeling?

While researching these questions, Shatz and her colleagues made another major discovery. They were exploring the mechanisms by which the brain selects which connections get discarded throughout the developmental process and which ones are preserved through adulthood. They showed that when neurons fire simultaneously, the result is stable connections, while unsynchronized neurons get pruned. She coined two memorable phrases to describe these phenomena: "Cells that fire together, wire together," and "Cells that fire out of sync lose their link."

The breakthrough was in showing the non-random nature of signaling from the eye to the brain. Instead, neurons nearby fired together, and coordinated firing strengthens connections that are used at the same time. This indicated that signaling was happening much earlier in brain development than commonly believed—even before birth and before vision. (It had been thought to start with learning and experience of the world after birth.)

That discovery begat yet another discovery, as Shatz and her colleagues began to research how the brain implements these processes. They discovered that a family of molecules known as MHC class I, which were previously known to be essential to the function of the immune system, were involved in pruning the synaptic connections between neurons during activity-dependent development. (This is known as the "out of synch" rule.) The conventional wisdom at the time was that these molecules did not play a functional role in the brain. The finding was so counterintuitive that when Shatz and her colleagues wrote up their discovery and submitted it to a respected journal in 1997, the editor wrote back and insisted that she must have made a mistake. "He said, in so many words, that everybody knows MHC class I molecules are only found in the immune system and they're certainly not in the brain and they're certainly not in neurons." The paper found a home in *Nature* the following year, and MHC-1 has continued to feature in her research. In 2012, she and her colleagues discovered that suppressing the molecules could mitigate the brain damage caused by a stroke.

Looking ahead, Shatz is optimistic about the future, pointing to the potential for a pharmaceutical product that would return the brain to some earlier version of its sponge-like self, with the capacity for neuroplasticity and reorganization seen in development. She says it's now possible to identify molecular mechanisms that seem to control the pruning process. As part of the MHC-1 research, she and her colleagues looked for genes that interacted with MHC-1 based on precedents of MHC-1 function in immune cells. They found a candidate, which they call PirB. The "r" stands for "receptor," and receptors are the favorite molecules of drug companies because it's possible to target a receptor and block its function with a medicine.

> We can make a little proto pill based on our knowledge of PirB structure, and we can actually block the signaling from PirB. Instead of genetic engineering, we can prevent the PirB receptor from working. Then we can give this proto pill to the mouse and we can ask what happens to plasticity in the mouse brain, and what happens to the synapses in the mouse brain.

Shatz and her colleagues tried this with an adult mouse—giving it a version of the proto pill for seven days. They found that new synapses were appearing in the brain of the adult mouse—an outcome she calls "extremely promising." They also found that the adult mouse brain became more "sponge-like," reminiscent of a young mouse brain. She cautions that "we don't know really how this pill works" and that there's still a lot of work ahead. Nonetheless, "it's possible that I could take some future version of the pill and finally learn French without an accent. *Incroyable!*"

UNDERSTANDING THE MYSTERIES OF AGING

Anne Brunet, the Michele and Timothy Barakett Professor of Genetics at Stanford, studies a condition that affects every living organism, contributes to the onset of many different diseases, and ultimately leads to death. That condition is aging, which she describes as "one of the greatest mysteries in biology, and arguably its next frontier."

Brunet and her colleagues seek to pinpoint the intrinsic mechanisms that convert a young, vigorous, healthy organism into an old, frail organism with increased susceptibility to many diseases. They are also interested in how environmental stimuli—such as diet, sexual interaction, and environmental stresses—impinge on the aging pathways. In their research, they pursue a variety of questions, which include:

- What mechanisms occur during the aging process?
- Are stem cells more susceptible or less susceptible to aging than other types of cells?
- How does the aging process differ between vertebrates and invertebrates?

One area of research is focused on animals with compressed life-spans (since this allows more experiments to be completed in shorter periods of time).

One of the favorite organisms of her lab (and many others) is the nematode worm. Just 1 millimeter long, it lives in the soil and it goes through all the phases of life—beginning, growth, vitality, vigor, decline, and death—in just 30 days. The genes that regulate the worm's aging have the same function in mice and even humans—a discovery made more than 25 years ago that has "pried open the genetics of aging," says Brunet. For example, the insulin-FOXO pathway regulates life-span in nematodes, and it is involved in life-span modulation in mammals as well, including humans.

Brunet also studies the nematode because it's one of the animal species in which a curious environmental interaction plays out. Males accelerate the premature aging of the opposite sex—hermaphrodites in nematodes (mostly female-like but with the capacity to self-reproduce). This phenomenon is called *male-induced demise*. In addition to dying faster, the opposite sex exhibits severely premature decrepitude. Part of the detrimental effect of males is via pheromones, so their mere presence (even without mating) affects the life-span of the opposite sex.

But nematodes have limitations as research subjects: they don't have bones, blood, stem cells, or an adaptive immune system. Brunet's lab has generated a tool kit to use the African killifish as a new vertebrate model to study aging. The killifish reach sexual maturity in as little as two weeks, reproduce in captivity, and recapitulate the aforementioned life phases in the span of four to six months. The killifish also engage in what's known as "suspended animation." They live in ponds that tend to dry up once the rainy season has ended. The species is nonetheless able to survive because the embryos can go dormant (akin to hibernation) for months, and sometimes years, and emerge intact. Brunet says she is "very intrigued" with this exceptional form of preservation. "In biology, it's often by studying the extremes that one identifies things that can be helpful for understanding things in the mainstream."

The ultimate objective is to learn more about aging in humans, but one of the challenges to doing so, says Brunet, is a public policy issue: the U.S. Food and Drug Administration does not consider aging to be a disease. As a result, scientists and doctors cannot set up clinical trials to measure whether several hallmarks of aging could be improved. Instead, they must focus on a specific age-related disease. But as Brunet points out, aging is the prime risk factor for multiple diseases—including cardiovascular disease, diabetes, cancer, and arthritis—and it dwarfs all other factors.

Amid these challenges, there has been progress in understanding aging in many different organisms. Once considered to be an irreversible phenomenon, aging has in fact turned out to be malleable. The life-spans of some organisms have been extended by inhibiting high-nutrient-sensing pathways and activating low-nutrient-sensing proteins. Diet-based interventions (such as dietary restriction), coupled with pharmacological interventions, have also been shown to slow the aging process. While many "rejuvenation" interventions have been tested on mice, Brunet and her colleagues have recently summarized in a review several approaches that have been shown to benefit human health and longevity, including four-day cycles of low/normal caloric intake, repeated twice per month [29].

There is much more to learn, though. "Our understanding of aging is still rudimentary," says Brunet. "We really only understand the tip of the iceberg. It is an extraordinarily complex process that defies many of the conventional rules in biology" [30]. Brunet, who grew up in France, is occasionally asked about her preferred antiaging strategy for humans. She has a simple answer: "Red wine."

Tony Wyss-Coray, a professor of neurology and neurological sciences at Stanford, is another pioneer when it comes to deepening our understanding of the aging process. His research has explored the way in which blood impacts the brain during the aging process. He's been particularly focused on identifying measures that can help prevent the effects of conditions closely tied to aging.

Wyss-Coray was trained as an immunologist in his native Switzerland. He came to the United States for postdoctoral work and wanted to understand Alzheimer's better, but he was frustrated by the inability to get a molecular understanding of the disease until an individual with the disease had died. This led him to study whether blood might hold untold secrets about the disease. "The brain has about 400 miles of blood vessels," says Wyss-Coray. "It's one of the most highly vascularized organs and uses about 20 percent of the whole blood supply that the heart pumps out."

This research showed that the composition of blood changed not only with disease but, more dramatically, with aging alone. Chance had it that Wyss-Coray's neighbor laboratory, belonging to Stanford neurology professor Thomas Rando, had a model to test if the changes in blood influenced the brain or were merely a correlate of aging. As part of a study, Rando paired the blood circulation of a young mouse and an old mouse by suturing them together at the flank, which resulted in the blood vessels growing together and sharing blood circulation (a process known as *parabiosis*). After a few weeks, something miraculous had happened: the old muscle stem cells resembled young stem cells, having regenerated muscle again like a young muscle.

To test his question, Wyss-Coray teamed up with Rando—conducting the same mouse experiment, with a young mouse (equivalent to a 20-year-old human) and an old mouse (equivalent to a 65-year-old human) but looking at the effect of the young blood on the brain. "The results were really surprising," says Wyss-Coray. "At multiple levels, from molecules to cells to electrophysiology to cognitive function, there were beneficial effects from young blood and specifically the liquid fraction—plasma—on the old brain." There were also negative effects on the young brain. The experiment upended the accepted thinking that cells in the aged brain were the only mechanism that reduced synaptic plasticity and hampered learning and memory. In fact, soluble factors, such as proteins in aged blood, were also the culprit.

In 2014, a study coauthored by Wyss-Coray revealed that these effects could be realized even without the shared circulatory system that was engineered for the mice. In the study, old mice benefited after receiving injections of plasma from young mice. That opened up the possibility of a similar approach being used with humans. In a 2015 TED Talk, Wyss-Coray elaborated on the findings:

> We find there are more neural stem cells that make new neurons in these old brains. There's an increased activity of the synapses, the connections between neurons. There are more genes expressed that are known to be involved in the formation of new memories. And there's less of this bad inflammation. But we observed that there are no cells entering the brains of these animals. So when we connect them, there are actually no cells going into the old brain in this model. Instead, we've reasoned, it must be the soluble factors, so we could collect simply the soluble fraction of blood, which is called plasma, and inject either young plasma or old plasma into these mice, and we could reproduce these rejuvenating effects [31].

Wyss-Coray's research ultimately led him to become the cofounder of a company, Alkahest, that is seeking to translate his discoveries into therapies that will combat many of the cognitive challenges that arise with aging. The company, which had 70 employees at the start of 2019, is particularly focused on treatments for Alzheimer's. Its research has uncovered specific proteins that accelerate aging and age-related diseases and others that have the opposite effect. The company conducted a clinical trial that involved treating 18 Alzheimer's patients, and once a week they were given one unit of young plasma. The infusions did not have any negative effects, and Phase 2 trials started in 2018, focused on both Alzheimer's and Parkinson's.

It's too early to tell what the outcome will be, but the research raises the possibility of eventually reaching a point where patients with these neurodegenerative diseases could, for the first time, experience a slowing or even reversal of the disease process.

Looking ahead, Wyss-Coray is researching how the brain and blood vessels interact with each other. He and his colleagues are particularly focused on trying to find molecules in the blood that influence the brain as people age. They are following hundreds of people who are experiencing cognitive impairment or who are at risk of such impairment.

Wyss-Coray emphasizes that we're a long way from a magic pill that will slow—if not reverse—the effects of aging, but his research does hold the promise of mitigating the debilitating consequences of Alzheimer's. It's a condition that affects five million people in the United States and is the sixth-leading cause of death—with no known cure. "We know so much more today than we did as recently as 10 years ago," he says. "There is still a lot we need to learn, but I am optimistic that this is a battle we can eventually win."

REVEALING THE ROOTS OF REGENERATION

Helen Blau is the Donald E. and Delia B. Baxter Foundation Professor at Stanford's School of Medicine and director of the Baxter Laboratory for Stem Cell Biology. Since earning her PhD from Harvard in 1975, she has accomplished multiple research breakthroughs. Blau's work provided the first definitive evidence that mammalian cells specialized for function in a given tissue are not irreversibly differentiated but are subject to change. This discovery of cell plasticity opened the door to novel ways to enlist cells in the repair of tissue damage. (Blau's work is featured on the School of Medicine's Discovery Walk, which commemorates advances in medical science made by scientists at Stanford.)

The theme running through much of Blau's work has been regeneration, which has fascinated her since the early part of her life. Her father was chief historian for the U.S. government in Europe, which resulted in Blau's growing up abroad and attending different schools, including high school in Heidelberg, Germany, and college in York, England. She also had other eclectic experiences. She spent summers living with an Austrian family at age 9 and French families at ages 14 to 17, as well as numerous months enrolled in an international school, the Ecole d'Humanité, in the Swiss Alps. She has written, "Clearly, these diverse locales changed me: my tastes, behavior, and language. So why shouldn't the environment of the cell do the same" [32]?

Regeneration was the focus of her undergraduate thesis, which was devoted to one particular feature of the liver: its striking ability to regrow after injury.

> I was fascinated by the fact that when you removed the two large lobes of the liver, the liver regenerated, and the small lobes became large. The proportions of the liver completely changed, yet the final mass remained the same because somehow the liver knew when to stop growing. To this day the mechanisms by which this occurs elude us.

Blau joined the Stanford faculty in 1978 and soon thereafter began researching an idea considered sacrosanct in human biology: the differentiated state of human cells was considered irreversible. Blau wondered if this was really true, and here is how she wrote about her thought process and what followed:

> "There's a divinity that shapes our ends, rough hew them how we will," wrote Shakespeare in *Hamlet*. But is anatomy indeed destiny? As an assistant professor at Stanford University in the 1980s, and after years of growing cells in culture and staring at them under the microscope, I could not believe that once cells differentiated, their fate was sealed forever. Why was differentiation "one way"? I still remember my excitement when our heterokaryon experiments, in which human differentiated cells were fused with mouse muscle myotubes, demonstrated that the "terminally" differentiated state of human cells could be reversed. The revelation of cell fate plasticity was thrilling [33].

This was a landmark discovery—"a paradigm shift in biology," according to the National Academy of Sciences in 2016 [34]—that garnered the cover of the "Frontiers in Biology" issue of *Science* in 1985 [35]. Today, it is a fundamental principle of cell and developmental biology, which laid the foundation for the current era of stem cell biology and regenerative medicine.

To test the plasticity of human differentiated cells, Blau designed experiments to investigate if human muscle genes could be activated in cell types that would normally never express muscle genes, including representatives of all three embryonic lineages: epidermal keratinocytes of the skin, mesodermal fibroblasts, and endodermal hepatocytes of the liver. When mouse cells (muscle) were fused with human cells (non-muscle), the activation of previously silent human genes was detected as the novel expression of human muscle proteins. Crucial to this discovery was a clever means she devised of fusing disparate cell types together to form stable non-dividing multinucleated heterokaryons. The absence of proliferation was key to circumventing changes in gene expression due to a confounding loss of chromosomes that accompanied division of bi-species cells. This loss would have made it difficult to discern if newly expressed genes resulted from the loss of transacting repressors or the presence of transacting activators. An ingenious feature of the heterokaryon design was the skewing of nuclear ratio, such that the mouse muscle nuclei outnumbered the human non-muscle nuclei. This nuclear ratio and shift in gene dosage to favor muscle was crucial to the activation of the silent muscle genes in the non-muscle cells.

The results of these experiments revolutionized our understanding of the state of specialized cells as fixed and irreversible. It demonstrated the plasticity of which highly differentiated cells were capable. Moreover, it showed that differentiation was dictated by the balance of regulators at any given time. Blau's discovery that gene dosage was key—that an excess of reprogramming nuclei relative to reprogrammed nuclei was necessary—paved the way for the finding by Shinya Yamanaka two decades later that overexpression of four embryonic transcription factors could activate a pluripotent gene expression profile in differentiated cells [36]. The derivation of induced pluripotent stem cells (iPSCs) now enables stem cell utilization in the modeling of human diseases, drug discovery, and stem cell therapies.

In the years that followed, Blau continued to advance our understanding of regeneration. In an elegant essay written with Nobel Laureate David Baltimore, Blau extended the principles of cell plasticity beyond humans to all phyla. This powerful duo highlighted the fact that the maintenance of gene expression in specialized cells is not the result of a passive mechanism, but instead requires "active management" and ongoing control. Their ideas, which were published in the *Journal of Cell Biology* in 1991, advanced the unorthodox notion that the differentiated state requires continuous regulation in order to be maintained [37]. This revolutionary concept is now dogma.

Blau has applied these findings to understand the most common form of muscular dystrophy (Duchenne), and explore why mice with the same genetic defect as humans—an absence of dystrophin—get only mildly weaker and do not develop the progressive muscle wasting and heart failure that kill humans. Duchenne results from the absence of dystrophin, a structural protein that connects the cytoskeleton with the extracellular environment and is critical to contractile function. Blau noted that for unknown reasons, mice have much longer telomeres (protective caps on chromosomes) than humans and wondered if this could be a factor in the observed species difference. When her lab created a mouse model of Duchenne with humanized telomere lengths, they were excited to find that all the features of the disease were manifested for the first time.

This discovery yielded novel fundamental insights: the longer telomeres of mice are protective against severe human degenerative diseases like Duchenne, and shorter telomeres lead to a reduced stem cell reservoir necessary to fuel the continuous repair of chronically degenerating skeletal muscles. In other words, the longer telomeres of mice make it possible for muscle stem cells to continue dividing and regenerate damaged muscle well beyond the point at which human cells stop dividing. Additionally, Blau's research revealed for the first time that skeletal muscular dystrophy is a disorder of stem cells. Blau said afterward, "The results suggest that treatments directed solely at the muscle fiber will not suffice and could even exacerbate the disease. The muscle stem cells must be taken into consideration" [38].

In other research, Blau drew lessons from evolutionary biology, learning from the newt, an animal not often associated with medical research. But newts have a biological characteristic that mammals lack: their hearts and limbs can regenerate by a mechanism known as *dedifferentiation*: reentry of cells into the cell cycle [39]. If part of a newt's heart is removed, it can regrow. This is known to occur by inactivation of the retinoblastoma (Rb) protein, which is a brake on the cell cycle. As Blau explains,

> In response to damage, skeletal and cardiac muscle cells of the newt reenter the cell cycle, divide, and make copies of themselves, regenerating the tissue. By comparing gene expression profiles of newts with mammals, we realized that in mammals another brake on the cell cycle arose in the course of evolution, known as p19, that is not present in the newt. Using single cell laser capture catapulting, we could follow single treated cells and show definitively that once both Rb and p19 functions were eliminated, specialized mammalian muscle cells could replicate in culture as in the newt.

Blau has pointed out, "If we extend these principles of dedifferentiation, we might be able to regenerate cardiac tissue and prevent heart failure."

Additionally, Blau's strategy for rejuvenation "could restore function to muscles of those who are immobilized." This work derives from her current passion to understand how muscle stem cells can be maximally stimulated to build strength of muscle tissues.

> We've developed a novel approach that entails activating the muscle stem cells that are resident within the tissue in a quiescent state to boost muscle mass and function. In our aging mouse models, a single injection of the drug regimen can lead to a long-term robust increase in strength.

Blau is particularly interested in potential clinical applications, noting that millions of people suffer from progressive muscle wasting and weakness as they age, especially after disease or injury that renders them immobile. Currently, there is no molecular therapy to treat muscle atrophy, a debilitating disorder. Combined, muscle disorders impose a significant economic burden in the United States exceeding $18 billion in health care costs annually. She is the cofounder of a company called Myoforte. It is focused on developing her recently discovered drug combination that leverages the body's own healing mechanisms to strengthen the regenerative process.

Regeneration is also at the core of research undertaken by Michael Longaker, the Deane P. and Louise Mitchell Professor at Stanford, as well as codirector of the Institute for Stem Cell Biology and Regenerative Medicine. Among his many interests—he is an inventor on more than 40 issued patents and patent applications—one is arthritis and the wearing down of joints. This is partly a product of the wear and tear he experienced as an athlete. He was a long jumper in high school, as well as a basketball player—a sport he also played at Michigan State University (where his team won the national championship and one of his teammates was future NBA star Earvin "Magic" Johnson).

Longaker went on to graduate from Harvard Medical School, and he joined the Stanford faculty in 2000. Given his interest in arthritis, he'd wondered if it was possible to regenerate the cartilage that gradually erodes from overuse and the aging process. That question led him to focus on skeletal stem cells, which are the cells that enable the creation of bone, cartilage, and stroma (the sponge-like material inside bones). One of his landmark discoveries was published in *Cell* in 2015. He and his coauthors spelled out their discovery of the skeletal stem cells in mice that create bone, cartilage, and stroma [40]. They also identified the chemical signals that have the potential to create skeletal stem cells. When the paper was published, Longaker described the possible applications connected to the discoveries: "Millions of times a year, orthopedic surgeons see torn cartilage in a joint and have to take it out because cartilage doesn't heal well, but that lack of cartilage predisposes the patient to arthritis down the road. This research raises the possibility that we can create new skeletal stem cells from patients' own tissues and use them to grow new cartilage" [41].

Longaker and his colleagues built on their findings to search for skeletal stem cells in humans. Their research, which utilized the FACS technology I describe below, identified gene switches that are activated in the skeletal stem cells of mice. They observed that the cells expressed genes found in cells that typically appear in humans just a few weeks after conception, and that are the foundation of bones, cartilage, and certain connective tissue. A Stanford Medicine article summarized the significance of their research, which was published in *Cell* in 2018 [42]:

> The finding is the first to show that mammalian adult stem cells can march backward along the developmental timeline in a process called de-differentiation to become more primitive in response to environmental signals. … The results suggest the possibility of using naturally occurring adult stem cells, which are usually restricted to generate only a limited panel of closely related progeny, to carry out more extensive regeneration projects throughout the body—much in the way that salamanders or newts can replace entire limbs or tails [43].

Upon publication of the paper, a stem cell biologist at the University of Southampton in the United Kingdom who was not involved with the research told the *Scientist*, "For many years there's been this debate about a true human skeletal stem cell. This study unequivocally demonstrates that it's there and that it is self-renewing. There's still a lot to do, but this is a tremendous step forward for the field" [44].

In related research, Longaker and his colleagues discovered that they could turn human skeletal stem cells into bone or cartilage by manipulating the micro-environment in which the cells exist. (This manipulation involves reprogramming human fat cells or induced pluripotent stem cells so they take on skeletal features.) Although Longaker's discovery has not found its way into the clinic yet, it has the potential to deliver far-reaching benefits. Arthroscopic procedures—millions of which are conducted annually—could be the gateway to injecting a skeletal stem cell that grows new cartilage.

Longaker hopes that human skeletal stem cells will be a "game-changer" in arthroscopic and regenerative medicine. "The United States has a rapidly aging population that undergoes almost two million joint replacements each year. If we can use this stem cell for relatively noninvasive therapies, it could be a dream come true" [45]. The potential does not end there. Longaker says the discovery is an opportunity to rethink long-standing ideas about the development of the skeleton, tissues, and organs. "Can we go back in time after an organ is formed to trigger more extensive regeneration? This at least opens the door to that possibility" [46].

BREAKTHROUGH TECHNOLOGIES AS A CATALYST FOR BIOMEDICAL DISCOVERIES

The development of new technologies often precedes and enables transformative, paradigm-shifting discoveries in biomedicine. The flow from a technological breakthrough to a series of novel discoveries about living systems is often seamless, with many of the innovative scientists and engineers responsible for the technology being the same people who use the technologies to make the discoveries. Indeed, the quest for knowledge is usually the motivation for seeking a breakthrough technology. I describe several of these examples below.

Development of Methods to Sort Cells and Make Drugs

Sometimes discovery is enabled by a marriage of the quest for knowledge and the need to overcome adversity. Consider the case of Len Herzenberg. For much of his life, he suffered from an inherited eye problem that made everything appear blurry when he looked in a microscope. This led him to wonder if a machine could be built that would allow him to track what everyone else saw under the micro-scope—but go one better and let him and everyone else see quantitatively what's in and on the cells (and without eyestrain!). How, he asked, could we measure differences in cells that might help to illuminate their function?

At the time, antibodies were already known to be remarkable targeting agents—able to specifically bind to only a single protein shape even when faced with the complexity of tens of thousands of proteins on or in a cell. Herzenberg also knew that if you attached a fluorescent molecule to those antibodies, and then used them to label cells, the cells would glow only if they contained or expressed the protein or other molecule that the fluorescent antibody was designed to detect. This led him to wonder how a machine could be developed that could automatically determine whether a cell being examined contained certain proteins or other molecules that were labeled with fluorescent antibodies, as this could be used to measure the relative amount of that protein in the cell.

Herzenberg knew that fluorescence detectors existed, so he talked to people about them and began pushing the idea of building a machine that would flow cells past such a light detector at a rapid pace and measure their level of laser-induced fluorescence. Since cells passing through a low power laser beam would also deflect light, Herzenberg realized he could simultaneously record other information from the cell and record other light-deflecting characteristics, such as the size of the cell and internal granules. With this information, his dream for the next stage of his invention was clear. He could determine whether a cell had desirable traits and use another technology, cell sorting, to purify the cells he wanted from blood and other kinds of tissues. "That was crucial," recalls his wife, Lee Herzenberg, his partner in the lab and who is now also a professor in Stanford's genetics department.

> To Len's mind, it was not science to look down a microscope and get an impression of the cells. He believed in two key principles when it came to biochemistry and cell biology. You need to be able to measure molecules and changes in cells quantitatively, and you need to be able to separate cells from complex mixtures so you can study them in isolation.

In the early 1960s, he learned that scientists at the U.S. government's Los Alamos National Laboratory in New Mexico had built a machine that could examine and sort large numbers of cell-sized particles, based on particle volume. He made a trip to Los Alamos, but the two key individuals told him there was no plan to have the machine measure fluorescence. But he persisted, as he would later recall:

> They finally agreed to give me a set of engineering drawings and the permission to use them as the basis of a machine designed to distinguish cells labeled with fluorescent antibodies. Little did I know when I brought these plans back to Stanford that I was starting on a lifework that continues today as a major activity in our laboratory [47].

"That's what science was like at that time," recalls Lee Herzenberg. "People did wonderful things like that. They felt they had a responsibility to share their knowledge."

Len Herzenberg used the drawing to develop a machine, which became known as a fluorescence activated cell sorter, or FACS. An article published by the Stanford School of Medicine provided an apt description of the machine's value:

> Like a coin sorter that separates a jumble of change into neat stacks of quarters, nickels, dimes, and pennies, the FACS sorts cells according to fluorescent tags attached to their surfaces and keeps cells viable during the process. Because researchers can couple the fluorescent tags that home in on and attach to molecules produced only by certain cell types, the sorter can pluck out rarer-than-rare immune stem cells for further study, or identify stem cells and other populations of cells that are waxing and waning in diseases such as cancer or HIV. The possibilities of the technology, also known as flow cytometry, are limited only by the creativity of the users [48].

The Herzenbergs partnered with a medical technology company, Beckton-Dickinson, which began marketing the FACS machines for commercial use in 1976—and, several years later, produced the commercial fluorescent-labeled monoclonal antibody reagents that made widespread, quantitative FACS use possible. The FACS technology found its way into laboratories throughout the world—in 2013, it was estimated that more than 40,000 of the machines were in use [49]—and the technology made possible the birth of modern immunology, stem cell research, and proteomics. It also improved the diagnosis of leukemia and significantly advanced the clinical care of people with diseases such as cancer and HIV infection.

FACS machines were also at the heart of several other scientific breakthroughs. In the late 1970s, the Herzenbergs began working with the monoclonal antibody technology, developed initially by Dr. Cesar Milstein in Cambridge, England, which enabled the culturing of immune cells to produce hybrid cells producing what are known as monoclonal antibodies. Further, they had the insight to apply the FACS technology to developing and producing monoclonal antibodies. As a result of these advances, more than 70 monoclonal antibodies have been approved by the FDA for clinical use in the United States. This FACS and monoclonal antibody technology contributed to progress in diagnostics and therapeutics. It enabled researchers to recognize that HIV led to the loss of T lymphocytes, which are fundamental to immunity. The technology also came to be widely used to track the growth and clinical status of HIV in individual patients.

The Herzenbergs later developed a process for generating functional antibodies, which was used by companies to produce chimeric antibodies to treat a wide variety of diseases, including products for rheumatoid arthritis and Crohn's disease, as well as for respiratory syncytial virus. Their work received a Stanford patent in 1998, and the royalties have exceeded those generated by any other patent connected to the university (including the Google patents). Those royalties were just one more contribution to helping fund research and advance science.

"Without the Herzenbergs, tens of thousands of people now alive would not be," said Irv Weissman, a Stanford professor of pathology and developmental biology, following Len's death in 2013. "Without Len, the entire conceptual framework of how to evaluate single cells by their 'FACS' signature, and to identify and isolate them from a tissue like bone marrow or a cancer like leukemia, may have never happened. Len and Lee weren't just the central players in the field; for decades they *were* the field" [50].

Len and Lee Herzenberg also helped train future scientists. One of them, Garry Nolan, has become one of Stanford's most prolific innovators. He's the founder of eight companies and holds 45 U.S. patents. His work spans many different dimensions (he's currently exploring the immunopathology of the Ebola virus)—and all of it rests on a foundation of basic science.

Nolan is the Rachford and Carlota A. Harris Professor at Stanford. One of his first innovations stemmed from his work exploring how to find where drugs might act in the complex environment of a cell. He started from a simple premise: "Drugs are just shapes that fit in the pockets of proteins and cause them to change their function." His other premise was that "the only purpose of viruses is to make more copies of themselves."

> This is the selfish gene theory of Richard Dawkins. That is, viruses don't care about the cell or the state of the cell they're invading. They only care about proliferating and whether the target cell can support such replication. My idea was to say, "Let's reverse this process and make it to the benefit of the virus to make the cell healthier." We could engineer an evolutionary bottle for the virus, and make the virus understand that there will be more copies of it, but only if it takes a sick cell and makes it healthy. That would force the virus to basically search through evolutionary space for incremental advances to itself to correct the biology of the cell [51].

By analyzing the virus in the healthier cell, researchers would be able to determine what led to the improvement. "It was a very hands-off way to create novel drugs," says Nolan, "because you let biology find the answer. A virus that previously would kill people is reengineered to make cells better. It was akin to running evolution backwards."

The success of this process led Nolan to launch Rigel, in 1996, which sold protein targets for conventional drug design. Today, Rigel is a publicly traded company focused on discovering, developing, and providing novel small molecule drugs for patients with immune and hematologic disorders, cancer, and rare diseases. (In 2018, the FDA approved the company's first drug, Tavalisse, which is used to treat adults with chronic low blood platelet counts who have had an insufficient response to previous treatments.)

Next, Nolan set out to develop something akin to a filter that would pinpoint the one cell made healthier in the process described above. He found a professor at the University of Toronto who had developed a mass spectrometer that could look at individual cells using antibody tags with isotopes rather than conventional fluorophores. This made it possible to boost the number of simultaneous tags per cell that could be measured—rising from about 5 per cell to about 50 and enabling the immune system to be profiled in a much more detailed and resolved manner. As Nolan describes it:

> Let's say there were only five ways of describing people: height, weight, hair color, gender, and race. If I had my wallet stolen, that might not be enough information in a police report to identify someone. But if I could draw on 100 different traits to describe the possible thief, I have much more information to identify the culprit or to profile. This basic technology allowed us to profile the immune system and cancer cells and any kind of cell in such explicit detail that it was head and shoulders above the prior generation's technology.

Nolan describes the technology, known as *mass cytometry* (CyTOF), as an "attempt to make a better FACS" (Nolan had worked on the original FACS in the Herzenberg lab). Soon after the technology started to be publicized, in 2011, a French scientist wrote, "I have never been so awed by a technological advance: in my eyes, mass cytometry is to fluorescence-activated cell sorting (FACS) analysis what a modern computer would be to a typewriter" [52]. CyTOF has brought greater precision to immunology, and today it is used in hundreds of labs to help decipher immune signals associated with conditions such as leukemia, ovarian cancer, and rheumatoid arthritis.

A TOOL PROVIDING NEW INSIGHTS ABOUT BIOLOGICAL SPECIMENS

Basic science has also greatly advanced our understanding of molecular structures. In the not-so-distant past, the only way to get an accurate picture of them was to make a crystal, which fixed them at a particular shape (known as *conformation*). But a technology called *cryogenic electron microscopy* (cryo-EM) is enabling enhanced visualization of biological specimens and potentially unlocking valuable information for drug discovery.

Cryo-EM is used to create 3-D images of viruses, molecules, and complex biological machines either inside or extracted from the cell—such as the ribosomes, where proteins are synthesized. This is achieved by freezing them in their natural or specific biochemical environments, and it gives scientists a much clearer picture of how they are built and what they do. One writer has pointed out that this process of stitching thousands of images together through computational methods is akin to creating stop-action movies and even taking virtual "slices" through cells, much like miniature CT scans [53].

This is critically important, says Wah Chiu, a professor of photon science, bioengineering, and of microbiology and immunology at Stanford. "In biology, everything is dynamic, always moving around and changing. Cryo-EM lets you capture snapshots of proteins and other biological nanomachines as they assemble, carry out their work, and disassemble again" [54]. This makes it possible to observe the conformations that may be present only a small fraction of the time but are critical for the action of the machine. For instance, when an enzyme undergoes a catalytic reaction, it binds with its substrate and undergoes shape changes. Cryo-EM can capture what is being changed in atomic detail. Such information is essential for designing potent drugs to alter the enzyme activity that may affect the health of the cell.

There's been extraordinary progress in cryo-EM in recent years, and in 2017 three scientists who are focused on the field were awarded the Nobel Prize in Chemistry. In announcing the award, the Nobel Committee observed that thanks to cryo-EM, "researchers can now freeze biomolecules mid-movement and visualize processes they have never previously seen, which is decisive for both the basic understanding of life's chemistry and for the development of pharmaceuticals" [55].

Cryo-EM is emblematic of how technology drives discovery. The microscopes used for cryo-EM have become progressively more powerful over four decades of research into biomolecular imaging. But even more important has been developing the ability to process enormous quantities of data. With crystallography, data are revealed for one crystalline structure, all at once. But with cryo-electron microscopy coupled with image processing, data are being generated in thousands, or even hundreds of thousands, of increments. It's now possible to synthesize that data and draw conclusions from it.

Chiu points out that the enhanced molecular images provided by cryo-EM benefit two different constituencies.

> One is academic scientists who want to understand the fundamental chemistry of molecules in different chemical environments that affect their functionalities. The other is pharmaceutical companies. They are drawn to the ability of cryo-EM to help visualize molecules carrying out their most critical functions, since that can help them develop more effective drugs.

Cryo-EM has been a critical technology in building understanding of viruses and degenerative neurological diseases. Research published in 2018, based on cryo-EM, revealed the potential for the Zika virus to contain drug-binding pockets, which will help with the development of antiviral compounds and potential vaccines [56]. And in 2017, cryo-EM was used to visualize misfolded tau proteins that had been taken from the brain of a deceased 74-year-old with Alzheimer's disease. The research, published in *Nature*, revealed the structure of tau isoform that is associated with Alzheimer's and could help lead to more precise treatments [57].

The discoveries described in this chapter are a reminder that the history of discovery is a history of people. To ensure continued discovery and maximize the opportunities connected to those discoveries, we must stay focused on training the next generation of leaders. That means supporting faculty who are conducting discovery-based research but also nurturing a passion for discovery among our students.

TRAINING THE NEXT GENERATION OF LEADERS IN BIOMEDICINE

For those who will devote their lives to basic science, it's important that they have the maximum freedom to explore fields of inquiry and areas of discovery without arbitrary constraints imposed by vicissitudes in funding mechanisms. In the United States, the traditional model of funding graduate education in the biosciences has involved covering the costs associated with the first one to two years of a student's enrollment from training grants and institutional resources. Students are then responsible for providing their own support or for finding faculty mentors who can support their tuition and other expenses from the faculty members' research grants.

This system is fraught with difficulties and perverse incentives. A student may have interests that align well with the areas of focus of a prospective faculty mentor, but that faculty member might not have a slot on his or her grants to support the student. It's not uncommon for students to have to choose their research project based on the availability of funding rather than pursuing their interests and attraction to a particular field or area of study. Even for students in a lab closely aligned with their interests, the support for the student from the mentor's grant is often linked to a specific project, making it difficult for the student to change projects if interests evolve.

My Stanford colleagues and I found this status quo for supporting graduate students in biosciences to be unacceptable. In 2013, we made the commitment to fund the four years of graduate education entirely from training grants and philanthropy. The results have been transformative. The number of incoming students who accept admission has risen from around 50 percent to the mid-60s range. The initiative has also aided the School of Medicine's goal of diversifying the student body.

Basic science education is important not just for the next generation of those who devote their lives to understanding the fundamental truths of living systems. It is also of critical importance for the next generation of physician-scientists. To help ensure that they develop an understanding of basic science and a passion for discovery, two of our Nobel laureates (Paul Berg and Brian Kobilka) spent three years studying basic science education and biomedical research at Stanford and at other medical schools and then led efforts to create a novel solution. In collaboration with other colleagues, they developed a Discovery Curriculum that, starting in 2017, became an option for all entering medical students. These students can now enter a "split curriculum pathway" that maximizes the time for longitudinal research by spreading the basic science curriculum over three years instead of two. This opens up two summers and an academic quarter for full-time research, plus an additional four quarters that are 50 percent research.

Students who pursue the Discovery Curriculum can model future careers as physician-scientists by spending time at the bench and in the clinic. They can also do this without increasing student debt, by utilizing subsidies available through the Medical Scholars program. Students can even elect to add a sixth year to pursue a master's degree through the new Berg Scholars program, funded by a grant from the Burroughs Wellcome Fund, or they can enter the MD/PhD program (Medical Scientist Training program). Innovative approaches like this need to be developed and tested to ensure that a critical mass of physician-scientists exists to deliver Precision Health.

"The goal is to matriculate and nurture students who want to be leaders and want to be researchers down the road," says PJ Utz, a professor of medicine who has been deeply involved in the evolution of the Stanford curriculum. Our focus on getting students immersed in research cuts against the grain of what's happening at many other medical schools, where coursework is being consolidated from four years into three—often at the expense of student research. Stanford medical students have had a long history of pursuing fields of study and often other degrees in addition to the MD degree while they are in medical school.

I am acutely aware that the twin pressures of time and money can lead students—and administrators—to press for more accelerated medical school coursework. But I also know that physicians with research experience can be more effective in their clinical work. As Utz explains,

> The students who understand the molecular underpinnings of medicine and who are able to think like a scientist almost become detectives when they get into medical wards. Think about a patient who comes in with a bunch of symptoms. The physician has to take a history, then formulate a hypothesis, then design an experiment—X-rays, lab tests, CT scan, etc.—to test that hypothesis. When the data come in, the physician sees if his or her hypothesis is correct. I've observed that our MD-PhD students, who are really well grounded in molecular medicine, tend to be very curious when they get on the wards. They don't just accept that a patient has something. They're asking, "Why do they have this? Is there a way that we can come up with a way to precisely treat them based on what we know about their disease or their genes associated with this that we could design, and can we then use specific drugs?"

The key, he says, is to get people excited about science as early as possible—whether that's during medical school, the undergraduate years, or even high school (for the past 20 years, Utz has run a summer research initiative for high school students). If they don't get the "research bug," he says, quoting a phrase commonly used by Brian Kobilka in his own presentations about physician-scientist development, "it's very unlikely that they're going to come back to science later in life," as they'll be consumed with whatever career they've chosen. "That's why we've designed our curriculum to get students to develop that bug, but also to give them the molecular foundation and the scientific foundation to ask questions that will make them much more effective physicians."

* * *

There have been remarkable gains in life expectancy since the start of the 20th century, as I noted in chapter 1. At the time, the average age of death in the

United States was 47. Globally, it was just 31. In 2017, U.S. life expectancy was 78.6 years, and the global average was 72. While several different factors have contributed to this progress, the dramatic improvement in medical therapies is among the most important, along with developments such as improved sanitation and higher per-capita income.

But amid great progress, we also receive daily reminders from throughout the world of how much remains unknown about the human body and how to treat disease when it arises. That underscores the need for individuals—and the institutions where they work—to continue to invest in basic science. If that investment is diminished, warns Roger Kornberg, "we will lose the capacity to accomplish any of the things which were the basis of modern medicine today. We will also lose the ability to find solutions to the great problems that remain, which include cancer, Alzheimer's, and so many other medical concerns. The solutions to those problems await the discoveries that will only come from having researchers continue to focus on basic science."

As I noted at the start of this chapter, basic science often competes with a desire to provide immediate solutions. Finding the right balance and ensuring that we are planting the proverbial seeds that can sprout years—or decades—in the future is going to be one of the critical issues facing the medical and scientific communities in the 21st century.

CHAPTER *5*

PEERING INTO THE FUTURE: LEVERAGING THE POWERS OF PREDICTION TO HELP PREVENT ILLNESS

Prediction is fundamental to Precision Health—and a tool to aid in prevention. If physicians, and indeed all of us, can draw on data and other evidence to predict where individuals' health might be headed, they can work on precise interventions that will help prevent illness and promote wellness. The earlier we can pinpoint the deviations, the bigger the payoff, in terms of illnesses that are diagnosed earlier and therefore treated more effectively—if not averted altogether.

The powers of prediction are steadily improving—and they're much better than when I first entered the medical field. But they're far from perfect. Current diagnostics are so intermittent that the information they provide is akin to watching a movie but only getting to see seconds-long snippets every 30 minutes. Knowledge about what predisposes each of us to disease should not be limited to medical professionals—it should be widely accessible and actionable.

With Precision Health, I envision a future in which we are continuously monitoring our health. This monitoring could begin before birth, with analysis of the genetic profile and family profile of every fetus and prediction of disease risk. The monitoring could then continue, with devices worn to collect data on each individual's environmental and behavioral conditions, as well as psychological and biochemical. The resulting data would generate something resembling a real-time movie, offering biofeedback and guidance that could be acted upon by each individual as well as their health providers.

By leveraging that data, in tandem with scientific advancements, and while maintaining the important doctor-patient bond, it would be possible to go beyond treating disease after the fact. Instead, health providers and individuals alike could focus on prediction—identifying trends and markers of future disease—as well as prevention.

Discovering Precision Health: Predict, Prevent, and Cure to Advance Health and Well-Being, First Edition. Lloyd Minor and Matthew Rees.

WHAT MEDICINE CAN LEARN FROM AVIATION

Sanjiv "Sam" Gambhir, who is the Virginia and D. K. Ludwig Professor for Clinical Investigation in Cancer Research at Stanford, and chair of the radiology department, points out that when it comes to predicting illness, modern medicine and health can learn valuable lessons from other industries, like aviation.

In decades past, airplane engines would be inspected every few months for maintenance and possible repair. As the engines became more complex, the maintenance became more frequent, to the point that the engines were inspected every time the airplane was on the ground. Today, it's almost constant, including during flight.

Modern planes often contain hundreds of sensors, which measure many different parameters—not just temperature and pressure, but even the debris (e.g., nanoparticles) coming out of the exhaust. The data from sensors can be analyzed every 30 seconds while the plane is in flight, and those data are fed to a "health" portal on the ground. If something is amiss, maintenance crews will address the problems once the plane lands. Tweaks can even be made by the health portal without the pilots being involved. If a serious issue is detected, the pilots can be notified and, if necessary, safely bring the plane to the ground. The improvements in monitoring are one reason there were no fatalities in the United States linked to commercial airline passenger jet crashes from 2009 through 2017. Health care and medicine can learn valuable lessons from the aviation industry's focus on prediction.

For more than a decade, researchers at Stanford's Canary Center for Cancer Early Detection (which Gambhir founded and leads) have been focused on trying to improve their ability to predict the onset of cancer. They have wanted to shift the focus away from simply developing better therapies, since those therapies are often applied too late, when cancer is relatively advanced.

For most cancers, if caught very early (stage 0 or 1), the survival rate over 5 to 10 years is 95 percent. Regrettably, very few people have their cancer detected early—most are caught at stage 3 or 4 (about 70 percent, in the case of ovarian cancer). As cancer evolves, it becomes more heterogenous—each cell looks different from every neighboring cell. As a result, no matter what treatment is applied, it can't kill every cancer cell, since all cells are different. But if cancer is caught early, it's more homogenous. As a result, therapies are more likely to succeed because more cancer cells are likely to be destroyed.

Prediction and detection present an enormous challenge. Consider that the human body is estimated to have more than 30 trillion cells. If just one of them has mutated and become cancerous, there is no simple way of knowing that. Even if the mutated cell is detected, what's really important to know is whether that cell is a bad actor (since some mutated cells are likely harmless) and will lead to more cell mutations that can prove fatal. One key goal of early detection is finding those cancers that are prognostically important—in other words, those that will go on to harm the subject. This underscores the importance of early detection, as well as the tools that help enable that detection.

DON LISTWIN'S CAMPAIGN TO ADVANCE EARLY CANCER DETECTION

Many billions of dollars were devoted to cancer research in the 20th century, but there was relatively little emphasis on something that was known to save lives: early detection. Because it was viewed as an intractable problem, it attracted little attention from scientists. That stalemate has started to change over the past decade, and while there are many different reasons why, much of the credit goes to Don Listwin. He is the founder of the Canary Foundation, which has helped give early cancer detection the prominence it deserves in the scientific and medical communities.

For most of his career, Listwin worked in the technology sector. He was the founder of technology companies, and at one time he was the second-highest-ranking executive at Cisco. His interest in cancer detection was a product of his mother having been misdiagnosed with a bladder infection—twice. She was actually suffering from ovarian cancer, which had reached an advanced stage by the time it was detected—resulting in her death in 2001.

That experience prompted Listwin to make the modern-day equivalent of cold calls to cancer centers—he emailed them—and ask about their work on early cancer detection. One reply came from Pat McGowan, a development director at the Fred Hutchinson Cancer Center in Seattle. He described their work in a new area called biomarkers, which involves developing a "fingerprint" of early tumors by looking for atypical patterns of proteins or gene activity in blood samples. Listwin eventually contributed $2 million to support ovarian cancer research by one of Hutchinson's scientists, Nicole Urban, and later made a $10 million gift to start a center of excellence at Hutchinson.

In 2004, he left the technology industry and started the Canary Foundation, which is focused on early detection diagnostics. (The name is based on the role played by canaries in helping coal miners detect dangerous gases.) The foundation's website describes how he has approached cancer "as a technology and market development problem waiting to be solved."

> As an engineer and entrepreneur, he thought just about any problem could be fixed with the right amount of leadership, intellect, and time. He saw cancer, and the way we studied the disease, as a series of network failures. And he believed that a systematic approach that involved researchers from many disciplines and institutions sharing information and working together would give us the edge on the disease. He had an "ah-ha" pattern-match moment when he recognized that the approach to fighting cancer was not that different than the breakthroughs in his tech career from building the essence of the mobile internet to the access business at Cisco and more. "Instead of fiber optics, it's genomics, and instead of switching, it's a focus on imaging," said Don in explaining the logic behind how new technology and a shift in funding could upend the entire cancer field [1].

Recognizing the importance of academic medical centers in generating the ideas that lead to new therapies, Listwin wanted to deepen links between academia and industry, and to have professors launch startups. To help advance that objective, in 2009 his funding led to the launch of the Canary Center at Stanford. Its focus is researching and developing minimally invasive diagnostic and imaging strategies for the early detection of cancer. In just the past few years, five companies have been founded by Stanford faculty members. Multiple Canary affiliates, focused on early cancer detection, have also been (or are being) established, at institutions such as Harvard, MIT, Oxford, Oregon Health & Science University, the University of Washington, and the University of Calgary.

Listwin says that when he first started exploring cancer research, there were about five scientists focused on early detection. "Today there are 500, and in a few years it will be 5,000." He cites this as his biggest achievement.

Listwin also wants to upend how cancer research funding is allocated. He points out that about one-third of cancer outcomes are attributed to prevention, one-third to early detection, and one-third to therapeutic improvements. Yet only 10 percent of the money invested in research goes to prevention and just 5 percent goes to early detection. The remaining 85 percent goes to therapeutics. Part of the problem, says Listwin, is that because early detection was viewed as intractable, "people simply didn't believe that there was potential progress. But that's changed in the past 10 years."

Even with the progress, one of the early detection challenges is access: cancer screening typically requires a battery of tests that can be time-consuming and expensive. The Canary Foundation hopes to change that.

> What if someday soon, cancer screening was as simple as a urine or blood test or an inexpensive imaging test at your annual doctor's appointment? Signs of cancer could be exposed before they technically became cancer. And treatment would be so minor, you might even forget you ever had it. That's the world we envision. We want early cancer detection tests to be commonplace—and always the first line of defense for cancer [2].

Today, the foundation is focused on funding research in two primary areas: blood-based biomarkers and molecular imaging. The biomarkers are designed to reveal whether individuals are at risk of developing cancer or if they already have it. The imaging offers precision in identifying types of cancer and whether they are benign or malignant. The foundation also supports clinical programs that explore five types of cancer: breast, lung, ovarian, pancreatic, and prostate. The research is organized along interdisciplinary lines: material science, engineering, biology, computer science and technology, and biology and medicine. "All of these disciplines have critical thinking to contribute," says Listwin.

A key indicator of Canary's progress is that venture capitalists have invested in companies that are focused on early detection of cancer. Listwin hopes these companies succeed and that more research centers emerge to develop even more precise technologies. "I would like nothing more than to have a 'going-out-of-business' party in the next 15 years, confident that our mission of enabling early cancer detection in routine medical practice has been achieved."

THE EMERGENCE OF NEW AND IMPROVED DIAGNOSTIC TOOLS

Central to predicting the onset of illness and disease is the ability to identify deviations in health. But this ability—known as *diagnostics*—has long been a shortcoming of the U.S. health care system. As a 2015 National Academy of Medicine report pointed out, "The delivery of health care has proceeded for decades with a blind spot: Diagnostic errors—inaccurate or delayed diagnoses—persist throughout all settings of care and continue to harm an unacceptable number of patients" [3].

Amid those shortcomings, new diagnostic tools have been emerging that can be used in a predictive and preventive way. At Stanford Medicine, some of these tools are being developed as part of the Precision Health and Integrated Diagnostics Center (PHIND), which was launched in 2017. "We want to be proactive, not reactive," says Gambhir, the center's director. "My thinking here was, 'What can we do so that the whole diagnostic field better aligns with Precision Health?' I think the way to get the biggest gain—although it will take several decades to play out—is to lead the charge on proactive health care research across multiple diseases in a broad-picture kind of way" [4].

The backdrop to PHIND's work is that every person has a specific set of biological determinants that influence his or her likelihood of developing disease. Not all of those determinants are fully understood, but new knowledge about them is being gathered all the time. Taking a variety of metabolic tests, and also looking in detail at genetic makeup, enables measurements for each person's relative risk of contracting certain diseases. With the revolution that's occurring in advanced diagnostics, hopefully it will be possible to develop a precise preventive regimen for every individual.

Back to Basics with Blood Tests

The importance of early detection, particularly related to cancer, has given rise to several procedures and tools that have contributed to progress. But many of them also have downsides. Protein biomarkers (such as a PSA test for prostate cancer) and imaging (mammography) can lead to many false positives. Medical procedures are typically invasive, which can lead to complications, and they may not be accessible to those who are without health insurance or living in an under-resourced community.

But we are also seeing important breakthroughs in prediction using a very elementary procedure: the blood test.

A pioneer in this area has been Stephen Quake, the Lee Otterson Professor of Bioengineering and a professor of applied physics, at Stanford. His research was spurred by his pregnant wife having to submit to an amniocentesis to check for fetal chromosomal abnormalities: "It was somewhat shocking to me that we had to risk the life of the baby to ask a diagnostic question" [5]. He began exploring whether a blood test could be a substitute for amniocentesis, which involves inserting a needle into the uterus to extract a small amount of amniotic fluid from the sac surrounding the unborn baby.

A team of researchers led by Quake used next-generation sequencing to measure the genome of a fetus and distinguish it from the maternal DNA, which is dominant in the blood sample. From there, they figured out how to measure for aneuploidy, which refers to the existence of an abnormal number of chromosomes in a cell. (Down syndrome is the most common, followed by trisomy 18 and trisomy 13.) The breakthrough involved being able to count chromosomes, based on fetal DNA found in the mother's blood. They published a paper on the topic in 2008, demonstrating the effectiveness of a blood test [6].

Just three years later, clinical trials were complete, and commercial versions of the blood test were made available to the public. Since then, millions of women throughout the world have used the test (and about three million do so annually). According to Quake, the test's adoption rate may be the fastest in the history of medicine, among molecular diagnostics. One reason why is safety. The blood test caries no risk, but approximately 0.6 percent of all amniocenteses result in a miscarriage, and the procedure can be dangerous for the mother as well. Another benefit is accuracy. A 2015 study published in the *New England Journal of Medicine* showed that when nearly 16,000 women were tested in the first trimester of their pregnancy, the blood test identified all 38 women who had a presence of trisomy 21 (the marker for Down syndrome), while standard screening tests only detected it in 30 women [7]. The test can also detect chromosomal abnormalities as early as 10 weeks into a pregnancy.

One expectant mother, interviewed by the *Washington Post*, described what she liked about the test. "It was an easy blood draw and we didn't see a downside. My husband and I hadn't discussed what we would do if we got a bad result, but I thought if we did, wouldn't we want to know as far in advance as possible" [8]?

In 2017, the director of the National Institute of Child Health and Human Development, Diana Bianchi, crystallized the impact of the blood test: "Just like Google or Airbnb changed how research and booking a room works, noninvasive prenatal genomics is altering the obstetrician profession around the world" [9]. And while amniocenteses are still offered, their usage has plummeted. In 2008, the Perinatal Diagnostic Center at Stanford Children's Health performed 1,122 amniocenteses. In 2018, they conducted only 183, according to Jane Chueh, a professor of obstetrics and gynecology at Stanford.

Although chromosomal abnormalities cannot be reversed, the blood test empowers the parent(s) with information. Specialized programs and resources can be provided to their baby immediately after birth, as research shows that this early intervention leads to improved outcomes [10]. And the information from the blood test can also be used by doctors, who look for organs that are often affected by chromosomal abnormalities, with treatment ready to be provided shortly after delivery. Without the knowledge of the abnormalities, interventions will be triggered only by a medical emergency or developmental delays.

In 2018, Quake achieved another blood-test breakthrough. Working with researchers from Stanford and other institutions, he developed a blood test that predicts, with 75 to 80 percent accuracy, the likelihood of a pregnancy resulting in premature birth. Globally, there are approximately 15 million such births every year—a number that has held steady for decades, as researchers have never developed a reliable approach to identifying women at risk. In the United States, about 9 percent of all births annually are premature—making it the country's largest cause of infant mortality.

Quake's research involved analyzing the blood of 38 American women who had already experienced early contractions or a preterm delivery. The women provided one blood sample during the second or third term of their pregnancy— and 13 of them ultimately delivered prematurely. The chief predictor of premature deliveries was the level of cell-free transcript RNA from seven genes found in the mother and the placenta. In announcing the breakthrough, one of the researchers, Mads Melbye, a visiting professor of medicine at Stanford, said, "I've spent a lot of time over the years working to understand preterm delivery. This is the first real, significant progress on this problem in a long time."

Blood tests are also being used as a tool to predict cancer. One test, developed by Max Diehn, an associate professor of radiation oncology at Stanford, reveals a biomarker called circulating tumor DNA, which stems from a tumor but is found in the blood of a person with the tumor. Among patients with cancer, healthy DNA is mixed with a little bit of cancer DNA. What's new is the ability to conduct a sensitive measurement of that cancer DNA.

Cancer researchers like Diehn see circulating tumor DNA as a transformative biomarker for Precision Health. An important advantage of circulating tumor DNA over prior biomarkers is its specificity, since it's possible to identify pieces of tumor DNA by the mutations present only in cancer cells. "Having a biomarker that tracks the actual cause of cancer is ideal," says Diehn. He points out that this is different from a PSA test for prostate cancer, which is a protein *made* by cancer, but *not the cause* of prostate cancer.

There are two other noteworthy features about circulating tumor DNA. First, it can be applied to any cancer, since all cancers are driven by mutations. As a result, it accelerates the pace with which biomarkers can be developed for any given disease. However, cancers that tend to have a higher number of mutations, such as melanoma and lung cancer, are easier to detect using circulating tumor DNA than cancers with fewer mutations.

Second, circulating tumor DNA can potentially be applied at nearly any point along a patient's care continuum—even as early as cancer screening and early detection. Thus in the future when individuals have their blood drawn, discovery of circulating tumor DNA could lead to a work-up to identify the source and determine whether it is a cancer that needs treatment. That would have the biggest impact, because the easiest way to cure a cancer patient is to catch the cancer before it spreads.

A blood test that looks for circulating tumor DNA can also be used to predict disease recurrence. In a study of 40 patients with lung cancer by Diehn and his colleagues Ash Alizadeh (a Stanford hematologist and oncologist) and Aadel Chaudhur (a Stanford radiation oncology resident), a blood test enabled them to distinguish between those who had been cured and those in whom the disease would recur. They were able to detect the circulating tumor DNA about five months before the recurrence was visible on scans. The earlier detection is critical, as it means aggressive treatment can begin sooner; delays in treatment are linked to worse outcomes. The focus on DNA also means that different treatments can be tailored for different patients—a hallmark of Precision Health, and all of it enabled by a simple blood test.

A blood test is also at the center of a massive effort focused on detecting cancer earlier, since early detection is fundamental to treating cancer and preventing it from becoming a disabling—and deadly—condition.

GRAIL is a company founded in March 2016 and focused on the development of diagnostic tests for early cancer detection. Its founding chief executive, and today the vice chairman of its board of directors, is Jeff Huber. He brims with the can-do attitude of someone who spent 13 years at Google, where he was the senior engineer for the company's trailblazing initiatives around advertising, apps, and maps.

GRAIL's scientific advisory board features leaders from several different industries, including one of my colleagues at the School of Medicine (Christina Curtis). It has raised more than $1.5 billion, from investors like Jeff Bezos, Bill Gates, and Google Ventures, and the money is helping fund two of the largest clinical studies ever undertaken—involving approximately 100,000 people.

Huber, who is on the advisory board of the School of Medicine's Precision Health and Integrated Diagnostics Center, says that some of his optimism stems from the existence of genome sequencing and the ability to digitize biology. But he's also candid about the challenge ahead:

> At GRAIL, we've debated how much of fundamental cancer biology is really understood. And the most ambitious, the most aggressive that anyone has ventured so far is maybe 2 percent. There's so much more that needs to be learned.

Huber approaches cancer with two powerful weapons. First, he's an outsider. Although he worked in life sciences at Google, he's not trained as a scientist, much less a cancer researcher. Second, he has a personal connection to the disease. In 2014, his wife, Laura, was diagnosed with Stage 4 colon cancer. She died 18 months later, at the age of 47.

We treated my wife's case aggressively. We were at Stanford, we had the best doctors, and we assembled a team of experts from around the country, and around the world. It was a full court press of being able to find a cure. But even with the state of technology and the best experts in the world, it was ultimately a losing battle, because it had spread and become so complex. By the time we were done, Laura was probably the most individually studied case of cancer in the world. But the whole experience showed how far we are from a cure or anything like it today, even with the billions of dollars that have been invested in developing cancer therapeutics.

The experience highlighted the fact that a fundamental challenge with cancer is detection. Screening procedures for most cancers are imprecise, which is one reason why about 80 percent of them are diagnosed at Stage 3 or 4—often too late to save the patient's life. This unfortunate reality is now embedded in the medical system, says Huber, creating what he says is an "intentionally reactionary system."

Doctors are trained that you don't treat something that "doesn't exist." Patients must have a problem or a symptom. They have to come in and complain. Otherwise, you leave them alone. And that's why so much cancer is diagnosed so late, when the outcomes are 80 to 90 percent negative, and people die. And because that's where cancer is diagnosed, that's why the pharmaceutical industry and therapies spend billions and billions of dollars on treatments—after the cancer has been caught.

To address this, GRAIL's signature product, which is still under development, is a blood test that is being designed to detect many cancer types at early stages, when treatment may be more successful. The test will leverage next-generation sequencing to look for fragmentary DNA that's been shed by the cancer from its earliest stages. The test results will be designed to tell patients not only if they have cancer, but where it is in their body.

One of the many challenges with detecting cancer is accuracy. Mammograms, for example, miss about 20 percent of breast cancers, according to the American Cancer Society [11]. Huber recognizes this, and he believes GRAIL can address the issue by developing tests with error rates below 1 percent.

The underlying analyte that we're looking at is altered DNA that leads to cancer development and progression. And that is really the signature of cancer. Nothing else has that behavior around it. Given that the thing we're detecting is the unique signature of cancer, we believe that we will not have the false positive challenges that others have had.

GRAIL's goal is for their blood tests to become deeply integrated into the medical system. Here's how Huber envisions it:

When you go in for an annual physical exam, you get a blood draw, where they tell you basic measures like your cholesterol and glucose, and then they will administer the GRAIL test. With the GRAIL test, we'll be able to tell you if you have cancer and where it is. Our hope is that you've gotten the test early enough to detect cancer at an early stage when it can make a big difference on prognosis and outcome, and save your life. The primary intervention today for solid tumor cancers is surgical recision.

In the future, with significant progress in understanding of cancer biology and immunotherapy based in part on the data we're generating and the work of others in the field, we hope the intervention and experience can be akin to receiving a personalized immunotherapy prescription or vaccine, where you might feel like you have a flu for a couple of weeks while your immune system wakes up and does its job. If we collectively succeed, getting a cancer diagnosis in the future could be about as eventful as having the flu.

I can't predict how successful GRAIL will be, or even whether it will succeed. Like all innovations, GRAIL is partly at the mercy of the third "C" of innovation I discussed earlier—chance. That is, by definition, impossible to predict, and it can certainly prove elusive. But the focus on what Huber calls "finding a different playing field" suggests that whatever progress GRAIL realizes may look very different than the progress achieved by others.

One thing is clear: progress is needed. Even after decades of research, and billions of dollars devoted to research, cancer remains a leading cause of death in the United States and throughout the world. It's precisely the situation that calls for innovative thinking, and if GRAIL can chart meaningful progress, their approach may be a model for combating other deadly diseases.

FORWARD THROUGH THE PAST

The blood test is not the only new predictive tool rooted in old procedures. Another tool being developed draws on a discovery made more than a century ago by the inventor of the telephone, Alexander Graham Bell.

Bell's research revealed that if sunlight was chopped up and allowed to hit dark materials, those materials would not only absorb the light but also slightly heat up and emit sound waves. It was an important discovery, but not one that seemed to have any practical applications until about 15 years ago, when it began to be applied to biological problems.

For example, it is used in connection with technology for detecting prostate cancer that relies on what's known as *transrectal photoacoustics*. A device is placed in the patient's rectum, and it pulses light waves into the prostate. The device then "listens" for sounds coming back from the prostate, drawing on both optical imaging and ultrasound imaging, since blood vessels feeding a cancer can absorb light and produce sound. The device, which took seven years to develop, involved the work of engineers, imaging experts, computational people, doctors, and surgeons, working under the auspices of the Canary Center at Stanford.

The imaging that underpins transrectal photo acoustics has also been used to aid in the diagnosis of breast and ovarian cancers. As these imaging techniques become more standardized and more broadly used, the hope is that they will reduce the need for the more invasive techniques that are used today to make a diagnosis.

Another advance in imaging of tumors, made by Sam Gambhir and the late Jürgen Willmann, who was a professor of radiology at Stanford, relied on something known as *targeted microbubble ultrasound*. It involves the use of technologies that send the equivalent of molecular spies into the body. They conduct a cell-to-cell search, and the "bad" cells give off signals detected by instruments that listen for those signals.

These techniques have led to the use of substances known as *microbubbles*, which are smaller than human cells. These bubbles have been chemically modified on their surface, and they are designed to attach to blood vessels that are feeding a very early tumor. For the tumor to grow, it needs to feed on blood vessels. The microbubbles navigate around the human body, and when they encounter blood vessels that are feeding a tumor, they latch on to those blood vessels. As this process plays out, an ultrasound device sends sound waves into the body—akin to a yell—and the researchers wait for the bubbles to yell back. When they do, the technicians create an image of where the bubbles are located. They then superimpose that on the body's anatomy—enabling them to identify cancerous cells at a very early stage.

In the Willmann/Gambhir study, published in 2017 in the *Journal of Clinical Oncology*, 24 women with ovarian tumors and 21 women with breast tumors were intravenously injected with the microbubbles. The bubbles only latched on to the blood vessels that were feeding a tumor [12]. This precision was noteworthy. "The difficulty with ultrasound right now," said Willmann, "is that it detects a lot of lesions in the breast, but most of them are benign. And that leads to many unnecessary biopsies and surgeries." He said that reducing the number of unnecessary biopsies "would be a huge leap forward," with benefits for people throughout the world [13].

BRINGING NEW PRECISION TO RISK MANAGEMENT AND SCREENING FOR BREAST CANCER

Sylvia Plevritis, professor and chair of the Department of Biomedical Data Science and professor of radiology at Stanford, develops computational models to study cancer biology and cancer outcomes. Her research has helped illuminate the value of different approaches to breast cancer screening, while also developing a valuable tool that brings new precision to risk management associated with improved breast cancer survival outcomes.

Plevritis has an unconventional background for someone immersed in biomedical research. Her undergraduate major and her PhD were in electrical engineering (EE). Her doctoral adviser, Al Macovski, ran a laboratory in Stanford EE, which housed a clinical-grade MRI scanner for research-only use. Through her studies, Plevritis applied principles in information theory to reconstruct images of early metabolic changes in human tumors using MRI. Some of her early research involved how MRI could help advance early detection of breast cancer. That work led her to pursue a master's degree in health services research at Stanford, which she earned in 1996. During this period, she collaborated with Alan Garber, who was a Stanford health care economist at the time (he's now the provost at Harvard), to develop a simulation model to predict how a then-hypothetical MRI exam, particularly for women with dense breast tissue, could be effectively applied to screen for breast cancer.

This research led Plevritis to develop a model to simulate a variety of MRI breast cancer screening strategies. She targeted her analysis on younger women who had an inherited mutation in BCRA1 or BRCA2 genes. She simulated a trial where women would get randomized into an MRI screening arm or mammography screening arm, and then estimated the additional mortality reduction for those in the MRI screening arm. She concluded that MRI could be an effective screening test despite its costs and false positive findings. This work was the basis of a paper she published in the *Journal of the American Medical Association* in 2006 [14]. The following year, the American Cancer Society cited the paper when issuing a recommendation to support breast MRI screening for high-risk mutation carriers [15].

Plevritis came up with an idea, based on this research: to create a decision-support tool that would help women make more individualized decisions, based on their specific risk and changes in their risk with age. The tool, which was developed with clinical colleague Allison Kurian, faculty in Stanford Oncology, and launched in 2011, can be used to determine the likelihood of different health outcomes for women between the ages of 25 and 69 who carry a BRCA1 or BRCA2 mutation. The assessments are based on factors such as a woman's age, the age at which MRI screening began, and whether she has had surgery such as a prophylactic oophorectomy or a prophylactic mastectomy. The predictions generated by the tool are based on data derived from clinical studies of BRCA mutation carriers on cancer incidence and the efficacy of screening, preventive surgeries, and treatment. It also draws on U.S. population data about surviving breast cancer, based on the stage of the cancer, nuclear grade, and hormone receptor expression.

The tool—the first mechanism to help women at high risk for breast cancer to calculate the risks they face—has been cited by the National Comprehensive Cancer Network, the American College of Obstetrics and Gynecology, and the American Society of Breast Surgeons (ASBrS). As of April 2019, it had been used by more than 44,000 women. "I receive emails from women across the country thanking me for this tool," says Plevritis. "It helps women think about their mutation in new and different ways. It's one of the most satisfying projects I've ever done."

Plevritis has also conducted pioneering research on how screening mammography and adjuvant treatment have impacted breast cancer mortality rates over time. She coauthored a 2005 paper that revealed that mammography and adjuvant treatment reduced breast cancer mortality by 37 percent, with the relative reductions about evenly split between the two [16]. In 2018, she was the lead author of a paper that featured updated outcomes, showing that screening and adjuvant treatment reduced overall breast cancer mortality by 49 percent in 2012. For all breast cancers, treatment accounted for 63 percent of the reduction and screening just 37 percent [17]. In addition, the study also demonstrated significant differences in the relative contributions of screening and treatment by molecular subtype.

Plevritis says the gains from treatment are a product of the many new technologies to help interpret the tumor at the time of diagnosis.

> We are reverse-engineering the biology of tumors in ways that are unprecedented. By understanding intrinsic and extrinsic factors driving tumors, we can pinpoint their vulnerabilities and attack them. This is helping with new approaches to not only cancer treatment but also early detection, which holds the greatest promise in reducing mortality, because if we can detect a tumor earlier, when it's less complex, we have a greater chance at curative therapy.

Plevritis also points to "transformative" progress in disease imaging, saying that "we're resolving human tumors at single cell and subcellular scales." Known as highly multiplexed *in situ* imaging, it enables researchers to see the different cell types that create so-called tumor neighborhoods—making it possible to understand the tumor not just from the malignant cells, which provide a limited view, but also from the spatial organization of other cell types that intermix with the malignant cells and influence their behavior (Garry Nolan, whose work is described in chapter 4). "This information is going to be absolutely critical to more fully understanding cancer and more effectively combating it," says Plevritis. She's also enthusiastic about the potential for the cell atlas initiatives being undertaken in the Chan Zuckerberg Biohub and the Human Tumor Atlas. Merging single cell genomic data with imaging data enables an unprecedented view of normal tissue and disease. She is confident that with this information, we will be able to resolve the cell-cell communication within the tumor microenvironment that underlies tumor initiation, progression, and treatment response. "I think that is going to be a game changer," she says.

NEW UNDERSTANDING OF GENETICS AND NEW POTENTIAL TO PREDICT, PREVENT, AND CURE DISEASE

The mapping of the human genome opened a new chapter in our understanding of human heredity and of hereditary propensities to disease. This chapter is still being written, based on our increased understanding of the interactions between the genome and environmental factors and other determinants of health. The mapping process began at the National Institutes of Health in 1990, with a $3 billion budget, and it was among the most comprehensive biological research projects ever undertaken. The goal, said Francis Collins, who served as the director of the National Human Genome Research Institute, was to "enhance the ability to understand hereditary factors in all diseases as quickly as possible" [18]. When the genome's first draft was published 11 years later, Collins spoke to what had been achieved:

> It's a history book—a narrative of the journey of our species through time. It's a shop manual, with an incredibly detailed blueprint for building every human cell. And it's a transformative textbook of medicine, with insights that will give health care providers immense new powers to treat, prevent and cure disease [19].

Indeed, there has been an accumulation of knowledge and understanding over the past 15 years that would have been unthinkable a few decades ago. With the cost of sequencing each human genome dropping dramatically—from $100 million for the first one to about $1,000 today—it's possible for people throughout the world to gain unprecedented insights into their genetic profile.

Genome sequencing is also enabling dramatic improvements in prediction. Euan Ashley, a professor of medicine and genetics at Stanford, is a leader in the field and points to the potential of predictive genetics:

> We now understand so much more about the genetic basis of the most common diseases in our society—cancer and cardiovascular disease. We can use genetic testing to provide better estimates of patients' future risk. With a better idea of who might be at risk, we can then intervene early, with precision, and help to prevent disease before it takes hold.

An example of the power of prediction and the power of sequencing comes from a baby delivered in 2013 at Stanford's Lucile Packard Children's Hospital. As related in a gripping article published in *Stanford Medicine,* doctors had detected an irregular heartbeat while the baby was in utero, which led to an emergency C-section being conducted 10 weeks before the due date. The baby, named Astrea, went into cardiac arrest soon thereafter and was diagnosed with a rare heart problem called long QT syndrome, in which part of the heart's rhythm is longer than normal, which can trigger erratic heartbeats, fainting, and sudden cardiac death. She had a pacemaker and defibrillator implanted. The mystery was that just 8 percent of her cells carried the mutation for long QT syndrome (an example of what's known as *mosaicism*), and it was unknown how long she'd live and what was causing her heart to stop.

A team of researchers—spread across universities and private companies—eventually conducted a rapid sequencing of her genome to determine the cause of her heart problem. At the age of just eight months she had a heart transplant, which helped stabilize her health. Soon thereafter, the researchers partnered with a genetic testing company to inquire about the frequency of mosaicism when looking at genes that caused arrhythmia. The answer was 0.1 percent.

Astrea's case may have answered a question that had eluded researchers: genetics don't explain approximately 30 percent of heart arrhythmia patients.

"Maybe there are additional mutations that are in the heart only," said one of the researchers, James Priest, an assistant professor of pediatrics at Stanford. "Genetic tests are nearly always done on blood or other easily acquired tissues. So it's easy to imagine a mosaic gene variant that occurs only in the heart and doesn't show up in the blood." The same reasoning, he said, could apply to other parts of the body. "And that really is a brand-new phenomenon," said Priest, noting that mosaic gene variants had not been looked to as the cause of these kinds of diseases [20]. One of the takeaways from this episode, says Ashley, is the ability to predict and treat long QT syndrome more precisely, given that the genetic basis of this cardiac disease is now understood.

More Precise Interpretation of Genetic Testing

One of the challenges associated with genetic testing is deciphering the results. This is of particular concern when the results reveal gene mutations known as *variants of uncertain significance*, since the effects of these mutations are unknown. "This is a really big problem," says Joseph C. Wu, who is director of the Stanford Cardiovascular Institute and the Simon H. Stertzer Professor of Medicine and of Radiology at Stanford. "If someone tells me I have a genetic variant that could cause sudden cardiac death, I'm going to be very scared. The result could be a lifetime of unnecessary worry for a patient when, in fact, the variant may be completely benign" [21]. Wu has been a leader in showing how gene-editing tools, coupled with stem cell technology, can help predict whether individuals are at risk from specific gene variants.

In a paper published in June 2018 in the *Journal of the American College of Cardiology*, Wu described how he and his team of researchers determined whether a 39-year-old patient with a variant of unknown significance on the KCNH2 gene was at risk of developing long QT syndrome. The patient was referred to Wu and his team, and they explored whether the variant was pathogenic or benign by studying cells derived from the patient. They used CRISPR—a gene-editing tool—to fix the mutation, which involved a defective nucleotide in the KCNH2 gene, and they also introduced the defective nucleotide into a healthy control gene. Their tests revealed that the features of long QT syndrome appeared only in the cells with the mutation—thus confirming that the patient was afflicted with the syndrome.

The use of gene editing enables researchers like Wu to determine the pathogenicity of variants in three to four months. Without that technology, physicians would have little option but to ask any of their patients with a variant of unknown significance to monitor their health over many years—and hope that the variant would turn out to be benign.

The results, said Wu, "will help improve the interpretation and diagnostic accuracy of gene variants, especially in the era of personalized medicine and precision health. The goal is to optimize the decision-making of clinicians in their choices of therapy by providing a much clearer result for the 'variant of uncertain significance' carriers" [22].

Predicting Disease through Genomic Testing

Another example, showing how the genome can help predict disease, comes from a member of the Stanford faculty. Michael Snyder is the Stanford W. Ascherman Professor at Stanford and chair of the Department of Genetics. He was an early adopter of wearable devices that monitored his health (he'll often wear eight or nine of them simultaneously). He was also fascinated by the potential of the human genome to serve as a predictive tool. In 2010, he worked with a team of researchers to have his entire genome sequenced—at a level of detail that had never been done before. (The researchers also tracked almost 20,000 distinct transcripts coding for 12,000 genes and measured the relative levels of more than 6,000 proteins in Snyder's blood.) The genome sequencing revealed that he faced an increased risk of developing high cholesterol, coronary artery disease, basal cell carcinoma, and type 2 diabetes.

The diabetes prediction was particularly surprising, given that there was no history of diabetes in Snyder's family, he was not overweight, and he had no other risk factors. Over the next 14 months, he had his blood analyzed 20 times to better understand his own immunity, metabolism, and gene activity. At one point, his blood glucose level shot up following a viral infection, and he reached a level that classified him as diabetic. The apparent nexus between the infection and the rise of his blood glucose was an unexpected discovery. "We have not been generally associating viral infection with this type of diabetes," he said later. "It is possible that the viral infection added additional stress" [23].

For Snyder, there was great significance attached to the real-time finding that he'd become diabetic. "Normally I go for a physical exam about once every two or three years. So under normal circumstances, my diabetes wouldn't have been diagnosed for one or two years" [24]. At that point, the diabetes could have already damaged his kidneys and nerves, and increased his risk of suffering a stroke or heart attack. Instead, he improved his diet, doubled his bicycle mileage, and started running. Over six months, the changes reduced his blood sugar level and eliminated the need for diabetes medication.

"It was the first time someone had used their genome to predict risk for disease, and then took action to reverse the effects of the disease," says Snyder, who later published his finding in *Cell,* an academic journal [25]. "And it showed the potential for Precision Health, with health care tailored to each individual's unique circumstances."

Detecting Atrial Fibrillation through Genetic Testing

To see the potential of genetic testing, consider how it is being used to help predict and treat a condition called atrial fibrillation. Afib, as it's known, affects about 1 percent of the general population and contributes to about 130,000 deaths and 750,000 hospitalizations annually, in the United States alone. It often leads to blood clots, and it's responsible for 15 to 25 percent of all strokes in the United States.

Atrial fibrillation is characterized by an irregular heartbeat, a misfiring of the heart's electrical signals that causes it to, in the words of the American Heart Association, "work as if it's enduring a marathon, even if the patient is relaxing in a chair." Atrial fibrillation goes undetected because many of its symptoms—like fatigue or shortness of breath—don't make us think our heart is beating with a dangerous cadence. Atrial fibrillation is also a condition that may not present symptoms in the moment of a diagnostic medical test, the primary one involving an electrocardiogram (ECG), which uses electrodes to detect the heart's electrical signals. This underscores the value of predictive measures.

Given that afib leads to very chaotic electrical activity in the top chambers of the heart, the effects interfere with everyday life, as do the most commonly recommended treatments, such as medications with significant side effects and invasive procedures.

In recent years, more precise clinical genetic testing has enabled researchers to learn that many genes are linked to abnormalities in the structure of the heart muscle, and these abnormalities are leading to the electrical disorder. That's significant because knowing that somebody has the potential to develop abnormalities in the heart muscle has implications for what kind of treatments they will receive.

The experience of a student in her 20s showcased the value of genetic testing. She developed afib, and when her cardiologist discovered that her brother also had the condition, she was referred to the Stanford Inherited Arrhythmia Clinic. A comprehensive genetic test revealed that she had a genetic disorder that had been previously well described in other families in a gene called RBM20, which was linked to a severe heart muscle disorder that could trigger sudden cardiac death. Although she had not demonstrated any clear muscle abnormalities, her genetics made it clear that she was susceptible to them. She was treated for the afib, but she also had a defibrillator implanted, which could potentially be life-saving. Genetic testing made this possible. Digital health tools can also play a valuable role in detecting afib, which I describe in more detail later in this chapter.

Genetic Testing to Predict How Patients Will Respond to Specific Drugs

Just as the mapping of the human genome has enabled new insights about genetic abnormalities, and opportunities to treat them, it has also spurred extraordinary progress in pharmacogenomics—a branch of medicine that uses each patient's genetic information to predict the effectiveness and safety of specific drugs. By using precise measurements of patients to make precise decisions about which drugs to prescribe for them, pharmacogenomics plays a critical role in advancing the Precision Health vision. Indeed, in its strategic plan for 2016–20, the National Institutes of Health singled out pharmacogenomics for helping to advance one of its fundamental objectives: "[to] accelerate and expand upon its efforts to encourage development of more precise, individualized ways of managing and preventing disease" [26].

Underpinning pharmacogenomics is a little-known fact: Each individual's response to certain drugs is an inherited trait—just like height, disease risk, and many other things. More than 90 percent of humans have a genetic finding that can affect how our body will react to taking a drug. Without any knowledge of an individual's genes, there's a risk that a given drug will prove ineffective in certain segments of the population. For example, approximately 7 percent of all people of European ancestry don't have the enzyme that turns codeine into morphine, thus rendering it no better than a placebo. Drugs used to treat about 90 percent of common conditions in the United States—including asthma, arthritis, high cholesterol, high blood pressure, acid reflux—are affected by the user's genetic profile.

The importance of pharmacogenomics, which has existed in different forms for 40 to 50 years, was underscored by a landmark report issued by the National Academy of Sciences in 1999. The report asserted that between 44,000 and 98,000 people died in U.S. hospitals each year because of medical errors, and it cited a study documenting the fact that in 1993, about 7,000 people died from medication errors alone [27]. Today, there are no definitive figures on medication error, but a 2016 study by the Johns Hopkins University School of Medicine concluded that more than 250,000 people die each year in the United States from medical errors [28]. That makes medical error the third-leading cause of death, following heart disease and cancer. With medication error undoubtedly responsible for some amount of death and disability, the need for the kind of knowledge uncovered by pharmacogenomics is clear.

The ultimate goal for pharmacogenomics is for doctors to draw on each patient's genetic makeup to make prescribing decisions—decisions that maximize the probability that each patient is going to benefit from the drug and minimize the probability that the drug will trigger toxic side effects or adverse reactions. To help turn that vision into reality, a key step has been determining the genes that matter, figuring out which variations predict good or bad responses, and making that information available to physicians in a database.

That work began at Stanford in 2000 with an NIH-funded knowledge base called the Pharmacogenomics KnowledgeBase, or PharmGKB. One of its founders was Russ Altman, a leader in the field of pharmacogenomics and today the Kenneth Fong Professor, as well as a professor of bioengineering, genetics, medicine, and biomedical data science (and computer science, by courtesy) at Stanford. PharmGKB catalogs published information about how human genetic variation affects response to medications. Although it started as strictly a research tool, over time physicians began to seek guidance on different drugs. That spurred Altman along with colleagues around the world to begin developing guidelines for the prescription of certain drugs.

In 2017, PharmGKB launched a pharmacogenomic clinic at Stanford. Patients are checked for the approximately 200 spots in the genome that are most important for modulating drug response. A doctor then meets with each patient for an hour, explains his or her pharmacogenomic profile, and makes recommendations about which drugs are likely to be effective and which drugs could prove toxic (particularly if certain drugs are taken together). Sometimes patients or their providers have questions or concerns about specific drugs that they are considering. For example, a patient with a rocky history of pain relief after surgery might seek advice about which pain medications are most likely to work.

PharmGKB is supporting the introduction of pharmacogenomics into many different areas of medicine. For the treatment of cancer, clinicians will choose medications that have proved effective based on mutations found in specific cancer cells. Altman points to the example of the breast cancer drug Herceptin. "If the cancerous cells don't have a specific genetic profile, Herceptin is ineffective. But if the cells do have the right genetics, Herceptin can be a miracle cure."

Psychiatry has been one of the most enthusiastic adopters of pharmacogenomics, which reflects the fact that the profession receives minimal guidance about which drugs to use and to avoid. "If I can tell a psychiatrist that the patient is going to excrete an antidepressant very rapidly, or it's going to hang around in the body for a long time, that's very useful information to have when making a prescription," says Altman.

But there are a few challenges associated with expanding the adoption of pharmacogenomics. One is that the patient tests—which cost about $300 to $400—are rarely covered by insurance. Another challenge is getting more doctors to embrace the findings in those tests. As Altman points out,

> Most physicians have a group of 20 to 30 medications that they use all the time. They get very familiar with them. Now we're asking them to expand their repertoire because we are saying, "The medications you like to use for an individual patient might not be the right ones. So, I'm going to need you to increase the array of meds that you're willing to consider." That's stressful for them because then they have to go to some computer system that's going to give them advice. It could slow them down and take away their autonomy. And with many primary care physicians having a maximum of one minute to make prescribing decisions, any pharmacogenomics system needs to be able to deliver what they need in 30 seconds. That's a challenge.

A related issue, says Altman, is many doctors don't feel equipped to make decisions based on genetics. "Many of them don't remember what they learned from med school, and even if they did, so much about genetics has changed that their knowledge is likely outdated."

One possible solution, he says, is to remove physicians from the decision-making about prescriptions and hand responsibility to pharmacists. "This would be an exciting expansion of their professional domain. They have the time. They naturally understand the importance of pharmacogenomics because they think about drugs all the time." While this would require some states to modify their laws on allowing pharmacists to prescribe, it has already started to happen in Canada. "In my opinion, it just makes sense economically," says Altman. "Time. Workflow. Everything."

Either way, the influence of pharmacogenomics is likely to grow. PharmGKB has at least one piece of genetic information for nearly 1,000 FDA-approved drugs, which leaves another 3,000 to explore—a process that is well underway, though Altman projects that it will be another 10 to 20 years before the process is complete. His goal is for genome sequences to become part of every patient's medical records, for clinical use, and for clinicians to choose drugs informed by genetic variations in drug targets, transporters, and metabolizing enzymes. "PharmGKB holds the knowledge to enable this vision," says Altman.

In the meantime, drug companies have a clear incentive to look for genetic influences early in the discovery process. That means designing their trials to include a test to make sure that the right people get in the trial who are likely to benefit. Then, when submitting the drug for approval, they can specify that it should only be used in people who pass specific genetic tests. If they learn about a genetic influence late in the process, the effort may be aborted, since the drug won't be approved. This means, says Altman, that more and more drugs are likely to be approved with all the pharmacogenetic background in the initial application. That could accelerate the drug approval process and contribute to drug safety and effectiveness.

FEELING THE BENEFIT OF PHARMACOGENOMICS

There is a portion of the population that does not properly metabolize certain kinds of pain-relief medications. Debbie Spaizman, who lives in Northern California, is one of those people.

About 10 years ago, she was hospitalized after experiencing severe intestinal distress. She was given Vicodin (hydrocodone/paracetamol) in the emergency room, but it did nothing to relieve her pain. "It left me loopy and fuzzy-headed, and itchy all over my body," she recalls. "I assumed I was allergic to it and was determined never to take it again."

But in August 2018, she was scheduled for nasal surgery. The surgeon emphasized that after the procedure she would need to take very strong medication to relieve the pain. "I was really concerned about the pain and how it would also interfere with my ability to heal."

Spaizman's concern led her to meet with her primary care physician, Megan Mahoney, who is a clinical professor of medicine at Stanford. Mahoney told her about pharmacogenomics and suggested that she be tested to see why she had responded so negatively to Vicodin in the past. The testing, which was part of a pilot program at Stanford, involved a cheek swab.

Once the results came in, she met with Russ Altman, who explained to her that she lacked the enzyme to convert hydrocodone—an element in Vicodin—into morphine. Altman recommended that she take a different drug, call Dilaudid (hydromorphone hydrochloride), since that type of drug does not require metabolization to activate pain relief.

I took that information to my surgeon, who then prescribed Dilaudid for me. I took it immediately post-op and it was amazing. I didn't have any of the swimmy, fuzzy-headed, drunken experience that I had with other narcotic drugs. I was clear and sharp and awake. It also did exactly what it was supposed to do: It took away my pain.

Spaizman is now an enthusiastic booster for pharmacogenomics—"It's life changing research"—which is a result of not only her smooth recovery from surgery, but also realizing that her pharmacogenomic profile is now part of her medical records. "Knowing that anytime I'm diagnosed with something that requires medication, and that the doctor will be able to see what I shouldn't take, or which medication or dosage will be the most effective for my particular genetics, means I have one less thing to worry about when it comes to my health and wellness. That's a huge relief."

New digital tools are being developed to help chart progress in genetics and other issues of human health, which I will turn to next.

THE EMERGING DIGITAL HEALTH REVOLUTION

Digital health is a key component of Precision Health, and it is unlocking myriad new ways to predict the potential for disease and promote well-being. There are a wide variety of digital health devices and tools, and they can be sorted into two primary categories: those that involve consumer-focused devices and technologies and those that involve artificial intelligence (AI) and data science to improve the delivery of health care. The two categories are closely related, given that the consumer-focused devices and tools are typically generating data—data that may be interpreted by analytical approaches and methods.

The consumer-focused devices are responsible for some of the most innovative digital health deployments—aimed at developing care for individual patients, with an emphasis on predicting disease before it strikes. These are often so-called wearable devices. One such device, which the *New York Times* highlighted in early 2019, is a small patch that adheres to the skin. It contains tiny valves that channel the wearer's sweat to sensors, which analyze that sweat and measure the presence of things like chloride, glucose, and lactate. The resulting data can provide a snapshot of an individual's health—and help predict the onset of different conditions. The developers of the device are testing its ability to screen for cystic fibrosis [29].

The Apple Watch is another wearable device, and its ability to predict medical conditions has been the subject of a landmark study. The study—a collaboration between Stanford and Apple—was designed to detect atrial fibrillation in people wearing the watch. The Apple Heart Study app intermittently checked the heart rate pulse sensor for measurements of an irregular pulse. More than 419,000 people agreed to participate in the study—the enrollment period ran from November 2017 through July 2018. If an irregular pulse was detected, they received a notification and were asked to connect with a study health provider virtually. They were then sent a patch monitor, which recorded the electrical rhythm of their heart for up to a week.

The study's findings were published in the *New England Journal of Medicine* in November 2019. They indicated that wearable technology like the Apple Watch can safely identify heart rate irregularities. Key findings included the following:

- Only 0.5 percent of participants received irregular pulse notifications.
- Of those who received a notification and were monitored by the ECG patch about two weeks later, 34 percent were found to have atrial fibrillation.
- During ECG patch monitoring, participants' Apple Watches continued to monitor pulse irregularities. If a participant had an irregular pulse detected, 84 percent of the time this was confirmed to be atrial fibrillation on the simultaneous ECG patch [30].

The results highlighted the potential role that innovative digital technology can play in creating more predictive and preventive health care. Also, the study design provided several valuable insights regarding patient engagement and interventions that will prove helpful in designing further studies. The study's completely virtual nature eliminated the need for participants to be physically present and allowed for the implementation of a massive recruitment strategy in a relatively short period of time. Moreover, the study opens the door to further research into wearable technology and how it might be used to prevent disease before it strikes.

The Uses of Artificial Intelligence and Data Science

The powers of prediction are also central to one of the most exciting, and potentially transformative, developments in medicine and health care: using artificial intelligence (AI) and data science to advance human health. A tremendous amount has been written about AI in just the past few years—books like *AI Superpowers: China, Silicon Valley, and the New World Order*, by Kai-Fu Lee; *Life 3.0: Being Human in the Age of Artificial Intelligence*, by Max Tegmark; *The Sentient Machine: The Coming Age of Artificial Intelligence*, by Amir Husain; and *Deep Medicine: How Artificial Intelligence Can Make Healthcare Human Again*, by Eric Topol.

But what exactly is meant by "artificial intelligence"? Like many terms that become part of our vernacular, AI means different things to different people. Jennifer Widom, the Frederick Emmons Terman Dean of the School of Engineering at Stanford and the Fletcher Jones Professor in Computer Science and Electrical Engineering, has provided a crisp and thoughtful description of relevant terminology:

> Artificial intelligence involves developing systems that automate human-level performance on tasks thought to require intelligence. Data science involves developing tools and methods that can be applied to large bodies of

data to gain insights, make discoveries, and advance knowledge. Machine learning is used in both AI and data science and involves computational methods that leverage existing data sets to "learn" operations or functions, without their need to be programmed explicitly.

Data's importance in today's economy is often compared to oil's importance a century ago—and that certainly applies to its importance to health care. Data-enabled artificial intelligence, coupled with data science, is playing an increasingly important role in medicine: enabling decision support for care providers, reducing the likelihood of physician errors, and analyzing massive data sets to yield valuable insights about human health.

AI is also improving our ability to predict the onset of disease, and it can play a particularly valuable role in addressing one of the biggest knowledge gaps related to personal health throughout the world: millions of people are at risk from diseases triggered by a single gene disorder (so-called Mendelian disorders), but they are not being detected or diagnosed. Carlos Bustamante, a geneticist and professor of biomedical data science and of genetics at Stanford, says that smart deployment of artificial intelligence would help identify those who are at risk from Mendelian disease but are not being diagnosed precisely, if at all. AI could be used to help identify the candidates for such testing and sequencing—drawing on a history of medical information that's part of the digital registries that have been built up over the past decade, as the use of electronic health records has become more widespread.

Artificial intelligence can also help predict which individuals are going to account for a disproportionate share of population-wide health care spending in a subsequent year. This is significant for three reasons, according to Arnold Milstein, a professor of medicine at Stanford and director of the university's Clinical Excellence Research Center (CERC). He points out that 10 percent of the population typically consumes 70 percent of the dollars. Second, the people in this 10 percent are not static—the majority of them are new each year, since most in the current year's top 10 percent either get healthy or die. Third, if identified in advance via predictive algorithms, many of a subsequent year's predicted highest-spending patients can be protected from otherwise costly and dangerous health care crises via proactive clinician intervention.

Milstein worked with another faculty member in Stanford's School of Medicine, Nigam Shah, to develop the required multiyear comprehensive health database, drawn from the entire population in Western Denmark, spanning 2004 to 2011. Using AI, they and PhD student Suzanne Tamang applied AI tools to build an algorithm that proved 30 percent more accurate than today's best available prediction tools—a finding reported in an article they coauthored for the *British Medical Journal* [31]. Their work is now the foundation of a new company that licensed the technology from the university. The company will allow health care organizations and health insurers to anticipate the individuals likely to consume the largest share of health spending and help clinicians target interventions that contain costs by preventing costly and dangerous health crises.

Milstein and CERC have also been at the forefront of applying a form of AI known as "computer vision" to monitor activity in hospitals. He and some of his Stanford colleagues led a study that used computer vision to monitor something that's fundamental to reducing infections in hospitals: the frequency with which physicians and nurses wash their hands. (About 4 percent of hospital patients develop health care–associated infections while in the hospital.) This involved training a neural network, via deep learning, to recognize when individuals washed their hands or applied sanitizer. Sensors attached to the hand sanitizers captured de-identified images of whether a sanitizer was used before someone entered or exited a patient's room. The images were then entered into an algorithm developed by Stanford researchers. It was 95.5 percent accurate in assessing images at Stanford's Lucile Packard Children's Hospital, and 84.6 percent accurate at Intermountain LDS Hospital in Salt Lake City.

Many potential benefits are associated with computer vision, as explained in a 2018 *New England Journal of Medicine* article coauthored by Milstein and some of his Stanford colleagues.

> If successfully developed and deployed, ambient computer vision carries the potential to discern diverse bedside clinician and patient behaviors at super-human performance levels and send user-designed prompts in real time. Such systems could remind a doctor or nurse to perform hand hygiene if they begin to enter a patient room without doing so, alert a surgeon that an important step has been missed during a complex procedure, or notify a nurse that an agitated patient is dangerously close to pulling out an endotracheal tube. The use of computer vision to continuously monitor bedside behavior could offload low-value work better suited to machines, augmenting rather than replacing clinicians [32].

Computer vision has also been central to important research that involves teaching software how to assess the skills of surgeons. The program was developed by having the software watch videos that captured all the activity in the surgical field.

Machine Learning Moves into Detection and Prediction

The potential for artificial intelligence and machine learning to generate new insights, and greater precision, across medicine is now being realized, with four recent studies previewing the future potential of health care.

One study, published in *Nature Medicine* in January 2019, showed how artificial intelligence can be deployed to diagnose genetic disorders with greater accuracy than the diagnoses delivered by clinicians. In this study, the AI program examined photos of patients with and without a condition called Cornelia de Lange syndrome, which leads the eyebrows, ears, and nose to take on distinctive features. The program detected the syndrome with nearly 97 percent accuracy, while a group of 65 experts examined the same images and had 75 percent accuracy [33]. This AI program is connected to an app, Face2Gene, which is available at no cost to health care professionals. As more professionals uploaded photos of different conditions, the program's detection abilities expanded—from 200 conditions to more than 1,000, in the span of a bit more than a year.

Another study, published in 2018, involved a team of researchers at Google who were looking at predictions around risk of mortality, hospital readmission, and prolonged hospital stays. The team, which included senior Google executive Jeff Dean, wanted to explore the accuracy of predictions in each of these categories, using data from patients' electronic health records. They drew data from more than 215,000 adult patients during a four-year period at UC San Francisco and a seven-year period at the University of Chicago. The total included nearly 47 billion data points.

But the challenge with developing predictive models, the study's authors pointed out, has been the creation of a custom data set, with specific variables. Moreover, "80 percent of the effort in an analytic model is preprocessing, merging, customizing, and cleaning data sets, not analyzing them for insights. This profoundly limits the scalability of predictive models" [34].

Recent advances in machine learning and artificial neural networks enabled the Google team to overcome these challenges and draw insights from the data. (In machine learning, computers draw on large sets of information to make decisions or provide insights. A key contributor to machine learning is artificial neural networks, which are designed to mimic networks in the human brain and help with the learning needed to make decisions that resemble those made by humans.) And those insights were quite significant. The predictions had a higher level of accuracy than other EHR models in all three categories—particularly unexpected readmission and prolonged hospital stays. "Our central insight," wrote the paper's authors, "was that rather than explicitly harmonizing EHR data, mapping it into a highly curated set of structured predictor variables and then feeding those variables into a statistical model, we could instead learn to simultaneously harmonize inputs and predict medical events through direct feature learning" [35]. And that "feature learning" has the potential to help physicians diagnose patients and provide precisely tailored therapies.

Dean says that there's a "significant effort" underway at Google and its parent company, Alphabet, to address health care. Given the complexity of the issue, Dean says that Google can draw on many of its innate strengths to drive improvements throughout the system.

> Google's origins are in taking information in the world and then organizing it for people so that it's useful. And it's pretty clear that health care is a specific domain where there's lots of information available in distributed form, which translates to lots of complexities in the ecosystem. But being able to organize that information can make an amazing difference in patient care, it can lead to people living longer, it can lead to them getting better decisions, and it can lead to doctors feeling more confident in the decisions they make.

The third study, published as a paper in *Nature* in January 2017, explored the ability of machine learning to detect skin cancer, with the performance measured against the assessments of 21 board-certified dermatologists. The study's seven authors, many of whom are affiliated with Stanford, showed that the neural networks powered by machine learning could achieve accuracy matching that of dermatologists in three key categories: keratinocyte carcinoma classification, melanoma classification, and melanoma classification using dermoscopy. "This fast, scalable method," wrote the authors, "is deployable on mobile devices and holds the potential for substantial clinical impact, including broadening the scope of primary care practice and augmenting clinical decision-making for dermatology specialists" [36].

The study started with Stanford computer scientists creating an algorithm for skin cancer diagnosis, powered by machine learning. They built a database of nearly 130,000 skin disease images and then refined the algorithm to diagnose potential cancer. Sebastian Thrun, who is an adjunct professor in the Stanford Artificial Intelligence Laboratory and a coauthor of the paper, remarked, "We realized it was feasible not just to do something well, but as well as a human dermatologist. That's when our thinking changed. That's when we said, 'Look, this is not just a class project for students. This is an opportunity to do something great for humanity" [37].

Indeed, with skin cancer diagnoses typically being made visually, having another, easily accessible tool could help improve detection and treatment. This is no small matter. More than five million new cases of skin cancer are diagnosed each year in the United States, and the estimated five-year survival rate for skin cancer is 99 percent among those who detect it early, but only 14 percent when it is detected in its late stages.

The Stanford Center for Artificial Intelligence in Medicine and Imaging (AIMI) conducted the fourth study. It developed a deep learning algorithm to detect 14 different pathologies in chest radiographs. The algorithm was used to evaluate 420 chest X-rays, and its performance was measured against evaluations of the same images by nine practicing radiologists. An AIMI study published in 2018 showed that the algorithm's performance was equivalent to that of the radiologists with 10 of the 14 pathologies, worse with 3 of the pathologies, and better with 1. The biggest difference, though, was the time needed to evaluate the 420 images. The nine radiologists needed, on average, 240 minutes. The algorithm needed 90 seconds [38]. Matthew Lungren, an assistant professor of radiology at Stanford, explains the significance of this:

> The World Health Organization tells us that two-thirds of the world's population—more than four billion people—do not have access to a radiologist or radiology services. Shortages of medical imaging diagnostic expertise can be found everywhere, even in modern health care environments like the NHS in the United Kingdom and the Veterans Administration in the United States, with disparities of availability and access to this critical part of modern medicine disproportionately high in resource-poor countries. The kind of artificial intelligence used in our work could potentially represent a very low-cost way to accumulate and deliver medical imaging knowledge and expertise to the point of care in any part of the world. These diagnostic tools could serve in a variety of ways to improve patient care—as a screening tool so that

sickest patients receive quicker diagnoses and treatment or as a second opinion or "over-read" for clinical providers in environments where there is a shortage of radiologist expertise.

Another paper coauthored by Lungren and published in 2018 described how an algorithm predicted outcomes for knee MRI exams with a level of accuracy that matched that of radiologists. But the study had another noteworthy finding: when radiologists and orthopedic surgeons were given the algorithm's model outputs, they achieved a significant improvement in their diagnosis of ACL tears [39]. In some cases, the surgeons even outperformed the radiologists, which was a surprise. Those findings and others like them that demonstrate the first proof-of-concept of an "AI augmented clinician," says Lungren, will likely inform how the next 5 to 10 years of artificial intelligence in health care will roll out. The critical goals will not be how algorithms can replace specialists but how specialists can become more effective, reducing errors, making quicker decisions, and improving quality of care when paired with specific AI algorithms.

Similarly, the study shows how every clinician, not just radiologists, could potentially use imaging AI tools to interpret medical imaging examinations—potentially even achieving accuracy that matches that of a radiologist. If so, this paradigm shift could completely change how we deliver care, says Lungren.

> If doctors can immediately leverage the output of accurate AI models at the point of care for their patients, it will greatly assist them in their decision-making. For example, if someone shows up to an urgent care and the clinician is worried about pneumonia, they could use an AI model to help determine the presence of pneumonia on the chest x-ray rather than the typical workflow of waiting for a radiologist to interpret first and report back. This potential future of the "clinician-in-the-loop" for AI model deployment in patient care will, given the consistent and reliable performance of the AI tools, improve throughput and patient satisfaction, save time, reduce costs, and improve overall quality of care for all.

The Power of Data

Information derived from data has contributed to many of the astounding advances in basic research and promising new therapies of the past few decades, encompassing health records, health outcomes, drug discovery, and any number of other categories. Data is only going to grow in importance, as it is going to help enable an unprecedented level of understanding about health and health trends.

Data is also going to be essential in helping to predict patients who are susceptible to a range of conditions. Big data science is already being used at Stanford and many other places to identify patients at risk of high-cholesterol disorders, predict pediatric asthma attacks days before they occur, and understand the impact of genetics on drug response.

Data can help address a basic shortcoming of modern medicine: the disconnect between what we know about health and disease and the care that physicians deliver in the clinic. Physicians rely on their own limited, subjective experience, research, and memory to provide diagnoses and treatment. Even if clinicians have worked at the top of their game for 20 years, they will only be able to draw on the experience of about 10,000 patients. The result is decisions that are often not as strong as they could be, leading to potential side effects, adverse treatments, multiple drugs tried, and even inadequate care. But armed with deeper data—from health wearables, on-demand testing, better hospital software, etc.—doctors will be able to more precisely predict the onset of disease, help prevent it, and enable patients to navigate health decisions, from prenatal care to palliative care.

As useful as big data can be, it comes with some significant caveats: Thomas Robinson, the Irving Schulman, MD, Endowed Professor in Child Health at Stanford, and a professor of pediatrics and of medicine, points out that the usefulness of data depends on how well and from whom it was collected. As a result, the quality of the resulting predictions, and whom you can apply them to, depends on the quality of data being drawn on and the sources of that data. "If the data is not representative of all types of people, or at least the same types of people you wish to use the predictions for," says Robinson, "then you may be applying the wrong predictions or decisions to the wrong people. Applying a prediction or decision rule derived from data from one group of people to a different type of people could do more harm than good." He adds that if models are created from data drawn from people it doesn't apply to, there's a risk of widening disparities and contributing to discrimination.

The appropriate use of data is also a concern. "Certain subgroups of the population are at higher risk of being afflicted with certain conditions," says Robinson, "and that's going to make it very tempting for certain entities, insurance payers, medical care systems, and employers, for example, to try to stay away from potentially costly patients." All of this underscores the importance of generating enough data to go into these predictive models from a wide diversity of groups—nationally and globally—that represent all the different types of people they will be applied to. Further, argues Robinson, "not enough attention is being paid to where the data come from. There is a false belief that if you have lots and lots of data, that it will be self-correcting and make up for poor quality and any biases introduced in sampling. However, the reality is just the opposite. More data only exaggerates biases that were introduced by the measures and sampling."

Tools That Operate in the Background

Some of the most popular digital health tools are wearable devices that monitor a range of health conditions and can help intercept disease early, or even before it has been identified. While these devices have enormous value, studies also show that a large percentage of the people who use them eventually stop doing so. This reality highlights the value of prediction tools that operate in the background of everyday life.

For example, there is now a smart device being tested that attaches to one's toilet and analyzes an individual's urine and stool. The device identifies healthy indicators associated with specific biomarkers but also evidence of irregularities that could predict medical conditions. For example, trace amounts of blood in urine, which can't be easily detected by sight, can be a predictor of bladder cancer, and bacteria in urine can be a precursor to a urinary tract infection. As for the information transmission, the individuals don't have to do anything out of the ordinary. The data is sent by Wi-Fi, and the device can also distinguish between different individuals using the same smart toilet. It can be programmed to monitor for specific conditions based on the risk profile of a given individual.

A similar device is the smart bra. It will use photoacoustic and ultrasound technology to provide continuous imaging of breast tissue, using a combination of infrared light and sound for early detection of breast tumors. In the future, more clothing items will likely contain this imaging—providing continuous monitoring of the individuals wearing them. False positives can be minimized by having multiple measurements from the same individual, looking for trends in the data over time, and combining multiple data sets from different devices.

Some tools are already on the market, such as the so-called artificial pancreas, which the FDA approved for use in September 2016. This tool closely replicates the glucose-regulating function of a healthy pancreas, while also making modifications in how much insulin is delivered. That can help address both high blood glucose levels (hyperglycemia) and low blood glucose levels (hypoglycemia). This activity is triggered automatically—an individual outfitted with the device doesn't have to do anything, other than remember to wear it.

Another noninvasive tool, which delivers improved monitoring and detection of atrial fibrillation, is what's known as a "patch monitor." Roughly the size of one's palm, a monitor is affixed to an individual's chest, can be worn for two weeks, and then is mailed to a lab to get the results. There are even patches that can communicate with one's cell phone and transmit the data instantaneously. This is a dramatic change from the recent past, when monitoring meant that an individual needed to be hooked up to a contraption with five or six wires that had to be carried around at all times and could provide only 24 hours of continuous monitoring. These devices are particularly valuable, given that there are often no clear symptoms, and thus many people with afib may not know they are afflicted with it.

If the same form of monitoring existed for other diseases, we could see diseases differently. It would be possible to get continual updates on one's health—and make adjustments when needed. They would provide a much more comprehensive, and nuanced, view of health and wellness.

These tools demonstrate how technology can drive prediction and prevention—providing measurements and then creating closed-loop systems, like the artificial pancreas, that can deliver precisely tailored interventions.

Bridging "High Touch" and "High Tech"

For all the merits of the digital health tools I've just described, health care professionals cannot lose sight of the value connected to developing intimate bonds with their patients. This means seeking information above and beyond what is revealed through lab tests and radiological scans. It requires doctors to be skilled in not only knowing what questions to ask but also listening for precisely what is being said. As Bernard Lown, a celebrated cardiologist, wrote two decades ago, "To succeed in healing, a doctor must be trained, above all else, to listen. Attentive listening is itself therapeutic, for one encounters many fine tales" [40]. Indeed, the information that patients share is an essential ingredient in a holistic approach to health care. Armed with both the "high touch" and the "high tech," physicians can be more effective in helping to predict and prevent disease.

I saw an example of this with a 34-year-old woman who was being seen by Stanford Primary Care, which is part of the larger primary care network at Stanford Medicine. She had been working in the technology industry and then transitioned to a job with a startup. Recently married, she had no health issues, but her weight had been creeping up. In October 2017, her primary care provider performed various screening tests, such as cholesterol and diabetes, and they all came back normal.

She had agreed to participate in a Precision Health pilot project, and so she was given several devices to track her health, such as a blood glucose monitor, a blood pressure cuff, a scale, and a digital pedometer. She monitored the devices for many months, and eventually they all detected that she was in the pre-diabetes range. This wake-up call led her to make dietary changes, exercise more regularly, and get more sleep—and prevent the onset of diabetes.

* * *

The ability to precisely predict every person's risk of experiencing deviations from good health is one of the fundamental objectives of Precision Health. Meeting this objective—or just making progress toward it—would have the potential to dramatically improve the health and wellness of billions of people throughout the world. But delivering on the potential of prediction is closely linked to progress on another key component of Precision Health: preventing disease before it strikes, which is the focus of the next chapter.

CHAPTER 6

PREVENTION AS A PATHWAY TO HEALTH AND WELLNESS

Benjamin Franklin captured an important concept when he wrote in 1735, "An ounce of prevention is worth a pound of cure." While his statement was focused on fire safety—there were no organized fire departments in Philadelphia at the time—the principle is fundamental to Precision Health. Investing time and resources in prevention can deliver substantial benefits, such as illnesses and diseases being averted, and people are likely to be happier and more productive. The ultimate goal of prevention is to help people live longer and healthier lives, says Doug Owens, the Henry J. Kaiser, Jr., Professor at Stanford and chair of the U.S. Preventive Services Task Force. "We know there are many interventions and practices that do this, and the challenge is to make sure that people receive these interventions."

But prevention is a dramatically underutilized tool in the U.S. health care arsenal. The reasons for this are varied, though one factor stands out from the rest: "The profit motive generally doesn't align with prevention right now," says Bill Evans, CEO of Rock Health. For that to change, he says, "there needs to be a reimbursement model that allows a sufficient value capture back to the entity that created the value. With a drug, it's really easy because we know you're sick, and if it's clear that the drug worked, payment will follow."

The U.S. health care system's focus on treatment, rather than preventing treatment, has contributed to the country's poor state of health. Chronic diseases, which are largely preventable, contribute to 70 percent of deaths each year. Indeed, nearly half of all deaths in the United States from heart disease, stroke, and type 2 diabetes result from a bad diet, according to a study published in 2017 in the *Journal of the American Medical Association* [1]. While the cost of seeing loved ones handicapped by disease and experiencing premature death is inestimable, we do know the actual cost of treating people with these conditions each year: more than $2 trillion, which accounts for about 75 percent of all spending on health care.

Discovering Precision Health: Predict, Prevent, and Cure to Advance Health and Well-Being, First Edition. Lloyd Minor and Matthew Rees.
© 2020 John Wiley & Sons Ltd. Published 2020 by John Wiley & Sons Ltd.

Prevention represents one of the biggest challenges for the health care industry, given that the biggest commercial opportunities have traditionally come from providing treatment and developing new medicines. Shifting to a focus on prevention would require a dramatic rethinking of how the U.S. health care system operates. It would mean embracing preventive measures with the same energy and enthusiasm that's traditionally associated with the pursuit of cures. That would call for creating new business models focused on wellness and helping people to thrive. For this to happen, the health care industry, in partnership with other industries, needs to tackle the vexing issues of behavioral change as well as social and environmental factors that are the biggest determinants of health.

While there has been some movement toward prevention in U.S. health care, the pace of change has been slow. But as I will show in this chapter, noteworthy ideas about prevention—many of them focused on diet—are being studied and implemented.

COMBATING DISEASE THROUGH HEALTHY FOOD CONSUMPTION

In chapter 2, I discussed how a range of social determinants can have an outsized influence on the health of individuals and populations. Three particularly important determinants are income, housing, and education. There is also considerable evidence indicating that health outcomes would improve if there was progress on raising incomes, expanding affordable housing options, and improving educational performance. But none of those lend themselves to quick-fix solutions—and each is largely beyond the currently perceived scope of health professionals.

There are, however, a plethora of ideas focused on helping to prevent the onset of sickness and disease. Many of these ideas build on an idea expressed by Hippocrates more than 2,500 years ago: "Let food be thy medicine and medicine thy food." I would slightly modify that recommendation to say that the consumption of *healthy* food can not only help people *get* healthy—it can also help *keep* people healthy.

But how can people be encouraged to eat healthy food? Or, put differently, what can be done to decrease the consumption of the food and beverage products that contribute to so much disease in the United States and throughout the world?

The traditional approach has been to emphasize the benefits of healthy food—or the perils associated with regularly consuming unhealthy food. This approach has some obvious merits, but limitations as well. For starters, survey data show that in the United States, people believe "healthy" food doesn't taste good. (In one 2018 study of words to describe grocery products, "vegan" and "diet" scored the worst [2].)

A more fundamental challenge of simply emphasizing the benefits of healthy food has been summarized by Thomas Robinson, director of the Center for Healthy Weight, whose work I described in the previous chapter.

Almost all existing approaches to changing behavior start with the assumption that humans will act rationally in their own best interest—they will make explicit calculations of anticipated costs and benefits and make a rational choice among alternatives. In addition, the promised potential benefits to health (or avoidance of poor health) often are in the future, further discounting their values as motivators. This has led to countless interventions that focus on persuading persons to adopt and maintain new eating and physical activity behaviors for their own good. Unfortunately, this rational choice assumption has persisted despite several decades of contradictory findings from social psychology, cognitive psychology, behavioral economics, neuroscience, and related fields. This research has clearly indicated that human decision-making and behavior are far from rational, but influenced by contextual factors and cognitive biases and limitations [3].

The magnitude of the challenge associated with reversing unhealthy dietary habits was highlighted in 2013 by the then-head of the World Health Organization, Margaret Chan: "Not one single country has managed to turn around its obesity epidemic in all age groups" [4].

New Ideas about Changing Behaviors

The obesity epidemic speaks to the need for trying new approaches. Robinson has advocated for something he calls "stealth interventions," which tap into motivations that already exist in the individuals, with the health benefits being a beneficial side effect. "The word 'stealth' is not meant to suggest deception," explains Robinson, "but that, from the perspective of the participants, [the interventions] do not necessarily look and feel like health interventions. Rather than emphasizing health-related messaging, stealth interventions select strategies and incorporate design elements to increase the intrinsic motivation of participating in the intervention activities themselves" [5].

In one stealth intervention study, Robinson and his team worked with low-income African American girls ages 8 to 10 years and their parents or guardians, living in Oakland, California. One group was offered traditional health education, teaching them about healthy habits, physical activity, and nutrition. The other group was offered a stealth intervention in the form of culturally tailored after-school dance classes emphasizing traditional African dance, hip-hop, and step. (Classes were offered five days a week, though attendance was voluntary.) The idea was that the girls, and their parents, would be drawn to the classes primarily for fun, social, and cultural reasons, with any potential health benefits an added bonus. The "side effects" of participating in after-school dance classes were more physical activity and staying away from screens and snacking during a large discretionary part of their day. The two-year study showed that the group offered dance classes achieved significant reductions in lipid levels, prediabetes (characterized by moderately elevated fasting blood glucose or hemoglobin A1C levels), and depressive symptoms [6].

Another stealth intervention approach to spurring dietary improvements is to link them to participation in social and ideological movements. Robinson has identified several such movements that have behavioral goals that overlap with obesity prevention. For example, a focus on reducing climate change can be a catalyst for reducing (or eliminating) consumption of heavily processed and packaged food and meat (particularly beef), given the high level of greenhouse gas emissions associated with meat production. The social interaction and camaraderie that comes with participation in a movement can help ensure that individuals adhere to the movement's goals, with opportunities to see others who have changed and maintained their healthy behaviors. "Individuals participating in social and ideological movements," writes Robinson, "will likely make greater magnitude and more sustained changes than are typical in health-related interventions" [7].

His ideas about linking behavioral change to social and ideological movements were partly tested by teaching a class to Stanford undergraduates called Food and Society: Exploring Eating Behaviors in a Social, Environmental and Policy Context with a Stanford colleague, Christopher Gardner. The class explored issues such as the environmental impact of agriculture and livestock production, ethical issues around eating animals, labor factors in the food industry, cultural traditions related to food, and the politics of food and nutrition. The students read books such as Michael Pollan's *The Omnivore's Dilemma* and Eric Schlosser's *Fast Food Nation: The Dark Side of the All-American Meal*.

As part of a study later published in the *American Journal of Preventive Medicine*, the students in the class were asked to complete a survey of their eating habits—at the start of the quarter and at the end. Students in three other classes being offered that same academic quarter—focused on health psychology, community health, and obesity—were asked to take the same survey. The students in the Food and Society class reported changes in their dietary habits—eating more vegetables and fewer high-fat dairy products, high-fat meats, and sweets. In the other three classes, the students showed no improvements in their consumption patterns and were actually eating fewer servings of vegetables [8]. While behavioral change was not the point of the class and was never promoted to the students, the dietary changes observed reinforced Robinson's and Gardner's belief in the potential for the stealth intervention approach to improve nutrition behaviors. Recalls Gardner:

> I'd been teaching classes for years and explaining things like how much fiber should be consumed, and how many milligrams of antioxidants. I could see students' eyes glazing over with boredom. And then I taught this class and observed students talking about making positive changes in their eating behaviors almost overnight. The experience made me appreciate that my tool chest for supporting healthier eating behavior changes would benefit from having more tools. Interestingly, no one message worked for all the students in the class; different topics resonated more with different students. We found that personalizing the messages and aligning those messages with the values of your audience could lead to making a much bigger impact. That was one of my epiphanies.

Marketing Matters

Eating habits can, of course, be influenced by the way food is marketed and presented. Although most of the marketing that Americans experience is focused on processed food, it can work with healthy food as well.

In one 2016 study involving a Stanford cafeteria that served mostly undergraduate and graduate students, researchers made daily changes to the posted descriptions of seven different vegetables. The language fell into four different categories—"basic," "indulgent," "healthy restrictive," and "healthy positive"—but in no case were there any changes to how the vegetables were prepared or served. Carrots, for example, were labeled as "carrots" (basic), "twisted citrus-glazed carrots" (indulgent), "carrots with sugar-free citrus dressing" (healthy restrictive), and "smart-choice vitamin C citrus carrots" (healthy positive).

Researchers recorded the number of diners who chose a vegetable and weighed each serving selected. The study revealed many more people choosing vegetables with "indulgent" labeling and also consuming a much larger volume of the vegetables. The study's authors—who were associated with Stanford's psychology department—wrote afterward,

> Our results represent a robust, applicable strategy for increasing vegetable consumption in adults, using the same indulgent, exciting, and delicious descriptors as more popular, albeit less healthy, foods. This novel, low-cost intervention could easily be implemented in cafeterias, restaurants, and consumer products to increase selection of healthier options [9].

Higher Education and Healthier Eating

The study on the impact of marketing on food choices is a reminder of the valuable role that colleges and universities can play in advancing healthy habits. Stanford has been a leader in this effort, and the university's head of Residential & Dining Enterprises' Stanford Dining, Eric Montell, has been an advocate of rethinking the student dining experience.

> We look at college and university dining as a time in life when students are making decisions that will shape the rest of their life. Those decisions include what they eat and how they eat. We've calculated that the 4,400 students on our meal plan will consume around 250 million meals over their lifetimes. So the ability to influence changes in students' eating habits can have a big impact, and it can continue into future generations, since they will also influence the dietary habits of their children.

To drive change, Montell has implemented a form of behavioral economics known as *food choice architecture*. This builds on the earlier example of food marketing and presentation, and it involves making subtle changes to encourage healthier consumption. Thus in the buffet-style arrangements that are common in Stanford dining halls, healthy options are placed in the locations that diners are most likely to encounter first, thus making it more likely that they will choose those foods. Similarly, Stanford has reduced the size of the bowls and plates that are used in dining halls—building on the studies showing that when people are given smaller dishes, they tend to consume smaller portions of food [10]. Trays have been eliminated from dining halls—another way of encouraging less consumption.

Stanford has also sought to treat dining halls as more than simply places where one goes to eat. Arrillaga Family Dining Commons, which is one of the largest dining halls on campus, features classes on a variety of topics, from the basics of cooking to the science behind cuisine (taught by a chemistry professor). There are also exercise rooms, a garden, and even a beehive. The objective, says Montell, is to "weave yourself into the fabric of the university through strategic initiatives and collaborative programs, and to look for research opportunities that are strongly connected to the academic mission of the university."

The work at Stanford is aligned with ideas that have been advanced by Richard Thaler, a Nobel laureate at the University of Chicago, and Cass Sunstein of Harvard Law School. In their book *Nudge: Improving Decisions About Health, Wealth, and Happiness,* they advance an idea they call "libertarian paternalism," which is focused on maximizing choices but influencing those choices such that people will be better off. Their shorthand term for this is "nudge," which they describe as

> any aspect of choice architecture that alters people's behavior in a predictable way without forbidding any options or significantly changing their economic incentives. To count as a mere nudge, the intervention must be easy and cheap to avoid. Nudges are not mandates. Putting the fruit at eye level counts as a nudge. Banning junk food does not [11].

Public policy can still play a valuable role in advancing prevention, as I describe in the next section. But enacting new policies is typically a very difficult process that can be measured in years—if not decades. The kinds of nudges that Thaler and Sunstein describe, and that Stanford has implemented in its dining halls, can potentially spur behavioral changes much more rapidly than government-imposed policies.

Healthy Bodies via a Healthy Gut

While it's widely known that healthy eating helps prevent a range of diseases, what has not attracted as much attention is the nexus between diet and what's known as *microbiota*, which are the bacteria found in the human digestive tract (the "gut"). They are closely linked to metabolism and immunity, and they have a major influence on conditions such as cancer, diabetes, allergies, asthma, autism, and inflammatory bowel diseases. As Justin Sonnenburg (an associate professor of microbiology and immunology at Stanford) and Erica Sonnenburg (a senior research scientist at Stanford's School of Medicine) have written,

Our gut microbiota sets the dial on our immune system. Our immune system is central to all aspects of our health. When it works well, we fight off infections efficiently and extinguish malignancies at their earliest appearance. When the immune system operates suboptimally, numerous ailments can result [12].

Many Americans have weakened microbiota. The Sonnenburgs point out that there are hundreds of different forms of bacteria in the average American's gut. More bacteria are better for fighting off disease, and an Amerindian living in Venezuela—with a radically different (and healthier) diet and lifestyle—has about 30 to 40 percent more bacteria [13]. One of the primary culprits is the so-called Western diet, which is high in processed, calorie-rich, fatty foods and low in fruits, vegetables, and whole grains, thus depriving the body—and the microbiome in particular—of the fiber it needs. "What's happening over time," says Justin Sonnenburg, "is that we are losing microbial species in our gut, likely because we're not feeding them properly, and this corresponds with rising health problems" [14].

In recognition of the microbiome's importance to human well-being, the National Institutes of Health launched the Human Microbiome Project in December 2007. "The human microbiome is largely unexplored," said NIH Director Elias A. Zerhouni, in announcing the project's launch. "It is essential that we understand how microorganisms interact with the human body to affect health and disease. This project has the potential to transform the ways we understand human health and prevent, diagnose, and treat a wide range of conditions" [15].

The project leveraged the technology that had been used to sequence the human genome and applied it to microbes. This was no small task, given that the personal microbiome is more than 100 times bigger than the personal human genome [16]. But the research turned up some noteworthy findings. It revealed, for example, that there are more than 10,000 microbial species in the human ecosystem. Researchers also learned that the microbiome contributes approximately eight million unique protein-coding genes, which is 360 times more than the human genome contributes. Researchers at Washington University in St. Louis used microbiome data to develop tests that can be used to identify situations when antibiotics should not be used to treat children with fevers [17].

By studying the nexus between microbes, health, and disease, we can define a healthy human microbiome. The problem, says Justin Sonnenburg, is that "the healthy American harbors a gut microbiome that is probably pushing us toward all of our common and serious diseases. It's one of the predisposing factors for heart disease, cancers, and autoimmune diseases." The authors of a study published in *Nature* in 2018 examined microbiome development in infants and found an association between the development of type 1 diabetes and the species and functions in the developing microbiome of infants [18].

But just as the microbiome has changed for the worse, it can also change for the better—primarily through improved nutrition. That distinguishes it from the human genome—which has inestimable value as a predictive tool, but it's largely fixed, even amid changes in our environment. Therefore, argues Sonnenburg, "the answer to our health problems is not really to look at the human genome, which is just a conduit for the symptoms we experience. We should be looking at what has loaded the gun and cocked the trigger, and that's the environment in which we live and the food we eat, since these are the most likely culprits in causing a deterioration of our microbiome."

The microbiome may eventually become a precision diagnostic tool, says Sonnenburg. Patients could visit clinics, where health professionals would review their microbiome, their genetics, and their immunity. The information gathered from those reviews could be used to generate personalized recommendations about how to improve and maintain one's health.

Sonnenburg is already taking the next step into what he calls "synthetic biology." In one conceptualization, microbes are engineered to secrete an anti-inflammatory molecule if they sense inflammation, and then that genetic circuit will turn itself off when the inflammation is successfully treated. In this scenario, individuals never even know they've had inflammation—it's prevented prior to developing into an actual disease. It's not just an abstract idea—work carried out in Sonnenburg's lab is the basis of a startup company that's focused on engineering microbes to treat diseases.

There is also important research underway at the Center for Human Microbiome Studies, at Stanford's School of Medicine. Researchers there are conducting studies focused on changing the microbiome fundamentally through dietary modifications, and then using blood tests to monitor so-called predators of the immune system. They hope to learn what parts of the microbiome speak to what parts of the immune system. That way, individuals who are fighting specific diseases can be prescribed specific foods—in other words, treating food as medicine.

Michael Fischbach, an associate professor of bioengineering at Stanford, also studies the microbiome. His research is focused on chemicals produced by the microbiome, many of which enter the bloodstream and have a plethora of effects on human physiology. He notes that the microbiome can be a tool to engineer not only immune function but also metabolic function. He gives an example of two people eating precisely the same meal of a steak and a salad.

> Anytime you eat, there are carbon atoms that stay with you and there's bacteria that is excreted as feces. But it's highly unlikely that the partition between those two paths is going to be the same in the two people. As soon as we understand why that is, and can control it, there is the possibility of endowing you with a bacterial community that makes it possible for someone to eat exactly the same thing he or she has been eating but take on 5 or 10 percent less mass every time, voiding it as a larger stool. That would be striking because physiological differences like that add up when they happen three times a day for weeks or months.

One noteworthy development in microbiome research is a process called *fecal transplantation*. It involves taking a fecal sample from an individual, checking to ensure that it is free of parasites or pathogens, mixing it with saline solution, and then administering it to another person, through a tube that goes into the nose and empties into the stomach. The procedure is akin to an organ donation, but for the microbiome.

Its popularity has grown amid evidence of its effectiveness. In one clinical trial, conducted in the Netherlands, fecal transplants were used to treat *Clostridioides difficile*—a bacterium that can cause life-threatening diarrhea. The typical standard of care has involved prescribing antibiotics, though they are effective only about 60 percent of the time (and become less effective with multiple recurrences). In the clinical trial, a fecal transplant was effective for 15 of the 16 enrolled patients. (The *New England Journal of Medicine* published an article about the study in 2013 [19].) To date, there have been roughly 30,000 fecal transplants performed at medical centers throughout the world. Significantly, these transplants have resulted in very few acute, adverse events [20]. This is a surprise to Fischbach.

> It's a big shake-up to your system to have the whole roster of bacteria in your gut wiped out and replaced by a different roster of bacteria. I would have thought that 1 out of 100 or 1 out of 1,000 people would have come down with a fulminant immune response against one of the new bugs or something like that. That just hasn't happened. The fact that this modality seems to be unusually safe is a really big deal.

Also significant, says Fischbach, is that once the donor sample enters an individual's microbiome—a process known as *engraftment*—that sample stays there indefinitely. "Today, engraftment works quite well, indicating to me that getting it from there to being predictable in 80-plus percent of people who undergo this community transplant procedure is an engineering problem that has a very clear solution. That means we won't need a bespoke community for you and a different one for me. Instead, it means we can design one bacterial community that will probably engraft successfully in a large share of the population."

Given the apparent safety and predictability of fecal transplants, are they likely to become a widely prescribed therapy? Fischbach isn't so sure. "Feces cannot be scaled very easily, nor can they be tweaked, nipped, and tucked—and that refinement process is fundamental to the drug discovery process." He says that what's needed is to create something that's completely defined.

> You can't do that with feces, which is an "undefined" product—you don't know what's in there. The need is to rebuild the gut community from scratch, in order to be able to make one where you know exactly what's in there. That would enable specific changes to it that are done in a science-based way where you have a goal, and you're able to measure whether you've improved against that goal.

Fischbach and Sonnenburg are leading a project focused on building highly complex bacterial communities from scratch, with the goal of manufacturing them and testing them in people and endowing them with the stability of a fully intact fecal sample. "We are likely to be creating something that makes it possible to use the microbiome to treat diseases with bacteria specifically demonstrated to be effective," says Fischbach. The future also holds the prospect of adjusting the microbiome in ways that are shown to prevent diseases. These approaches represent entirely new ways of thinking about and leveraging the role of the microbiome in health and disease.

DEPLOYING A DIGITAL TOOL TO IMPROVE THE HUMAN DIET

The food we eat is fundamental to our health. But in the United States and many other countries throughout the world, poor food choices are contributing to a rising prevalence of chronic conditions. This speaks to the need for innovation that's focused on helping people make better dietary decisions. A San Francisco–based company called Zipongo is working to meet this need. It uses digital tools to deliver individually tailored recommendations to its subscribers, with a focus on trying to improve both the food they eat and the environment in which they make decisions about food.

Zipongo's founder, Jason Langheier, grew up near Buffalo, New York, and many of his relatives struggled with obesity. Strokes, heart attacks, and cancer diagnoses were commonplace. As he was growing up, his mother took him to Diet Workshop group sessions, where he learned about how difficult it could be for people to overcome obesity. He studied neuroscience at Williams College and later earned a medical degree at Duke and a master's degree in public health from Harvard. Before medical school, one of his formative experiences was helping Boston Medical Center (BMC) launch the Nutrition and Fitness for Life pediatric obesity clinic. About half of the kids who came to BMC were overweight or obese; and their approach of personalizing a family grocery list based on preferences, budget, and health improvement supported, for many of the prediabetic kids, reversal of disease. But what about the thousands more obese kids being seen by pediatricians who didn't have the clinic time, nutrition training, or health plan reimbursement to provide care? They asked: Could you connect home food delivery and digital prescriptions? That was the inspiration for Zipongo.

Langheier launched Zipongo in 2010, one year after completing medical school at Duke. He and his colleagues targeted their offerings at consumers, with the slogan "Eating Well Made Simple." But it became clear that a B2B2C (business-to-business-to-consumer) strategy was more appropriate.

> We found that it's really hard to get paid, because consumers don't really allocate money to spend on their health care. The money really comes from advertising, but the problem is that all the food advertisers want to pay you, but they want to pay you to feature brands that aren't always the best choice for the consumer.

In 2013, Zipongo shifted its focus to working primarily with health systems and health plans. While this brought its own set of challenges, he was encouraged by one basic fact: these entities have an incentive for their subscribers to be healthy. That typically means eating better food.

Zipongo, says Langheier, is "a food marketplace where there's a digital dietitian attached." Here's a shorthand description of how it works. Subscribers—typically the employees of companies that use Zipongo, but individual consumers as well—complete a questionnaire about their dietary preferences and also provide information regarding their weight and conditions like hypertension, hyperlipidemia, and diabetes.

From there, meal options are prepared, factoring in eating habits, preferences, and restrictions. Zipongo sends its subscribers notifications once a day, asking them whether they are planning to cook or eat out and then using the answer to make recommendations about what to cook or what to order in a restaurant. Zipongo offers integrated daily discounts that come from all the major grocery stores in the United States, as well as Instacart, Amazon Fresh, and meal kit companies like Sun Basket. The items needed to prepare meals can be added to an online shopping list (or the subscriber can have a list generated that can be taken to a retail store). For those not wanting to cook, Zipongo is also linked with restaurant ordering companies like GrubHub. Since many people often eat at least one meal a day at their workplace, Zipongo's tools are integrated with select corporate cafeteria providers like Eurest, Bon Appetit, and Flik.

Zipongo doctors and dietitians can also issue FoodScripts, which are meal plans for people with diabetes, hypertension, hyperlipidemia, or obesity. The individual's employer or health plan covers the cost of the meals for the first month, and then discounts are offered to the individual after that. The goal, says Langheier, "is to get people off really expensive diabetes or hypertension medications and to literally reverse their disease by going back to a normal state with food." Zipongo is collaborating with pharmaceutical companies to evaluate the impact of food-drug combination therapies to improve disease outcomes.

A fundamental objective of the Zipongo Foodsmart platform, says Langheier, is to "lure you away from the advertising that is built up into the food system of the food retail environment."

> Trade spend from the specific food manufacturers is what drives the profit margin of many grocers, and the way everything is merchandised in the store. So you're walking into one giant advertisement every time you buy food. There's not a single place in the United States or the developed world where you can buy food without it being an advertisement because of it—except the digital environment. Food marketers are now turning to advertise on Amazon and Instacart. But, just like GPS or Uber or Lyft can change your transportation environment, Zipongo can change your food environment, sparing you from food maker ads and nudging you instead with healthy food merchandising.

To that end, Zipongo does not accept food maker advertising revenue, which ensures that it never faces financial pressure to advocate for a particular company's products. Its FoodScripts default to a whole-food, plant-based diet—heavy on water, fruits, vegetables, whole grains, and legumes—because "that's the one with the strongest outcomes data," says the company's chief medical officer, Dexter Shurney, MD, MPH. Zipongo recognizes that many people aren't going to adopt that diet, but its recommendations are still much healthier than what's found in the standard American diet, says Shurney.

> We'll take something like the DASH diet [Dietary Approach to Stop Hypertension] and we'll enhance it with things such as blueberries and hibiscus tea and potassium load that we know can actually make that diet that much stronger. And in doing so, we'll also make it plant-forward. While it may not be an entirely plant-based diet, we'll try to push the users in that direction as much as we can.

Langheier points out that the recommendations go beyond the nutritional content of each food item.

> We also look at how food combinations can make a difference. For example, if someone is having rice as part of their main course, it turns out that there's a big difference in glycemic load of the rice, depending on whether or not the person say, drinks water, has a fiber-rich appetizer salad with healthy fats from olive oil, or just eats the rice first. So we're very precise in the recommendations we make to each of our subscribers.

But with most people understanding the difference between food that is healthy and food that is unhealthy, the Zipongo platform "is based on the principles of brain science as much as nutritional science," says Langheier—also a board director for the Partnership for a Healthier America, created by former first lady Michelle Obama and Bill Frist, MD, a former U.S. senator. Says Langheier:

> It's about more than saying, "Here's what you should be eating." We encourage understanding why you don't eat that already and providing decision support throughout the day. In other words, we make it as easy to eat super-healthy as it currently is to eat unhealthy.

According to Zipongo, 75 percent of its corporate participants say they have developed healthier eating habits since using the company's tools, with an average improvement of more than 11 percent in user NutriScores. A recent study with AmeriHealth and Drexel University showed that Zipongo use contributed to a 9/5 mm Hg drop in blood pressure, a 13 mg/dL drop in total cholesterol, and an average weight loss of nine pounds within six weeks. A more recent study involving an economically diverse population of health plan employees showed that Zipongo's Foodsmart platform led to 32 percent of them losing 5 percent of their weight or more at one year; most notably, weight loss increased with time over 18 months, whereas with most studies there is weight gain after initial weight loss within 18 months. The company has made considerable headway in attracting customers. As of February 2019, more than 200 companies had enrolled—including big names such as Google and IBM, as well as four of the six largest health plans in the United States.

But Langheier's experience selling Zipongo to potential customers has also highlighted the countless obstacles to improving nutrition in the United States. The hardest part, he says, "is that nobody budgets for nutrition programming, or systematic ways to help their people holistically change their food environment."

> Everybody knows nutrition is the biggest driver of death, disability, obesity, and everything else. But the fee-for-service system that has evolved drives us to default to high-cost drugs and procedures instead of digging in to help people change their food environments. Doctors unintentionally seem to look down on food as something farmers do, so it has taken some time for doctors, scientists, and actuaries to take food as medicine more seriously. But LinkedIn and *Forbes* highlighted health plans paying for groceries as one of the top 50 things to watch in 2019. The health care system and health plans take time to change, but it is starting to happen now.
>
> Still, day to day, employers invest most of their benefits dollars on their health plan and medical claims—with most money going to doctors, the surgeries, and the drugs. They don't have much left over to then spend on changing the environment; and new vendors get nickel-and-dimed, making innovation slower versus consumer innovations like Google or Facebook. CEOs, and COOs, and CFOs should be bold in helping their people change their food environment for their own sake and their children's.

Langheier does point to progress—ironically, from the federal government. Thanks to the most sweeping reforms of Medicare policy in a decade, insurers offering Medicare Advantage policies are now permitted to fund healthy food for members after they've been discharged from a hospital—or even just to counteract chronic disease. In select states, Medicaid recipients are being given healthy food at no cost, since it's now recognized that this can promote health and save the government money in the long run. "I think that is super-exciting and encouraging," says Langheier. "CMS [the Centers for Medicare and Medicaid] is going in the right direction, and people are trying to make a change."

But progress is not all about technology. Langheier also emphasizes the need for high-touch environments, marked by strong human-centered care.

> Technology can play a significant role in delivering personalization and helping to transform food environments. But progress also depends on the ability of people to help other people activate into those new digital environments—including friends, family members, community leaders, and health professionals. Do you use Uber or Lyft? How long did it take to set up your first ride? Now, have you ever been the one to create the very first online food order? There's a reason only 5 percent of people regularly buy their groceries online; but there's also a reason over 50 percent of people in the UK have used online food delivery. As with Netflix, Apple, and Amazon for movies (seen a Blockbuster lately?), the world is changing fast. But will

doctors and health plans just let people port over to the digital equivalent of the physical world dominated by advertising of food that is often unhealthy, or will they help shepherd people to safe zones for nourishing their bodies and their families?

PREVENTING PRETERM BIRTH AS WELL AS PERINATAL AND MATERNAL MORTALITY

Approximately 10 percent of all births in the United States are considered "preterm," meaning the baby is delivered before 37 weeks. These births can trigger severe health challenges in the newborns—respiratory problems, underdeveloped organs, cerebral palsy, life-threatening infections—as well as developmental and learning disabilities. Globally, preterm birth is the leading cause of neonatal mortality, having passed infectious disease a few years ago.

The United States has one of the world's highest preterm birth rates. Although the rate has fluctuated over the past 30 years, it is 30 percent higher today than it was in the early 1980s [21]. Yet "in about half the cases, no one knows exactly what's causing them," says David Stevenson, the Harold K. Faber Professor of Pediatrics at Stanford, and there is no test to help identify who might be at risk.

In 2011, the March of Dimes recruited Stevenson to lead a research initiative at Stanford focused on trying to understand the causes of preterm birth, with a goal of being able to identify at-risk women more effectively and then intervening with them. Stevenson organized a team of experts from Stanford to join him—but they were not experts in preterm birth, or even childbirth. As Stevenson explains,

> I assembled a team of scientists from across the university, put them into teams, and then said, "Our goal is to prevent preterm birth. I want the best scientists. I don't care if you've never thought about preterm birth or anything about it." We began to educate each other about our different areas of expertise, our technologies, the tools that we use, the mathematics and computational approaches we were using, and then began to focus on trying to solve this problem. We've pulled from genetics and different disciplines in medicine, but also the fundamental sciences, such as chemistry, physics, and engineering.

He draws a parallel with the Manhattan Project, except that "we're not making a bomb. We're working together to solve a very practical problem by using very fundamental approaches." The effort involves using many innovative tools and technologies to look at pregnancy in new and different ways. "We are trying to describe a woman during her pregnancy from just about every perspective that you might measure an individual," says Stevenson. Those tools and technologies include the following:

- Transcriptomics—Studying a mother's cell-free RNA molecules and drawing on that information to better understand messages expressed by the mother's genes, as well as those expressed by the baby and placenta.

(Steve Quake's work on preterm birth, which I described in the previous chapter, draws on transcriptomics.)

- Proteomics—Studying circulating proteins is one element of molecular approaches employed to detect aberrations in pregnancies.

- Metabolomics—Studying small molecule chemicals that help determine the biochemistry and physiology of full-term and preterm pregnancies.

Stevenson and his colleagues are also using a technology that enables them to look at how cells signal throughout pregnancy in the mother. This provides clues about certain gene pathways that are turning off and on throughout pregnancy and provide what's known as an *immune clock*. Because immune cells change how they express genes during gestation, disruptions in the normal patterns of expression can signal pathological processes. These processes can portend preterm birth and other pathologies of pregnancy, like preeclampsia. (Transcriptomic and proteomic clocks have also been described.) According to Stevenson, "All of the information we're collecting is converging, thanks to computational approaches that allow us to better understand the underpinnings of a normal pregnancy, as well as those pregnancies that end in preterm birth."

Another area of study is the microbiome, as described in the previous section of this chapter. Unique patterns of microbes called *community state types* that are deficient in certain *Lactobacilli* species, and contain other kinds of microbes, have been associated with preterm birth. Stevenson says that studying the microbiome, along with the elements mentioned above, helps him and his colleagues to understand the trajectory of pregnancy in tremendous detail: "We can predict which pregnancies are going to be going awry and then intervene to avoid that outcome."

The microbiome also factors into what's been identified as another contributor to preterm birth: inter-pregnancy intervals of less than six months. A 2015 paper coauthored by Stevenson revealed that one dimension of the vaginal microbiota changes following a pregnancy and that this change can contribute to a higher risk of preterm birth if another pregnancy follows within 12 months [22]. This finding has led physicians in California and entities like the March of Dimes to issue guidance stressing that the minimum interval between pregnancies should not be less than six months—and ideally at least 12 to 18 months.

The Stanford research team has made important progress in other areas as well, finding that maternal obesity, or a maternal diagnosis of PTSD in the year preceding birth, can contribute to preterm birth. They've also tested the immune cells of women who have had preterm births and found that these cells respond differently to induced inflammation than do the cells of women who have had full-term births. This finding makes it possible, says Stevenson, that at-risk women could receive immunotherapy to combat the factors contributing to preterm birth.

Amid the challenge of combating preterm birth, Stevenson has also been a champion of a statewide initiative focused on reducing maternal and perinatal mortality. There have been significant achievements: California is the only state with maternal and perinatal mortality rates that have been declining.

A key contributor to this progress has been two parallel initiatives headquartered at Stanford and connected to both the California Maternal Quality Care Collaborative and the California Perinatal Quality Care Collaborative, which Stevenson says are "fundamentally quality improvement organizations."

One of the initiatives is a comprehensive, multi-stakeholder effort to develop a more complete picture of the state's perinatal and maternal mortality trends. It was made possible by tying funding for hospitals throughout the state to their sharing of maternal and perinatal data, and then having that data integrated into databases. Today, these are the most comprehensive state-level databases in the country. Data is collected every 45 days, and the analysis that follows highlights performance trends, whether statewide or even at individual hospitals. In the event of worrying developments, experts can intervene, diagnose the situation, and propose remedies. "They have become an incredible tool for improving the quality of care for mothers and babies throughout the state," according to Stevenson.

The other initiative is a program that makes it easier for care providers throughout the state to access real-time information about treatments. These online tool kits deliver highly detailed guidance to care providers—best practices tools and articles, care guidelines, a hospital-level implementation guide, and professional education slide sets [23]. They were developed with input from experts across the state and focused on how to treat conditions such as pre-eclampsia, postpartum hemorrhage, and cardiovascular disease during pregnancy and postpartum. Each of these tool kits has been downloaded thousands of times—in California, across the United States, and throughout the world.

"We can implement change in what people do for various conditions," says Stevenson, "to improve health across the whole population."

> When we link it to other really unique things we're doing at Stanford, we can track specific communities in California and learn about their health and how they might be targeted for tailored interventions. This enables community-based approaches, neighborhood-based approaches, and even individualized approaches.

The progress has been remarkable. California's infant mortality rate is 4.5 deaths per 1,000 live births—down from 4.8 in 2011 [24]. (The national rate is 5.7 [25].) California was the only state that saw a decline in perinatal mortality from 2014 to 2016 [26]. The maternal mortality rate data is even more striking. In the seven years following the maternal care collaborative's founding in 2006, California's maternal mortality rate fell 55 percent, at a time when the national rate was rising [27]. In 2013, while the national average for maternal mortality was 22 deaths per 100,000 live births, in California, the figure was just 7.3 deaths [28].

The achievements in California have attracted notice. In a 2018 *Washington Post* article about the state's progress, the president of the American College of Obstetricians and Gynecologists said, "We all look to California because they have reversed the trend and decreased their maternal mortality rate significantly" [29].

USING PREVENTION TO BENEFIT CHILDREN

The incidence of preterm birth is one example of how some children in the United States begin to experience health disparities at a very young age. This handicap is often a product of the conditions in which they grow up. Studies show that children raised in homes plagued with a shortage of food experience health problems at two to four times the rate of children in food-secure environments. It's also been shown that these children often face challenges that prevent them from reaching their full academic potential.

The reasons for these disparities are complex, but Stanford's Lisa Chamberlain, whose work I described in chapter 2, has been working to remedy them. She points out that the medical system has nearly universal access to every child during the critical neurodevelopmental years of zero to five, since children receive episodic well-child care and immunizations, and are likely to see a doctor for various ailments. This repeated access to all young children presents an opportunity for the medical system to also function as "kinder-ready clinics" that help ensure that children will not be far behind their peers when school begins. (Stanford is involved with a "kinder ready" project—a collaboration between pediatricians, patients, families, and early childhood education communities.) Chamberlain points out that among low-income groups, pediatricians are more trusted than anyone else outside of the immediate family. "When we say something to a parent, it's really heard." Thus the access, coupled with the trust, creates an opportunity to supplement early childhood education in a way that's not happening today. The benefits from this early intervention are plentiful. Studies show not only improved educational performance, but also better health and a lower incidence of criminal activity, teen pregnancy, and drug use [30].

Children's health is closely tied to dietary patterns, as I've discussed, but another key factor is physical activity. Extensive evidence shows that most children do not get the 60 minutes of moderate-to-vigorous physical activity each day that's recommended in federal guidelines. The reasons for this are varied, and the prevalence of mobile phones and tablets is undoubtedly a factor, given that they offer entertainment and personal communication that can be achieved with little or no movement needed. But technology is also being used productively to help stimulate children to exercise.

Seda Tierney, an associate professor of pediatrics (cardiology) at Stanford's School of Medicine, developed a fitness program that was based on her own experience. While living in Boston, she had regularly exercised with a trainer. When she took a job at Stanford, she continued her training sessions with him, one-on-one, via live videoconferencing. That gave her the idea for a study, which involved having obese children participate in one hour of personal training by live videoconferencing (via an iPad), three times a week, for 12 weeks. The remote access to the trainer and being able to exercise one-on-one, said Tierney, was an attempt to overcome the challenges associated with getting children to come to a site for an exercise intervention, since that invariably is a burden for parents and reduces adherence. The tele-exercise study, published in the *Journal of Pediatrics,* resulted in an impressive adherence rate of 85 percent, strikingly higher than exercise interventions delivered on site (as low as 10 percent), and improved the health profiles of obese children, particularly those who had abnormal vascular health [31].

She also used the personalized training in a pilot project involving children who had had heart transplants, and who typically had no history of engaging in exercise or physical fitness. Parents have written to her and explained how the exercise has further improved the lives of their children. Some of the statements she has received:

- "This was an excellent program and I am so glad my child was able to participate."
- "This program helped our daughter not to be afraid to exercise."
- "Our child has increased confidence and stamina."
- "The role model of a personal trainer had positive effects on our son's thinking. To hear importance of exercise from people other than mom and dad is important. Working out at home with a live trainer removes so many barriers."
- "This program has been modeled so well it changed our child's life."

One of the children in the study wrote to Tierney and her colleagues and described the benefit she gained from participating in it.

Over the course of the duration of the study all of you have helped me grow stronger, build my stamina, and gain confidence in my abilities to start playing all the sports I wanted to. I finally have the strength, confidence, and physical abilities to start doing things I always wanted to, such as joining (and leveling up!) a competitive badminton league, biking to school on my own, playing with my dog, and playing mild sport games in P.E. with my friends. Without your help, I would never have been able to push myself to try new things, build stamina, and exercise regularly. I would never have been able to do the things I have always wanted [32].

"I really believe exercise is the best medication, but it's underprescribed and underused," says Tierney.

We, pediatric cardiologists, still don't think about exercise as prescription since we remain focused on keeping our patients, children with complicated heart conditions, alive. We send our patients to surgery and make sure their heart defect is fixed, but we frequently do not focus on the next step of making sure that they enter adulthood as fit as possible. Exercise is the golden key to a healthy heart and healthy arteries and should be instituted as routine care of these children as early as possible.

A POTENTIALLY NEW CHAPTER IN PREVENTION COMING FROM GENOME SEQUENCING AND DATA SCIENCE

While nutrition and exercise are the most far-reaching tools of prevention, many conditions call for other interventions, particularly if they involve genetic mutations. We are seeing the potential for progress via a thoroughly modern mix of genome sequencing and data science.

Consider familial hypercholesterolemia (FH), which affects about 1 in 250 people globally. It involves mutations in the genes for the LDL receptor, and the mutation reduces the ability to recycle the so-called bad cholesterol. The result can be circulating LDLs of up to 600 milligrams per deciliter, which is six times higher than what is considered healthy. Among those with FH, the risk for coronary heart disease is five times higher than among those without it. In the United States, it's estimated that fewer than 10 percent of those with FH have been diagnosed. They often don't learn that they have the condition until they have a heart attack, which strikes about half of those with FH.

Genetic research has made it possible to identify those people at risk, and there are now pharmaceuticals (PCSK9 inhibitor drugs) that can help those with FH. But with a list price of $15,000 annually for treatment, a confirmed diagnosis of FH is necessary to get their use reimbursed by insurance.

Data science offers a solution for helping to identify those patients with the highest risk. Genetic testing for high-risk patients is strongly recommended. Working with a patient advocacy group, the FH Foundation, two faculty members at Stanford, Nigam Shah and John Knowles, trained an algorithm that learns from the electronic health records of known cases to identify individuals at risk of FH—who can then be sequenced. In a validation study, the algorithm was correct 8 out of 10 times when it flagged a patient as a likely case of FH—a striking improvement over simple screening strategies that have a 95 percent false positive rate. Several variables not typically used to identify FH, such as triglyceride levels, are among the top 20 predictive concepts revealed by the algorithms [33].

Shah and Knowles describe the benefits in terms of bringing greater cost-effectiveness to FH screening.

> If FH occurs at a probability of 1 in 70 in a cardiology clinic with costs of $1,000 to do genetic counseling and testing, and 15 minutes to apply the screening criteria, for each case found we would need to spend roughly $70,000 in genetic testing and 1,050 minutes of clinician time. However, after applying EHR-based screening, the chance that an individual flagged by our algorithm has FH is 8 out of 10. Therefore, the cost to find one new case drops to $1,429 in genetic counseling and testing and 21.4 minutes of clinician time, and can massively improve the ability of a health system to find patients at risk.

Given such a massive change in post-test prevalence, it is now economically viable for pharmaceutical companies to pay for the costs of the genome sequencing to confirm the diagnosis of FH. If individuals with the mutation can be identified at or around the age of 18, the benefits are substantial. Over a 20-to-30-year timeline, the use of PCSK9 inhibitors, coupled with statins, may make it possible to avert 80 to 90 percent of the heart attacks and strokes that these people are otherwise likely to have before they're 50 and 60. That is a textbook example of treating and preventing disease precisely.

SCALING INNOVATION TO HELP MANAGE A CHRONIC CONDITION

Although much of this chapter has been devoted to preventing the onset of disease, the unfortunate reality is that for millions of Americans, disease is part of their everyday existence. In 2012, 117 million adults in the United States were living with a chronic condition. That's nearly half the entire adult population. The treatment of chronic conditions can be very costly, and small segments of the population account for a disproportionate share of spending on health care. A study published by the Kaiser Family Foundation and the Peterson Center on Healthcare showed that in 2015, 23 percent of total health expenditures were accounted for by just 1 percent of the population, and 51 percent of the expenditures were accounted for by 5 percent of the population [34].

The coordination and management of the care of these diseases poses a challenge in any health care delivery system. So when we talk about "prevention" in the context of health, we also need to focus on how to prevent those chronic conditions from worsening—and how to help ensure that those living with the conditions can still lead active, productive lives.

Livongo

Several digital health-related innovations are showing encouraging results. One dynamic company operating in this space is Livongo, launched in 2014. Its founder and CEO, and now executive chairman, Glen Tullman, had a background in health IT, but he wanted to focus more on promoting health outside the four walls of the hospital. A special area of interest was tackling chronic conditions (his son has type 1 diabetes and his mother had type 2 diabetes). He was discouraged by what he discovered: "You would think that the health system would make it easier for people to stay healthy, but in fact, everywhere I turned, we were making it harder for people to stay healthy. And that was the genesis behind founding Livongo."

The name grew out of early research by Tullman and others about how to get people with chronic conditions more engaged with their health. A common reply was along the lines of, "Actually, we do not want to be reminded of our condition. We want to be *less* engaged with our health. We just want to live our life and we're on the go all the time, so don't give us solutions that tether us to the hospital or a physician's office or even our own home." In other words, they wanted to live on the go—thus "Livongo."

The company's president, Jennifer Schneider, has had type 1 diabetes for over 30 years. She explains,

> No one actually wants to be more engaged with their health. They don't want to spend more time to become healthy. They just want to live. I don't want to actively spend more time on my diabetes. I never wake up and say, "Oh yeah, I'm going to spend a lot more time thinking about diabetes today." Diabetes is not the most important thing to me every minute of every day. I have little kids, and a big job. I also have friends and parents. What I want is to be able to live healthier by spending more time on life and less time on diabetes.

The company has been focused on trying to empower people and not simply treat them as patients. "People want to be in charge," says Tullman. "And they want to lead better, healthier lives. So we explored how we could help them do that while also helping them better manage that challenging part of their life."

Livongo's primary product is a cellular connected blood glucose meter. Whenever people use the meter to check their blood glucose, Livongo gets the results, conducts real-time analytics, and provides feedback on what actions can be taken. If the company sees that a user's blood glucose is dangerously low, that person will receive an instant message, via their meter, with a recommended action, such as drinking four ounces of fruit juice within 30 minutes. More than 200,000 different messages exist—they're based on clinical guidelines from the American Diabetes Foundation and the Endocrine Society and powered by a unique AI engine (called Ai+Ai). This helps ensure that the message that will drive the optimal behavior is delivered to each specific person, tailored on the basis of factors such as age, weight, and gender—and, importantly, on unique real-time experiences and personal history.

"We're providing real-time, actionable feedback based on the story the body is telling," says Tullman. Schneider characterizes the company's work as "behavioral precision health."

> It's around the delivery of the medical science for ongoing and continued motivational behavioral change. And that's critical, because so much of health is driven by behavior. We're giving people these nudges constantly, and then we're measuring whether they actually followed through. We can see if they came back to check their blood glucose in 20 minutes and whether we are actually changing behavior. We may not know what they did, but we can see the results. While everyone knows you should exercise and you should eat healthy, to make that happen sometimes requires making micro suggestions at the time the people are making decisions. And it's not a one-time recommendation. It's continuously suggesting and nudging and highlighting those actions that should be taken.

This continuous monitoring—and the real-time interventions—distinguish Livongo from the traditional medical system, where a person with diabetes might see an endocrinologist once every few months. Tullman draws a parallel between Livongo and OnStar, which can detect if a car has been in an accident and then sends emergency roadside assistance, while also communicating directly with the passenger. "We're doing that for your body and trying to make sure you treat it as well as you treat your car."

But the medical equivalent of emergency roadside assistance doesn't always happen. People with diabetes wearing traditional insulin pumps and glucose monitors don't necessarily experience a medical intervention even when the data shows a crisis. Schneider tells a story of going to sleep one night and waking with paramedics surrounding her, unable to move or speak. She was suffering from low blood glucose, and the issue was remedied, but the continuous glucose monitor (CGM) collecting her data did not provide an intervention.

Schneider is also a doctor—she did her residency in internal medicine at Stanford Medicine and served as an attending physician here—and the experience with temporary paralysis despite the massive data collection was a wake-up call for her—personally and professionally. When she met Tullman and heard about his vision, she came away even more convinced of the need to leverage patient data to help drive behavioral change and improve health outcomes. That's how she ended up working for Livongo.

She and Tullman, in tandem with others on the Livongo leadership team, have built a successful business by staking out new territory on the health care financing landscape. The traditional business model calls for having employers pay a monthly premium for each employee. Livongo decided to go in a different direction. Its customers—typically large, self-insured employers and health services organizations—only pay when employees are using the product, creating perfect alignment that employers love. Livongo also incorporated performance metrics into each product, measuring user satisfaction, clinical outcomes, and reduced costs per patient.

According to the company, the savings are about $83 per participant, per month, just in the first year [35]. "At a big company like FedEx," says Tullman, "where more than 10,000 people have diabetes, that can result in significant savings." In addition to FedEx, other large customers include Amazon, AT&T, Citigroup, Delta Airlines, Intel, Lowe's, Microsoft, PepsiCo, SAP, and Time Warner. (As of February 2019, the company counted 700 of the largest self-insured employers in the United States as customers.)

Studies have also shown improved outcomes among those using Livongo's products. One study, which involved Livongo, evaluated blood glucose data of more than 4,500 customers over a 14-month period. It showed a decline of more than 18 percent in the likelihood of having a day with hypoglycemia and a decline of more than 16 percent in hyperglycemia [36]. According to Schneider, individuals with three low blood glucose situations over a two-week period receive a customized message—with the result being a 43 percent reduction in the incidence of low blood glucose.

Tullman emphasizes that no one is mandated to use Livongo's products.

> That's unique, because a big part of the health care model is forcing people to use specific medication or see specific doctors. But we don't believe in any of that. We think if you're going to get anybody to change their long-term behavior, it has to be because they made the decision, not because they've been forced to make it. We're putting the people with the chronic condition back in charge, empowering them with information, tools, and support. It used to be that health care was done to you ... we're creating a future where you are in control and health is on your terms.

Livongo started by focusing on people with diabetes, but it has branched out to other conditions, such as hypertension, prediabetes, weight management, and behavioral health. Seventy percent of people living with diabetes have at least one other chronic condition, and of those, 70 percent have hypertension. To treat the whole person, says Tullman, a company like Livongo needs to address a range of conditions, with the ultimate objective of "making it easier for people stay healthy."

Omada Health

Omada Health, based in San Francisco, is another company experiencing robust growth in helping people at risk for, and with, chronic conditions, including type 2 diabetes and hypertension. It calls itself a "digital behavioral medicine company" and provides lifestyle interventions focused on changing the habits that lead to chronic disease. The company is the largest Diabetes Prevention Program provider to achieve full recognition by the federal government's Centers for Disease Control and Prevention [37]. It has worked with the American Medical Association to develop the first-ever digital-specific medical code (known as "CPT"), which is used for reporting and billing purposes throughout the U.S. health care system.

Omada embodies something I discussed in the introduction—the need for health care to be both high tech and high touch. Sean Duffy, Omada's founder and CEO, has a keen appreciation for the power of technology—he previously worked at Google on the People Analytics team—but he recognizes the need for health providers to have frequent contact with those whom they serve.

> There's extensive evidence to show that people with chronic diseases or risk factors can be supported through behavior change to lose weight. All the evidence prior to Omada were for very high touch programs. A caregiver would show up and provide support—helping customers think about their lives and their needs and help them set goals, all with the goal of helping people lose weight. Omada started with the ambition to take what was known in the evidence base and build on top of it, using the tools and technologies available in this digital era.

Those tools and technologies are introduced immediately when individuals sign up with Omada (typically through participating employers or health plans). They are mailed a scale that comes with a cellphone chip preinstalled. It does not require any setup—the user simply inserts the batteries and then steps on it, and the data is automatically uploaded to his or her account.

The high-touch part comes next. Individuals are paired with a group based on demographics, and each group has a coach who is a full-time Omada employee. The coach starts them on a timed program, where members of the group progress through the curriculum at the same pace. There are different lessons each week, and everyone can see the progress of others in the group. Omada places no limits on how much contact a user has with his or her coach; the contact is offered via secure direct message, chat functions within the application, and, where necessary, phone conversations.

Duffy talks about the Omada program by contrasting it with other popular ways to help people lose weight. One is controlling the diet through meal replacements. "But that doesn't help people reform relationships with food in a healthy way," he says. Another option is to eat less. "But the self-discipline required to do that is hard." A third approach is medical/surgical, "but that's usually a last-ditch option for individuals who have exhausted all other options."

The best approach, says Duffy, is to emphasize behavioral approaches because they tend to be the most sustainable. "Focus on painting a positive psychology of what foods you like that are generally considered to be healthy and how to incorporate more of them into your regimen." This can help with *wanting* to eat more of what's good for you and not yearning for the unhealthy options. He acknowledges that "there's tons of subtlety and nuance in it," which is one reason why Omada has a team of behavioral scientists that work closely with the product team on how to make every feature in the Omada experience as evidence-based as possible. This includes how to set goals, how to track food, and how to harness the power of social relationships.

Instead of calorie counting, Omada asks its customers to write a short note when they eat something. Was the item healthy? Did they eat the right amount or too much? The goal, says Duffy, is to "build awareness and an acceptance that in times you will eat things that you don't think are healthy, and you'll overeat them. But it's knowing that you're doing that, and not blaming yourself for it, but rather rolling with it like the ins and flows of life." He says success is "when someone tells us, 'I had this crazy experience. I was at the grocery store and I looked at the cart in front of me, and I found myself judging them for the food that they're putting in their family's body.' When it becomes part of your self-identity to try to eat with more thoughtfulness about the health attributes, you've won. That leap is very delicate and requires a journey and a narrative—and pulling people along in a very gentle way.

Although leveraging technology is central to Omada's offerings, Duffy says progress depends on not being captive to what he calls "the single instrument fallacy, where you think that that one thing will work."

> Some calorie-counting apps are good-quality products, but they're not enough. Similarly, you can't just get someone a coach, or a scale, or a great content experience, or an online social group alone and expect them to achieve a long-term improvement in his or her health.

For that reason, when it came to designing and building the Omada platform—the components, the food and activity recommendations, the coaching tools, and more—Omada chose to do all of the work itself. They wanted the instruments to function according to what the users do at each moment. "The secret sauce to Omada," says Duffy, "is that we built it all, and so we can control the layout of how everything fits together."

One of Omada's objectives is to minimize something that plagues most health-focused programs: attrition. "We work to make it so that the path of least resistance is to stay in," says Duffy. "We want people who may be wavering to think, 'I signed up because it looked really neat, but I have made this commitment, I'm really engaged, and I guess I'll stick with it.' It builds the flywheel."

As much as Omada has achieved—working with more than 500 employers—Duffy says "we're just at the starting line," noting that there are 84 million people in the United States with prediabetes. "The fact that Omada is getting any spotlight at all is a statement on how poorly we in the United States have been about preventing chronic conditions. We hope to change that, by helping to change the paradigm of how chronic disease is handled in this country."

PREVENTION AT WALMART

Walmart is the biggest company in the United States. Its revenues in 2017 were more than double those of the next-largest company, Exxon Mobil. It employs more than 1.5 million people, and one study estimated that in 2016, 95 percent of U.S. consumers made a purchase from Walmart—either online or in one of its stores [38]. The company's massive presence on the U.S. commercial landscape makes it the most powerful platform for being able to influence health and wellness in the United States. One example of that influence is the preventive health screenings that the company offers its customers and employees.

In 2014, Walmart started offering quarterly Wellness Events at its stores, where people can have their blood pressure, cholesterol level, and glucose level tested, and get flu shots and vision screenings—all at no cost. By the fall of 2018, Walmart had conducted more than 2.5 million screenings for people throughout the country. Many Walmart locations also feature health-focused kiosks, where customers can obtain personalized information about their health. Today, it's estimated that Walmart has done more blood pressure readings than any other organization. According to Alex Hurd, of Walmart's Health and Wellness Transformation business, "There have been many instances of customers, immediately after being screened, being referred to urgent care or a local emergency room. Lots of stories come back to us about people who are alive today because they were able to catch a condition before there was a major escalation."

Walmart has also stepped into digital health, with a particular focus on encouraging healthy behaviors among its employees, and doing so through shared experiences with colleagues. As explained by David Hoke, who leads Walmart's work on the health and well-being of its employees,

> We believe that most decisions are emotionally driven and intellectually rational. These decisions and behaviors are also consciously and unconsciously socially influenced. This social influence is strongest with individuals to whom we relate. Peer-to-peer influence builds confidence and self-efficacy, which leads to continued efforts to change. In order to bring this people-follow-people approach to life, we emphasized peer-to-peer storytelling. By amplifying and celebrating authentic peer stories, we use inspiration and aspiration to inspire and drive change.

Emblematic of this focus on peer influence, the company offers an app called ZP, where anyone—whether a Walmart employee or not—can participate in 21-day challenges in four different categories (food, fitness, family, money). Every time a user completes one of the challenges, he or she can enter a sweepstakes-style event that offers cash prizes. But first the user must answer the following question: "If you could inspire another person to lead a better life, who would it be and why?" Every six months, entries are evaluated, and 23 prizes are awarded, from $5,000 to $25,000. The stories of each "champion" are publicized throughout Walmart and distributed via social media.

The focus of the ZP Challenge, says, Hoke, is on "making one better choice today than yesterday."

> Following the work of B. J. Fogg, our message is that any change, no matter how small, matters. Steady progress leads to big results. We focus on the process of engaging in change and building self-efficacy. One of our goals is to shift the mindset from an arbitrary finish line to focus on the process of changing behaviors. Success is not indicated nor counted by the number of challenges completed, but rather the focus is on how a person can actually make any small change. By focusing on change, rather than the outcome, individuals build trust in themselves and grow their sense of self-efficacy. The intent is to help Walmart associates, friends, and family support each other in lasting improvements, rather than creating short-term winners and losers.

The approach seems to be working. The ZP Challenge has received more than two million entries, and the users self-report significant changes:

- 95 percent report increased exercise,
- 75 percent report improved relationships and more family time,
- 68 percent report increased financial savings.

There have also been striking improvements related to body weight. Nearly 80 percent report losing more than 20 pounds, 58 percent report losing more than 50 pounds, and 20 percent report losing more than 100 pounds.

Asked why he thinks the program has been so effective, Hoke emphasizes both the peer influence and the nonjudgmental approach.

> I think people are starved for connection. Shame and guilt are vastly underestimated. People want to feel better, but they don't want the expert telling them how to do it from Day 1. When you think about any time in your life you tried to change something, you're kind of embarrassed, and you're not sure even what questions to ask, and so you don't want to go talk to the expert on this thing. You really want to try to figure out some of it yourself, and so that leads to an increase in self-efficacy, and then you talk to other people like you. You realize that you're not alone, and that you feel connected in a way you didn't before. And then once you start making progress, you're willing to go the extra mile, which is what we see time and time again. There's this element of permission—we like to say it's almost like church, in that there's no judgment, there's no guilt, there's no shame. The idea is, "we're all here together." So there's a humanism in it that is lacking in many of today's clinical interventions, and it means connecting people and giving them the freedom to be who they are and know that failure is OK.

PREVENTION AT STANFORD

A primary objective of Precision Health is care and treatment that is precisely tailored to each individual. While, as Jennifer Schneider stated, some people want less engagement with their health, there are others who want more. There are many ways that can happen—such as the use of digital health tools—but engagement can also come about through something as general as primary care. At Stanford, we've structured our primary care system so that it drives engagement with health by empowering people with actionable information.

A few years ago, we started rethinking how our primary care could function, and as part of that process we conducted interviews with everyday consumers. Many of those consumers said their experience with health care consisted of a 15-minute visit with a doctor once a year. What they wanted, they said, was a continuous trusting relationship with their health care team. That meant continuous communication, and continuous access to information that was customized to them. We saw that as an opportunity—to intervene early and help prevent some of the downstream incidence of disease. To that end, our Primary Care team designed Primary Care 2.0—a program that is much more team-based (drawing on the knowledge of nutritionists, behavioral health experts, clinical pharmacists, and physical therapists), with time allocated for telehealth and for digital health. We've found that this promotes trusting relationships with our patients and helps deepen our connection with them.

One of the Primary Care initiatives was something called ClickWell. It was based on the idea that one segment of the patient population is very low risk and primarily interested in transactional health care. They want prompt access to care and something that is seamless, easy, and probably via the phone or video—maybe even via email or text messages. One of our discoveries, which came as a surprise, was that about half of patients using ClickWell wanted to be seen in person by a doctor, in a longitudinal relationship, though they also appreciated having access to "virtual" experts, such as a health coach and a nutritionist. ClickWell has now been integrated into all our clinics, and it's helping to drive the engagement that is essential to prevention.

Precision Health Pilot

Stanford Primary Care conducted a pilot called Humanwide through 2018. "It was the clinical implementation of Precision Health in a general primary care setting to identify high-risk patients in cancer previvor and pre- and early cardiovascular disease states for targeted, cost-effective treatments and interventions," according to Megan Mahoney, who oversaw the pilot in her role as the chief of general primary care in the Division of Primary Care and Population Health at Stanford. "We began with a nine-month design/thinking process, assessing patient and provider needs for comprehensive data and likely use cases in technology and genetics data-mediated care" [39].

From January to July 2018, 50 patients were recruited, taking care to include a diverse representation among ages, races/ethnicities, sexes, and medical complexities. Each patient started by sharing his or her health goals and a genetic assessment for disease risk and pharmacological interactions, which was used to design a customized care plan. We provided them with a blood pressure cuff, a glucometer, a pedometer, and a scale, to provide continuous monitoring. (All of the devices were Bluetooth-enabled, so that the data would be uploaded to their electronic health record.) The patients were connected to a health coach, which meant we could interact with them beyond the traditional doctor-patient relationship.

We found that the novelty and potential of the pilot was a draw for the participating patients, indicating promise for Humanwide's role in future patient-centered, precise care. Humanwide helped us develop the trusting relationship with the patients, since we were shifting away from a traditional "sick" model whereby we'd interact with them only when something was wrong. Instead, we were interacting with them 365 days of the year. Rather than starting conversations with a diagnosis and recommendation—"Your hemoglobin A1C and your diabetes is high, so I think you should go on insulin"—we would ask questions: "What are your goals?" "What's your understanding of diabetes, and how is it impacting your life?" We found that there's greater engagement in the care plan when it's been designed around patients' needs.

"Theresa" is the pseudonym of a woman in her mid-60s who has been a Humanwide patient. An international business executive for many years, she would hopscotch around the world helping her employer complete transactions. "I lived the grueling executive lifestyle. Too many hours, too much travel, not enough sleep, and a very haphazard diet." She also had a family history of heart issues and diabetes.

Eventually the family history and lifestyle caught up with her. She suffered congestive heart failure. She had to stop working in 2013 and had a heart transplant the following year (her doctors suspected that she'd already had a few heart attacks that went unnoticed). The transplant brought benefits, but, she says, "it was close to a year before I got to feel halfway normal, because I got several infections."

Still unable to return to full-time employment, Theresa enrolled in Humanwide in the fall of 2018, at the recommendation of her primary care physician, Marcie Lynn Levine, clinical assistant professor of medicine at Stanford. She took several DNA tests, as well as one that identified whether she was genetically resistant to any specific drugs. As part of the program, she also met regularly with a health coach, who encouraged her to eat more fiber and more vegetables. The health coach also reassured her. "She tended to be more mellow than I am and told me, 'Don't worry, everybody has issues like this.'" As a result of the changes in diet and encouragement of the coach, her lipid panel showed a reduction of approximately 40 percent in cholesterol and LDL—a development that lowered her risk for further cardiac events substantially.

Theresa said she would "definitely" recommend Humanwide to other people. "It will help people prevent disease, instead of needing to be treated for it." She points to her own experience as indicative of the program's value.

> My focus tended to be on working and not on health. If I had been more focused on my health and preventing disease, I would still be working. In order for people to be able to contribute to their fullest capability, they need to stay healthy. And this program will enable that.

* * *

The prevalence of chronic conditions in the United States and throughout the world, coupled with the cost of treating people who have succumbed to these conditions, underscores the need for renewed focus on prevention. This chapter has shown the challenges to changing the behaviors that contribute to, if not directly cause, chronic conditions. But it's important to remember that behaviors can change for the better.

Smoking in the United States was once prevalent (so prevalent that doctors were featured in cigarette ads). In 1964—when the American Medical Association first highlighted smoking's health hazards and the U.S. surgeon general issued a report on the nexus between smoking and lung cancer—42 percent of American adults were cigarette smokers. Today, only about 15 percent are. That's a tribute to a range of public and private initiatives focused on preventing the health risks associated with tobacco.

That battle is far from over, but it shows what's possible. With new knowledge emerging in areas such as the genome and the microbiome, and with new tools such as AI, there are new opportunities to advance more precise forms of prevention. Seizing those opportunities will be critical to advancing the vision of Precision Health.

CHAPTER 7

CURING DISEASE WITH MORE PRECISE MEDICAL THERAPIES

Medical breakthroughs over the past century have unleashed extraordinary benefits for people throughout the world—leading to longer life expectancy and better quality of life. Yet there are still thousands of conditions for which cures have not been identified. Donald Lo, a professor at the Duke University School of Medicine [1], has pointed out that while approximately 400 molecular targets have been addressed by FDA-approved drugs, that's only a fraction of the approximately 20,000 genes in the human genome [2].

As I highlighted in chapter 3, the quest for medical cures is typically quite complex and quite costly. Medicines are fundamental to medical cures, but other forms of medical research—some of which I describe in this chapter—also contribute to therapies that improve health and alleviate human suffering. Even with the long odds of achieving meaningful progress, the trial and error that's fundamental to the search for cures is a daily occurrence in labs throughout the world. Breakthroughs continue to happen, and there are exciting developments underway in many different fields. Approaches and advances described in this chapter make me optimistic that the future is bright for curative therapies.

OBSTACLES TO CURES—AND OVERCOMING THEM

One of the fundamental obstacles to progress in biomedical research, and in developing cures, is something basic: our limited understanding of human biology and how to cure diseases. This has far-reaching implications. Consider that neurological disorders are the leading cause of disability, and the second-leading cause of death, throughout the world. But most of these disorders lack effective therapies.

Discovering Precision Health: Predict, Prevent, and Cure to Advance Health and Well-Being,
First Edition. Lloyd Minor and Matthew Rees.

A Stanford faculty working group highlighted the knowledge gap in a 2017 report, "Leading the Biomedical Revolution."

> Reductionist molecular science has brought forth spectacular insights into the structures and dynamics of individual or small collections of biomolecules. And at the macro scale, we have a reasonable comprehension of what a healthy or diseased organ system looks like. But between simple molecular interactions and systemic organ dysfunction lies a knowledge vacuum that renders human diseases difficult to understand, diagnose, and treat. Indeed, the pharmaceutical industry is perennially frustrated by clinical failures with drugs that, by all preclinical measures, should have hit the mark. One is left with the conclusion that we simply don't have sufficient understanding of biological pathways and their interconnectedness in humans to make informed decisions regarding intervention in disease.

Addressing the "knowledge vacuum" that's referenced in the report is an ongoing challenge and one that's going to be remedied through a focus on fundamental, discovery-based research, which was the subject of chapter 4.

As that research moves forward, Stanford has also been developing partnerships and collaborations that we believe will contribute to improvements in human health. One of those steps was the 2013 launch of an interdisciplinary institute called ChEM-H. Its objective is to bring together Stanford's brightest minds from basic biology, clinical medicine, physical science, and engineering to help understand life at a chemical level and then apply that knowledge. (The "Ch" is for chemistry, the "E" is for engineering, the "M" is for medicine, and the "H" for is human health.) ChEM-H reflects the dynamic new opportunities to leverage the power of chemistry to deepen our understanding of human biology. ChEM-H is also focused on training scientists to be able to operate at the intersection of chemistry and biology, so that they can think like engineers as they recognize and address challenges relevant to medicine. Chaitan Khosla is the ChEM-H codirector, the Wells H. Rauser and Harold M. Petriprin Professor in the School of Engineering at Stanford, and a professor of chemistry. He explains,

> There is a breed of engineer that has evolved over the past 20 to 25 years and they consider themselves to be molecular engineers. They do everything that a mechanical engineer might be doing to an automobile, or an electrical engineer might be doing to a power system's device. But they do it at the level of molecules, and assemblies of molecules. So they're tweaking bonds that hold molecules together or get molecules to do calisthenics that then translate into macroscopic property. It is this breed of engineer that we are looking to harness in the mission of ChEM-H.

ChEM-H is particularly focused on recruiting faculty who have interdisciplinary backgrounds. An early recruit was Carolyn Bertozzi, who is one of the world's leading chemical biologists and who now serves as codirector of ChEM-H with Khosla, and as the Anne T. and Robert M. Bass Professor of Chemistry. She describes the individuals they're trying to hire as "the multilingual people who can speak to biologists and chemists, to engineers and clinicians. Some of those people are going to be physician-scientists. They'll be MD PhDs who spend time in the clinic and work with patients, and who can help us identify the most important problems we can mobilize around."

These individuals will help develop what Bertozzi envisions as "world-class knowledge centers." Research will be conducted in areas such as medicinal chemistry and metabolic chemistry, which are rare in academic medical centers but are central to the process of drug development.

Facilitating drug development is at the core of an entity within ChEM-H called the Alliance for Innovative Medicines (AIM). It is a partnership that began in 2017, initially between Stanford and Takeda, which is one of the world's oldest and largest drug makers. The purpose of AIM is to help accelerate the translation of lab discoveries into therapies that can treat human disease. The partnership is intended to remedy what is often a considerable delay between when researchers make a discovery and when drug companies begin exploring the discovery's potential. "There are some things that biologists and chemists know, while their industrial counterparts often know different things," says Khosla, "and that results in many discoveries never being translated. AIM is intended to allow the two groups to truly partner by letting their hair down and work as a single team."

The AIM leadership accepts ideas from Stanford faculty once or twice a year, and then a committee composed of four Stanford faculty and four senior managers from Takeda reviews those ideas; 30 to 40 are typically submitted. Ten proposals are chosen by the committee, which looks for the projects that have the greatest potential for medical impact. This committee ultimately chooses three to five projects, and each one gets two dedicated project managers (one from Stanford and one from Takeda). From there, they develop a timeline of 12 to 36 months, with a plan for realizing the project's potential.

One of the first AIM projects involves a potential treatment for lymphoma, developed by the team of Shoshana Levy, a professor in the Department of Medicine at Stanford. Her research has uncovered an antibody that combats tumor cells taken from human lymphoma specimens while sparing normal cells. Needing a system that would enable her to bear the risks associated with investigating the antibody's therapeutic effects, her work was a perfect fit for the partnership with Takeda. As of spring 2019, she was in regular contact with company scientists via bicoastal, biweekly phone meetings—and the company was gearing up for large-scale production of the antibody, aimed at conducting preclinical safety and efficacy studies.

Although all the approaches being pursued by ChEM-H are most applicable in the treatment and cure of disease, they also will provide benefits in prediction and prevention.

A MORE PRECISE CANCER TREATMENT: IMMUNOTHERAPY

The first recorded evidence of conditions that resemble cancer dates to 2500 BC [3]. But cancer's emergence as a leading cause of death is a relatively recent phenomenon. As Siddhartha Mukherjee points out in *The Emperor of All Maladies*, his masterful book about cancer, "In most ancient societies, people didn't live long enough to get cancer" [4]. It's a condition that tends to emerge with age, and many other conditions caused death earlier. At the start of the 20th century, when U.S. life expectancy was just 47, cancer was only the seventh-leading cause of death. The top three were tuberculosis, pneumonia, and diarrhea [5].

But as U.S. life expectancy increased, and as the ability to detect cancer improved, cancer rates began rising. By the 1940s, it was the second-leading cause of death. With that rise has been an escalation in the resources devoted to finding a cancer cure—something that has occupied the world's leading researchers, and research institutions, for decades. But cures—or even effective treatments—have been elusive. "America's four-decade investment in cancer research—a total of more than $300 billion (inflation-adjusted) in taxpayer spending, private R&D, and donations—has not stopped, or even substantially slowed, the soaring cancer burden," wrote Clifton Leaf, author of *The Truth in Small Doses: Why We're Losing the War on Cancer and How to Win It* [6].

Leaf's book was published in 2013. In the intervening years, there have been some remarkable advances in the precision treatment of cancer—and the apparent ability to cure it. But a 19th-century surgeon's characterization of cancer—"the emperor of all maladies"—is still true today [7].

A defining feature of most cancer treatments has been their lack of precision. Surgery sometimes involves the removal of an entire body part (such as the breast) in order to remove a small tumor. Similarly, radiation therapy involves applying radiation to a section of the body much larger than that occupied by the cancerous tumor, and chemotherapy targets cells indiscriminately, as the chemo drugs cannot distinguish between healthy cells and cancerous ones. A by-product of the imprecision is often a range of devastating side effects.

Researchers have sought greater precision through one particular technique: immunotherapy, which involves using the patient's immune system to fight cancer. It was first tried in the late 19th century by William Coley, a doctor in New York. Although it proved effective, it did not gain traction in the medical community amid excitement about the potential for radiation to treat cancer [8].

Interest in immunotherapy revived in the 1950s, thanks in part to Coley's daughter establishing a research outfit called the Cancer Research Institute, which was dedicated to exploring immunotherapy. Radiation oncology remained more prevalent for years, and it was a Stanford professor, Henry Kaplan, who delivered one of the critical radiation breakthroughs. He originated the use of a linear accelerator to target tumor cells, and he focused on one specific disease, Hodgkin's, because it tends not to have spread to other parts of the body. "Instead of trying to tailor the disease to fit his medicine," writes Mukherjee, "Kaplan learned to tailor his medicine to fit the right disease" [9]. Kaplan's insights led to extraordinary progress in the battle against Hodgkin's. "In the 1950s, when he began his work, Hodgkin's disease was considered a hopeless condition," according to his biographer, Charlotte Jacobs. "Today, almost 90 percent of patients survive, in large part because of his work" [10]. Jacobs has also pointed to the reach of Kaplan's influence on cancer research.

He not only co-invented the first medical linear accelerator in the western hemisphere, but he also set the standards for its use. He formed a multidisciplinary group of specialists to treat cancer—a model used at most cancer centers today. He and oncologist Saul Rosenberg ushered in the era of modern clinical trials with their studies. His influence extended beyond Hodgkin's disease; he changed the way cancer is treated [11].

The work of Kaplan and others helped drive the popularity of radiation-based therapy for decades, but the year 2010 marked an inflection point, says Crystal Mackall, the Ernest and Amelia Gallo Family Professor of Pediatrics (hematology/oncology) and of internal medicine at Stanford. There were reports of immunotherapy benefiting people with conditions such as lymphoma and leukemia [12]. "All of a sudden," she says, "immunotherapy became the reality. And it has been the source of the most impressive gains in cancer treatment over the past decade. I expect it is going to dominate the landscape for new therapies in the decade ahead." Emblematic of the excitement about immunotherapy's potential was its being named by the American Society of Clinical Oncology as the research area showing the most progress in the battle against cancer in both 2016 and 2017 [13]. Then, in October 2018, two cancer immunotherapy pioneers, James Allison and Tasuku Honjo, shared the Nobel Prize for the discovery of a highly effective approach to immunotherapy known as *checkpoint inhibition.*

A celebrated example of immunotherapy's promise involves a former U.S. president, Jimmy Carter. In August 2015, he announced that he had been diagnosed with metastatic melanoma in his brain and liver—conditions that would typically result in a life expectancy of about three months. He was treated with surgery, radiation, and a checkpoint inhibitor called pembrolizumab. Four months later, he made a startling announcement: "My most recent MRI brain scan did not reveal any signs of the original cancer spots nor any new ones" [14]. Treatment with the immune checkpoint inhibitor has been widely recognized as having played a significant role in Carter becoming cancer-free.

Contributing to the optimism about immunotherapy's future was the FDA's August 2017 announcement that it had approved the first gene therapy for use in the United States. The therapy, Kymriah (tisagenlecleucel), is a genetically modified autologous T-cell immunotherapy intended for certain pediatric and young adult patients with a form of acute lymphoblastic leukemia. In announcing the approval, the FDA commissioner at the time, Scott Gottlieb, MD, said, "We're entering a new frontier in medical innovation with the ability to reprogram a patient's own cells to attack a deadly cancer. New technologies such as gene and cell therapies hold out the potential to transform medicine and create an inflection point in our ability to treat and even cure many intractable illnesses" [15]. Tellingly, cancer immunotherapy drugs are now estimated to account for nearly half of the total oncology drugs market—an encouraging indicator that precision is becoming a hallmark of cancer treatment.

As noted above, immunotherapy involves using one's immune system as a weapon to combat diseases such as cancer. In cell-based immunotherapy, the first step is to extract a group of T cells from the patient being treated. These cells, which are fundamental to immunity, are then taken to a lab, where a disabled virus (known as a *vector*) is added to them—a process that takes two to four weeks and endows the cells and their progeny with a new gene. The new cells are then grown and injected into the patient. The new cells also multiply so that all the daughter cells have the gene as well, and they are there in perpetuity. The gene, if it has been engineered correctly, expresses a unique receptor on the surface of the T cells, and that receptor enables the T cells to recognize a cancerous tumor. Mackall draws a parallel to giving a bloodhound a scent to follow.

> The chimeric antigen receptor (CAR) uses a part of an antibody, and it uses the signaling domains that are present in normal T cells. When you express that on a T cell, the cell will fire at—and kill—every time it finds a target the antibody recognizes. So it's a completely new way of doing medicine. Patients are hijacking the power of their immune system to do their bidding.

This ability to trick the T cell into attacking the tumor has been transformational. Mackall points out that when a group of children with childhood B cell acute lymphoblastic leukemia were treated with this therapy, after showing resistance to all other modes of therapy, 70 to 90 percent of them had complete responses after just one treatment [16]. She is now overseeing a clinical trial in which a next-generation version of CAR-T cells are programmed to be able to respond to two different targets (CD19 and/or CD22) in an attempt to overcome the most common cause of resistance to this new therapy. She says she is "absolutely convinced" that immunotherapy is going to become progressively more effective for patients with leukemia, lymphoma, and brain cancer, and other conditions that are extremely difficult to treat. "It truly has been a game-changer," she says, "and it has ushered in a new optimism regarding the promise of cell therapy as a whole new area of medicine."

Another Stanford professor, Ronald Levy, is exploring different ways to marshal the immune system to fight cancer. In one approach, he is injecting antibodies, which wake up the immune system, directly into one site of a tumor in the body to trigger an immune attack on the cancer wherever else it is in the body. (This is known as "*in situ* vaccination.") He is also collaborating with colleagues in the Department of Chemistry at Stanford to deliver RNA coding for the unique genetic signature of each patient's tumor, again to trigger an immune response against the cancer. In a third approach, he plans to replace

CAR-T cells with CAR-T genes. By doing this, he hopes to eliminate the process of extracting cells from the patient's body and then having to engineer them in a lab. Instead, he wants this approach to become "off the shelf," with the entire process happening within the patient's body. That would expand access, reduce costs, and increase safety.

COMBATING GENETIC DISEASES

The excitement about immunotherapy's potential is matched by the enthusiasm arising from the insights being unlocked by the mapping of the genome. One example is the revolution in thinking about conditions caused by genetic abnormalities. These abnormalities have been recognized for years, but as Stanford's John Day points out, "The belief was that you couldn't manipulate them and wouldn't be able to manage them or treat them. And so they were dismissed." The attitude, says Day, was "diagnose and adiós."

But starting in the late 1980s, and continuing through the 1990s and the early 2000s, there was a proliferation of gene targets for neuromuscular disease. As a result, it became possible to identify hundreds of different genes that cause muscular dystrophy and nerve damage, as well as dozens that cause motor neuron damage. That, says Day, "has really increased our awareness of what, specifically, underlies these different disorders."

Making Headway Toward Conquering Spinal Muscular Atrophy

Over the past 30 years, neuromuscular neurologists have identified the underlying genetic mutations responsible for hundreds of different nerve and muscle disorders, all of which can now be identified with a simple blood test at birth. These conditions have not been part of traditional newborn screening tests, however, because treatments have not been available. As a result, infants have not been tested until they showed signs of the disease, which could be months into their life, and at a point after it was no longer possible to reverse the condition. In the case of spinal muscular atrophy (SMA), the genetic defect results in progressive deterioration of all muscles, and thus impairment of swallowing, head control, limb movements, and breathing. Eighty percent of children afflicted by the most common form of SMA (SMA-1) appear normal at birth but die before their first birthday. Despite this bleak picture, investigators realized that the availability of a definitive genetic diagnostic test, and the highly predictable prognosis for all infants with SMA-1, provided a rare opportunity to validate methods being developed to treat a genetic disease.

One out of 40 people in the general population is a carrier for SMA. It is a recessive disorder, meaning that one of four children develops the disease when both parents are carriers (who are all asymptomatic, thus having no indication of their carrier status). The primary gene involved in SMA (SMN1) is normally present on Chromosome 5. Everyone has two copies of Chromosome 5—one from each parent—and if both copies are missing SMN1, the individual will inevitably develop SMA [17]. This situation is similar to all recessive disorders, but unlike patients with those disorders, every patient with SMA carries a backup gene, SMN2, that makes the identical protein. However, every copy of SMN2 has a single-letter flaw in the genetic code that distinguishes it from SMN1 and which prevents it from working well; SMN2 makes a fraction of the SMN protein that each copy of SMN1 generates, not enough to protect motor nerve cells, which die early in life.

All patients with SMA-1 have this same genetic profile—no copies of SMN1 and two copies of SMN2, both of which contain the same single letter flaw. While there are many recessive genetic disorders in which the affected patient is missing a particular gene, typically each patient carries a different mutation in that specific gene; this makes genetic correction difficult to develop because the number of patients with exactly the same specific mutation is extremely small. All SMA-1 patients carry SMN2 genes with the identical genetic flaw, which provided a rare opportunity to prove the efficacy of gene correction methods, resulting in the first infant being treated at Stanford in May 2013.

That infant, Zoe, was the first child of her parents, John and Eliza Harting, of El Granada, California. They were happy that Zoe was a beautiful, healthy baby at birth, but then noticed that she wasn't developing at the same pace as her cousin, even though the two were born a week apart. As John later told the *Mercury News*, "Her cousin was very mobile: wriggling around, pushing stuff. Zoe wasn't doing any of that. She was very quiet" [18]. When Zoe was three months old, she was diagnosed by genetic testing with SMA. John and Eliza were told the condition would cause a steady erosion of Zoe's ability to move, eat, and breathe—and that she would likely die before reaching her second birthday. About three months after the diagnosis, Zoe's pediatrician met Stanford's John Day, and he told her that he was about to launch a clinical trial involving the first drug for SMA-1. Day then spoke with John and Eliza and explained what the drug was supposed to do but also cautioned them that the outcome was uncertain—it might or might not help, or could result in persistence of profound disability. They agreed to have Zoe participate in the trial, and she became the first infant treated with the drug, SMNRx, which is now being commercially prescribed as nusinersen (Spinraza). Nusinersen is an antisense oligonucleotide (a short strand of synthetic RNA) that specifically binds to the SMN2 gene and thereby increases production of full-length SMN protein.

Even with the injections of nusinersen, the next 18 months were very challenging for Zoe, as she repeatedly contracted pneumonia. But she eventually showed great progress, and by the time of her first birthday, "she was doing things that you just never see SMA kids do," said Day. Without treatment, SMA children always get progressively and relentlessly weaker, but Zoe's muscles continually strengthened, helping her breathe and swallow more forcefully, and reducing her tendency to develop pneumonia. Some muscles were already too weak to respond to nusinersen, but overall she continued to get stronger and physically develop, to the point where she could sit upright on her own by the time she was three-and-a-half, and can now propel herself in a manual wheel-chair. Another milestone came in August 2018: she started kindergarten.

"Having spent so much time around adults, Zoe loves to be with other kids," says her father, John, mentioning her propensity for goofing around and watching SpongeBob cartoons. Zoe now gets an injection of nusinersen every four months. She's not cured of SMA, but she's thriving in a way that was unimaginable just a few years ago—and in doing so, she's showcasing the value of research into genetic conditions, and the possibility for disease-modifying correction of a specific gene in every cell of an affected patient.

Concurrent with the trial involving Zoe, Day was involved with a Phase 3 study of nusinersen. It started in late 2015 and by the following summer was halted because the results were so positive. ("The data was as clean as any study I've ever participated in," says Day.) The FDA approved the drug in December 2016, just two months after the results of the trial were submitted for review—the first such approval for SMA or any neurodegenerative disease [19]. Over the next 24 months, more than 2,000 patients in the United States had been treated, as had another 6,000 patients around the world. But as Day points out, the drug's effectiveness depends on treating infants early in life before their muscles weaken, so newborn screening and detection are fundamental.

Asked about the outlook for correcting genetic disease, Day is enthusiastic, while remaining cognizant of the challenges.

> I don't think we can be so naïve as to think that all genetically defined diseases are now treatable. We're going to have to refine the targets and improve the methods for correcting each of them individually. However, knowing that these methods have worked with such tremendous success for one disease addresses many of our previous questions and concerns about treatment possibilities, and gives all of us working in the field a sense of confidence and optimism that gene modification treatments can now be developed that will penetrate and correct cells throughout the brain and body of patients harboring these devastating genetic conditions.

The Quest to Tackle Amyotrophic Lateral Sclerosis (ALS)

The progress in treating SMA has helped unlock new insights about treating a similar disease: amyotrophic lateral sclerosis—also known as Lou Gehrig's Disease, named for the Hall of Fame baseball player who was diagnosed with the condition in 1939 and died two years later. ALS, which leads to about 6,000 deaths in the United States each year, is a neurodegenerative disease that causes muscles to erode and interferes with communication between the brain and the rest of the body.

One of the breakthroughs achieved by the SMA researchers was creating a synthetic molecule—known as an antisense oligonucleotide (ASO)—that could target the central nervous system and make it possible to treat neurological and neuromuscular disease. That's provided a template of sorts for ALS researchers, says Aaron Gitler, Stanford Medicine Basic Science Professor and professor of genetics.

"The SMA breakthrough proved that once you figure out the mechanism of a disease, you can design a precision therapy for it." For SMA, in which patients have a dysfunctional SMN1 gene, the approach is to use the ASO to prevent the backup SMN2 gene from being degraded. For ALS, the ASOs may also be used to target and degrade the toxic mutant genes that cause some forms of ALS.

There is no cure for ALS, and progress in combating it has been elusive—when a new ALS therapy was approved by the FDA in 2017, it was the first such approval since 1995 [20]. But there have been discoveries along the way. In 2010, for example, Gitler and his colleagues were the first to discover a connection between ALS and mutations in a gene called ataxin-2. Because the mutations in ataxin-2 that increase risk for ALS seem to make the protein more abundant, Gitler and his team have proposed that targeting ataxin-2, for example with an ASO, could be an effective therapeutic strategy for most cases of ALS; in 2017, they demonstrated the efficacy of this approach in a mouse model of ALS [21]. More recent progress has been realized thanks to another study by Gitler and his colleagues, published in *Nature Genetics* in March 2018, which focused on the role of aberrant proteins in ALS [22].

The most common genetic cause of ALS is a mutation in a gene called C9orf72. "In this gene," says Gitler, "there is a stretch of DNA in which six letters are repeated several times—GGGGCC. Normally this is repeated two to five times in a row, but it can get expanded to several hundred or several thousand times. This massive expansion of the six-letter repeat causes a large portion of ALS, by several potential mechanisms, including a bizarre one that involves stimulating the production of toxic proteins."

Gitler and one of his Stanford colleagues, Michael Bassik, explored why these proteins interfere with healthy neurons and whether other genes impact how the proteins interact with the brain. They used the CRISPR-Cas9 gene-editing technology to select the genes that would help neurons counteract the toxic proteins. The process led them to be able to pinpoint some genes that protect the cell from the toxic proteins. This knowledge, says Gitler, will allow them to understand the disease process better and design new gene-based therapies to protect neurons from the rogue proteins that accumulate in ALS.

It was the first time CRISPR technology had been used to advance understanding of a neurodegenerative disorder. "I think we're really entering a new translational phase," says Gitler, "and thanks to these discoveries from the lab, in the next five years we're going to start to see other neurodegenerative disease genes targeted by these therapies, and that could lead to greater understanding of other neurological diseases, such as Huntington's, Parkinson's, and Alzheimer's."

Using Gene Therapy and Gene Editing to Treat Disease

SMA and ALS are two of about 7,000 diseases that are classified as "rare." But "rare" is a relative term—these diseases are present in about 30 million Americans and 350 million people throughout the world. About half of all people living with rare diseases are children—about one-third of whom die within the first five years of life. The mortality is partly a result of the overwhelming share of the conditions lacking any FDA-approved drug treatments [23]. It is against that bleak backdrop that professors at Stanford are pursuing research that's focused on curing conditions—and doing so precisely—by engineering cells to treat disease or even modifying DNA to fix genetic abnormalities.

Much of this work has traditionally been in the field of gene therapy, which involves treating genetic diseases at the molecular level. The new frontier of gene therapy is genome editing. In the simplest sense, it involves entering the genome and removing the defective piece of DNA. Every edit is unique to each individual, with the mutated gene converted into a gene that doesn't cause disease.

The progress on this transformational practice has been remarkable, says Matthew Porteus, a professor of pediatrics at Stanford. Speaking in February 2019, he said,

> Five years ago, if you had told me you could get 1 percent of your blood stem cells corrected, I would have said, "That's great." And I would have wondered if we could get to 2 percent. But we're now in an era where we're routinely getting 30, 50, 60, 70 percent correction. ... Similarly, the idea that one can go in and precisely change a single letter in the DNA code was conceptualized for decades. But now it's at our fingertips and we can do it. That's why I think this is a unique time.

Although the concept of genome editing has existed for about 15 years, it was not very advanced. That began to change in 2012 with the discovery of what's known as CRISPR (Clustered Regularly Interspaced Short Palindromic Repeats). Studies showed that CRISPR and the enzyme Cas9 could be used to modify specific DNA sequences in a test tube. In 2013, additional studies revealed how CRISPR-Cas9 could edit human DNA. It's a relatively simple process, says Stanford's Stanley Qi, an assistant professor of bioengineering and of chemical and systems biology:

> To fix a damaged gene, you begin by designing an RNA molecule that matches the mutated DNA sequence in that gene. You then combine the RNA with a Cas9 enzyme, which can cut through DNA like sharp scissors. The RNA acts like a very fast GPS—it guides the Cas9 enzyme to the mutated DNA sequence. The enzyme then binds to the sequence and deletes it [24].

The last step is taking a benign virus that will insert the correct DNA sequence into the edited gene. The result is a gene that no longer contains the disease-causing mutation.

The existence of these tools is "revolutionary," says Mark Mercola, a professor of cardiovascular medicine and a member of the Stanford Cardiovascular Institute. "With CRISPR, we can do genetic experiments that would have been unimaginable just a few years ago, not just on inherited disorders but also on genes that contribute to acquired diseases, including AIDS, cancer, and heart diseases" [25].

Extensive gene-editing research is being conducted at Stanford. It's a particular emphasis at Stanford's Center for Definitive and Curative Medicine

(CDCM), which was launched in 2017. The center is directed by Maria Grazia Roncarolo, the George D. Smith Professor in Stem Cell and Regenerative Medicine at Stanford and a professor of pediatrics and of medicine, and its focus is exploring rare diseases that today are uncurable. Before Roncarolo came to Stanford in 2014, one of her signature achievements had been serving as the principal investigator of a trial that is considered a landmark in gene therapy. It involved treating 18 children who were born without the ability to make an enzyme called adenosine deaminase (ADA). Children born without that enzyme don't have the immune cells that prevent infections, which forces them to live in sterile environments (the condition is sometimes referred to as "bubble boy disease"). In the trial, Roncarolo and her team inserted the gene for ADA into blood stem cells, and those cells were transplanted into the children. Once the modified blood stem cells could produce the enzyme, they were able to form the necessary immune cells and the children were cured—allowing them to live outside their sterile environments.

CDCM has plans to launch clinical trails in late 2019 or early 2020 that will be focused on fixing the genetic defect that causes type 1 diabetes, chronic inflammation disease, and eczema. The center's researchers will be utilizing a gene therapy approach in the blood immune cells, and if the "drug" is effective—it's actually a cell that delivers a gene—it will be able to be used to treat other conditions. Roncarolo says that "we see rare diseases as the entry door for the technology to prove that it's safe and effective and then broaden its use, so it can help cure more common diseases." That would be a major breakthrough, and it would showcase the potential of gene therapy to improve human health—and do so with extreme precision.

Ethical and Moral Issues Connected to Genome Editing

The ability to edit the human genome unlocks tremendous opportunities to make precise changes to individual genomes and may help prevent or cure medical conditions in those individuals. But genome editing also raises complex ethical and moral issues that members of the scientific community have been working through in recent years.

In January 2015, some of the world's leading scientists gathered in Napa, California, to discuss the scientific, medical, legal, and ethical implications of genome editing. A few months later, they published an article in *Science* and highlighted "an urgent need for open discussion of the merits and risks of human genome modification" [26]. That discussion, they wrote, should involve scientists, clinicians, social scientists, the general public, and relevant public entities and interest groups. The article contained four near-term recommendations, which are quoted below:

> *We recommend that steps be taken to:*
>
> 1. *Strongly discourage, even in those countries with lax jurisdictions where it might be permitted, any attempts at germline genome modification for clinical application in humans, while societal, environmental, and ethical*

implications of such activity are discussed among scientific and govern-mental organizations. (In countries with a highly developed bioscience capacity, germline genome modification in humans is currently illegal or tightly regulated.) This will enable pathways to responsible uses of this technology, if any, to be identified.

2. *Create forums in which experts from the scientific and bioethics commu-nities can provide information and education about this new era of human biology, the issues accompanying the risks and rewards of using such pow-erful technology for a wide variety of applications including the potential to treat or cure human genetic disease, and the attendant ethical, social, and legal implications of genome modification.*

3. *Encourage and support transparent research to evaluate the efficacy and specificity of CRISPR-Cas9 genome engineering technology in human and nonhuman model systems relevant to its potential applications for germline gene therapy. Such research is essential to inform deliberations about what clinical applications, if any, might in the future be deemed permissible.*

4. *Convene a globally representative group of developers and users of genome engineering technology and experts in genetics, law, and bioethics, as well as members of the scientific community, the public, and relevant government agencies and interest groups, to further consider these important issues and, where appropriate, recommend policies.*

In 2017, another distinguished group of scientists (including Stanford's Matthew Porteus) collaborated on a report issued by the National Academy of Sciences and the National Academy of Medicine, *Human Genome Editing: Science, Ethics, and Governance.* The book contained a comprehensive explo-ration of issues connected to human genome editing and identified and described seven principles that should govern such editing: promoting well-being, trans-parency, due care, responsible science, respect for persons, fairness, and trans-national cooperation.

More recently, Porteus co-authored an article in 2018 that noted the likelihood of many preclinical proof-of-concept studies being conducted, given the surge of interest in genome editing. The article emphasized the need for sev-eral key steps to be taken before the studies can be used to help patients.

First, more attention must be paid to validating proof-of-concept studies in clinically relevant situations. The base editing systems, for example, have been developed only in easy-to-manipulate and highly abnormal human can-cer cell lines. Unfortunately, we have learned that systems that work well in such cell lines, such as the published high-fidelity Cas9 nucleases, do not have high activity when applied in a clinically relevant fashion. Thus, it will be important to quantitatively validate approaches in systems that are relevant to clinical translation.

Second, for streamlined and efficient translation of preclinical work to the clinic, standards for evaluating safety and toxicity should be established. Regulatory agencies, within the boundaries that constrain them, should work with the field to establish such standards.

Finally, once clinical trials are initiated, they should be designed to generate more knowledge about the clinical applications of genome editing. The current standard "adverse events" that are monitored should be supplemented by assays that are directed toward understanding the specific potential toxicities engendered by either *ex vivo* or *in vivo* editing protocols.

The field of gene therapy has taught us that one can learn valuable lessons from the first trials that then enhance the safety and efficacy of subsequent clinical trials. It is the learning from past trials that has facilitated the renaissance of gene therapy. This lesson should not be forgotten as the transformative potential of genome editing is translated to the clinic [27].

Gene Editing to Treat Sickle Cell Disease

The gene-editing tool CRISPR has enormous potential to bring precision to the process of repairing harmful gene mutations that affect millions of people throughout the world. But realizing that potential is going to depend on the outcome of clinical trials focused on CRISPR's safety, as well as its efficacy in treating specific conditions. One of those trials is scheduled to be undertaken by Stanford's Porteus. It's focused on sickle cell disease—a common genetic disease of red blood cells, in which the patient has a single mutation in a single gene. In the United States, it affects about 100,000 people—the vast majority of whom are African American—and it typically results in premature death. From 1979 to 2005, the average life expectancy of those with the disease was 42 for women and 38 for men [28].

The clinical trial—the first of its kind—is going to use CRISPR to correct the mutation in blood stem cells and then return the corrected stem cells to the patient. In theory, that should result in the patient being cured. The clinical trial will be testing that theory. Porteus emphasizes that the treatment is highly precise, as only the mutation is being corrected—"modifying one letter of the six billion letter genetic code," as he puts it. And it's personalized. The change is being made only in the patient with sickle cell disease—and using that patient's own cells.

For those patients who meet the criteria for participating in the clinical trial and agree to participate, the first step will involve having their own stem cells harvested, and then using CRISPR to locate and delete the DNA mutation. Next, a virus will need to be engineered to deliver the correct sequence of normal DNA. Once that weeklong process is complete, Porteus and his colleagues will analyze the cells to see if they achieved the needed frequency of correction and to ensure that there was no detectable harm to the cells.

When the corrected cells are approved, the next step is returning them to the patient (in what's known as an *autologous stem cell transplant*). That involves the patient being hospitalized and receiving chemotherapy to kill all (or nearly all) of the hematopoietic stem cells residing in the bone, since those will give rise to the red blood cells causing the disease. This therapy is similar to that used commonly, and with high rates of success, in bone marrow transplantation.

Once the chemotherapy is complete and has washed out of the patient's system after 36 to 48 hours, the patient's own cells will be reimplanted. This is a relatively simple process, as the cells can be dripped into their blood through an IV. While waiting for the cells to engraft and start making blood, the patient will stay in the hospital and be enclosed in a functional bubble to protect against infections. The hope is that at some point within 10 to 21 days, the new stem cells will start making blood and the patient can be released from the hospital and then followed as an outpatient. Porteus and his colleagues would be following whether the corrected stem cells are starting to make red blood cells that don't have sickle cell disease. "That will be a very exciting and nerve-wracking time for a lot of people," he says.

If the first small trial proves successful, then a larger trial will be initiated in order to get the process approved as a drug to treat any sickle cell disease patient, not just those in a clinical trial. But it can take 10 to 15 years for approval of a new drug. The FDA has said it hopes to accelerate that process for innovative new therapies, such as genome editing.

Whenever that approval comes, it will mean that those with sickle cell disease in the United States—and perhaps the millions of others with the disease throughout the world—will be able to look forward to something that was thought to be impossible: living symptom-free for the rest of their lives.

GENE EDITING OF EMBRYOS

CRISPR has many different potential applications, and while there's broad public and scientific support for using it to try to correct conditions such as sickle cell anemia, other uses are more controversial. For example, a biophysicist in China revealed in November 2018 that he had engaged in gene editing of two embryos (which became twin girls) during in vitro fertilization. The disclosure led to widespread criticism of the biophysicist, given that the safety and efficacy of such editing has not been established. A few months later, 18 prominent scientists, representing seven countries, published a paper in *Nature* in which they called for a five-year "global moratorium" on the practice of editing DNA in human sperm, eggs, or embryos. The five years would be used, said the authors, to develop an international framework [29]. They raised several technical, scientific, medical, and societal/ethical/moral considerations. But there are differences of opinion within the scientific community about the value of a moratorium. Although one of the scientists signing on to the *Nature* paper was Emmanuelle Charpentier, a coinventor of CRISPR, one of the technology's other inventors, Jennifer Doudna, did not sign it. "It is a bit late to be calling for a moratorium," she told the *Wall Street Journal* [30]. More than two dozen nations have laws that directly or indirectly outlaw clinical uses of germline editing, but this issue is far from settled—and will only become more complex as the science advances.

Treating a Painful and Debilitating Skin Condition

A rare skin disease called epidermolysis bullosa (EB) is among the most painful and debilitating conditions ever diagnosed. "The word 'pain' itself doesn't even describe how bad EB is," said one courageous young man, Paul Martinez, living with the condition, in a 2015 film about EB patients called *The Butterfly Effect* [31]. "Your body is constantly on fire—it burns from the wounds from raw flesh, and it keeps repeating over and over and over. The cycle is never-ending" [32].

Approximately 1 in 200,000 babies is born with EB. There are different subtypes of the condition, but a common one is caused by the absence of a gene that results in the skin being unable to make something called *anchoring fibrils*. They are primarily composed of collagen and function like a staple—keeping the top layer of the skin (the epidermis) attached to the next layer (the dermis). As a result, for people with EB, virtually any force applied to the skin leads to blistering and that part of the epidermis falling away. These wounds never heal, resulting in mutations that trigger metastatic skin cancer and take the lives of many of these patients.

In the absence of any treatments for EB, most of those with the disease have not lived past their mid-20s. But in recent years, Stanford dermatology professors have been making steady progress in developing a treatment that can deliver life-changing wound-healing treatments for EB patients and potentially help remedy other, more common conditions.

One of those Stanford professors is Jean Tang. She and some colleagues in the dermatology department have been working on a therapy called EB101, whereby they take somatic keratinocyte cells off a patient's skin, use a retrovirus to reinsert the gene, and then graft those cells onto the patient. A Phase 1 clinical trial showed that these grafts are safe and lead to durable wound healing for up to four years and counting. A Phase 3 clinical trial was set to begin in mid-2019, and positive results would mark an important step toward one of the ultimate goals: securing FDA approval for a drug to treat EB.

Anthony Oro, the Eugene and Gloria Bauer Professor of Dermatology, is working on the next generation of therapy to treat EB. His focus is developing a product that would cover the wounds of EB patients and permanently heal those wounds—and do so at an early age so that they don't get skin cancer from the chronic wounding.

His research aims to develop a scalable manufacturing platform to make large amounts of corrected tissue stem cells. In 2014, Oro was one of the authors of a study with Marius Wernig, an associate professor of pathology at Stanford. The study showed that it was possible to create induced pluripotent cells from the skin cells of EB patients and then replace the disease-causing gene with a healthy version of the gene. ("Making science fiction come true," says Tang.) Oro described this development as enabling "an entirely new paradigm for this disease."

Normally, treatment has been confined to surgical approaches to repair damaged skin, or medical approaches to prevent and repair damage. But by replacing the faulty gene with a correct version in stem cells, and then converting those corrected stem cells to keratinocytes, we have the possibility of achieving a permanent fix—replacing damaged areas with healthy, perfectly matched skin grafts [33].

This process involves the use of autologous CRISPR corrected induced pluripotent stem (iPS) cells. These cells are made by collecting cell samples from someplace easy to access, such as skin or blood. The cells are then treated in a dish with a combination of genes that enable them to go back in time—a process known as *cell reprogramming*—so that they resemble the cells from which all tissues are formed. John Gurdon and Shinya Yamanaka were awarded the Nobel Prize in Physiology or Medicine in 2012 for this pioneering work in regenerative medicine.

"The CRISPR technology was very efficient," says Oro, "and it allowed us to develop a very robust, one clonal step manufacturing protocol to make the autologous CRISPR corrected iPS cells." (Previously these cells were being derived through multiple clonal steps, which brought more risks, as they were in culture longer and subject to more mutations.) The effect was to reduce cost and increase safety and to mark a shift from "this could be done" to "now it's being done less expensively and with more safety."

This process has also made it possible to grow the cells in much larger quantities. The next step is inducing activity of the cells to make the skin, which results in a thin sheet of skin cells derived from the iPS cells. Like EB101, these sheets are akin to a Band-Aid that's roughly the size of a smartphone. Each one is laid onto a patient's wound, and it then grafts onto the patient's skin. The benefits are realized almost immediately, says Oro, as the grafting heals the wounds. "Kids can walk around and not have to worry about what will happen if they accidentally bump into something."

Today, the grafts are small and only cover a small fraction of a patient's skin. The ultimate goal is to have the graft cover all of a patient's skin—and perhaps even for the product to come in a liquid form that can be sprayed onto the patient's skin.

As with so many other medical and technological discoveries developed for the treatment of a rare disease, the same technology can then be generalized to more common diseases. The iPS technology has a range of potential applications beyond EB. Oro points out that the therapy can be very effective for wounds that are slow to heal or don't heal at all—such as those caused by injury, burns, or diabetes. The technology of making tissue from iPS cells that have undergone genetic manipulation is also being used to make stem cells for other tissues. There is already research underway on the thymus, the bladder, and even the heart. Tang points out that much of the progress that's been achieved is the result of many years of basic research (particularly in the area of recombinant DNA) as well as powerful tools (like electron microscopy) and tests that reveal valuable information (like indirect immunofluorescence). "It's very gratifying when all of these elements come together to give a patient hope that their suffering can be reduced—if not eliminated."

The many potential applications for the skin grafts are encouraging, and we remain hopeful that there will be continued progress in developing a remedy for EB that can end the suffering of those with the disease. Paul Martinez, whom I mentioned at the start of this section, has participated in EB clinical trials, and he's said that the results have been promising.

> Even if I can't get any benefit from it ... I just want the disease to stop for the future. ... I've been blessed to live longer than most people with this disease. But it's kind of bittersweet. Thirty-five years is a long time to live with the pain that I go through. And I don't want any children to go through that. If I'm in a position where I can help the future of EB, then I'm going to do it.

INDIVIDUALIZING CELLULAR APPROACHES TO UNDERSTANDING DISEASES IN INDIVIDUALS

As we learn more about the general characteristics of disease, we've often seen that a therapy that works in one patient may not work in another patient. The process of trial and error in an individual patient, with many different therapeutic approaches, is time-consuming, expensive, and potentially dangerous (because of adverse reactions). The ability to manufacture iPS cells, which I described in the previous section, has helped to change that picture. Thanks to advances in iPS cell technology, it's now possible to use that technology to manufacture cells for most cell types in the human body. What follows are some examples of how the technology is being used to make organized, differentiated groups of cells that form tissues with many of the functional characteristics of organs and to test the effectiveness of therapies in these organoids made from individual patients.

The Brain

I wrote in chapter 3 about our limited understanding of the brain and how that knowledge gap has impaired the development of treatments for mental illness. Recently, however, there has been noteworthy progress in many areas of brain research. Many people have contributed to this progress (including those I have profiled), and there's another person who deserves highlighting: Sergiu Pasca, who is an assistant professor of psychiatry and behavioral sciences at Stanford. He's helping dramatically expand our understanding of how the brain functions—and what mechanisms contribute to the onset of neuropsychiatric disorders.

Although Stanford draws professors from countries throughout the world, Pasca is one of only two who grew up in Romania and attended medical school there (the other is his wife, Anca). He developed an interest in basic science at an early age—he set up a home laboratory when he was 11—and while in medical school he reached a conclusion that would shape his future plans: "I felt that psychiatry had a huge unmet need, in terms of breaking boundaries in understanding the human brain. I would go on the oncology ward and be surprised by the level of medical advances, and then go on the psychiatry ward and see little I was able to do for patients." He still sometimes jokes that he suffers from "oncology envy syndrome."

A fundamental challenge, as Pasca has pointed out, is that while human brain development occurs over a long period of time—before birth and years after—"it is largely inaccessible for direct, functional investigation at a cellular level. Therefore, the features that make the human central nervous system unique and the sequence of molecular and cellular events underlying brain disorders remain largely uncharted" [34].

That's begun to change, as Pasca and others have achieved several break-throughs. In 2011, he showed that induced pluripotent stem cells could be created in such a way that they would replicate key features of neurodevelopmental disorders. Today, his trailblazing, noninvasive technology can take any cell from the human body (using iPS cell technology)—whether from blood or from skin cells—and over a period of a few months transform that cell into functioning human brain tissue. That tissue, which is known as a three-dimensional brain organoid, grows into something resembling a ball of cells floating in a Petri dish, and it can represent different regions of the brain.

This enabled Pasca to introduce another revolutionary approach of putting together different brain regions to allow them to connect into circuits and observe how different cell types interact with each other. That's noteworthy because over time the cells from one brain region could migrate to the other region—just as they do in the brain of a living person. Or neurons from one brain region would send projections and connect by synapses with neurons from another brain region.

Pasca says he finds this exciting because "some of these processes are actually taking place at late stages of human gestation—second and third trimester, and soon after birth—which are periods of brain development and function that we have never really had access to. But now we can actually watch them live and study them in a noninvasive way. And we can see how they're moving and why they're moving the way they're moving" [35]. In recent years, Pasca has used these technologies to gain insights into neurodevelopmental disorders, such as genetic forms of autism and schizophrenia.

Pasca identifies the cells as brain-region-specific spheroids or organoids, and with their existence, he can pinpoint abnormal activity in the brain region that can be a trigger for disorders such as autism, schizophrenia, and epilepsy. "This is our doorway into personalized psychiatry," he says [36]. And he's energized about the potential to use these insights to treat—if not prevent altogether—these disorders.

> The technology will allow us, for the first time, to bring the power of molecular biology into psychiatry. And down the road, it can help us do a number of things, such as understand what makes human brain development unique. This could have implications for building better artificial intelligence. I believe it is also going to help us develop the next-generation model of disease and will help us develop new therapeutics for these disorders [37].

The Transformative Potential of iPS Cells

The applications of iPS cells extend beyond the brain and have far-reaching potential. Joseph C. Wu, who is the director of the Stanford Cardiovascular Institute and the Simon H. Stertzer, MD, Professor of Medicine and Radiology, says the technology underlying iPS cells "is not only revolutionizing science but will also fundamentally alter our health care system and the future of medicine by making it proactive, predictive, preventive, and personalized" [38].

Emblematic of the potential, says Wu, is the impact that iPS cells may have on therapies—transforming them from being one-size-fits-all to customized for each individual. Here's the situation as Wu describes it today for one common condition:

> When a patient shows up at a clinic with high blood pressure, the doctor will prescribe one of the popular anti-hypertensive medications. A week later, the patient may come back claiming that the medication isn't working and the doctor will switch to another drug, for example switching from a beta-blocker to a calcium channel blocker. When the patient does not come back or call back to the clinic, it probably means the prescribed drug is working. However, this is a hit-or-miss approach because we're operating on educated guesses. The reality is that we have a variety of drugs out there to treat the same disease, but we don't know which one works best for each individual. In this scenario, the patient is the guinea pig [39].

Wu's goal is to "eliminate the guesswork by personalizing medicine to each individual patient." iPS cells can make that possible, and a lot more. To illustrate the potential of iPS cells, Wu cites a condition called hypertrophic cardiomyopathy (a thickening of the heart muscle), which can cause people to collapse or can even result in death. When individuals are resuscitated, they can have their DNA sequenced for clues about their condition. However, although results can reveal numerous genetic variants, there's no reliable way to test for a variant that may cause hypertrophic cardiomyopathy.

That has led scientists to what seems like the next-best option, which is to breed mice to have the same mutation and see if they experience hypertrophic cardiomyopathy. But in most instances, mice will not be afflicted with the condition because they differ from humans in many key aspects.

According to Wu, generating iPS cells can help identify the key variants or mutations causing the hypertrophic cardiomyopathy. "We can see if your heart cells have hypertrophic cardiomyopathy. And through genome editing, one of the variants can be deleted to see if the phenotype with the hypertrophic cardiomyopathy goes away. The same variant can also be introduced into a control cell line in my iPS cell to see if the hypertrophic cardiomyopathy pops up." Wu sees this process, which can be replicated for several conditions, as a hallmark of precision medicine: "It's going to be a very different process for every person."

Wu has also been a leader of research he calls "clinical trial in a dish." It represents a break with the traditional model of clinical trials, in which a drug company has multiple drugs in its pipeline to treat the same condition without being able to test all of them because of the high costs associated with drug development and clinical trials. This means that sometimes the most effective drugs may be excluded or lost in the process. By contrast, under the "clinical trial in a dish" model, a company could skip many of the conventional steps and start by having all its drug options tested on iPS cells, and then use the clinical trial only for the most effective option. This approach should dramatically boost success in drug testing and approval, bringing new drugs to patients faster and at a fraction of the costs we pay today.

In addition to testing the effectiveness of drugs, iPS cells can be used to reveal which individual patients will have an adverse reaction to specific drugs. This can be of great benefit for cancer patients, many of whom develop heart disease because there is no reliable way to test whether chemotherapy will lead to cardiac toxicity for particular patients. For instance, the iPS cells would be generated, differentiated into heart cells, and then exposed to doxorubicin (a common therapy for breast cancer patients) to see how the body responds. Wu says that "it's probably the best test we have because it encompasses the genetic information, the transcript information, the protein information, the metabolic metabolism, and all of which is combined to generate a miniature cell readout." Wu led a seminal study that involved using the iPS-derived cardiomyocytes from breast cancer patients to predict which one of them would experience cardiac toxicity after treatment with doxorubicin [40]. He believes this technology will become a very popular platform to study the molecular and genetic basis of other types of chemotherapy-induced cardiotoxicity.

The iPS technology may also be used for regenerative purposes. Consider someone who has had a heart attack that devastated 25 percent of their heart muscle. That muscle is dead and can't be replaced. But with iPS cells generated from this individual's blood, billions of heart cells can be differentiated to be injected back into the individual, potentially replacing the dead tissue with the individual's own heart cells.

A major goal of developing iPS cells ultimately is to make precise medicine possible. In 10 or 20 years, says Wu, "we should be able to draw blood, make iPS cells, differentiate them into cardiac cells or other cell types, and expose these cells to different drugs to find out what would be the ideal drug for that patient. This is the future of personalized medicine" [41].

Exploring the Therapeutic Value of Organoids

Calvin Kuo, the Maureen Lyles D'Ambrogio Professor of Medicine at Stanford, is at the forefront of organoid research. In 2009, he published one of the first papers in an academic journal on the potential to grow intestines as organoids for extended periods of time [42]. That paper helped spark a dramatic expansion of research into the potential therapeutic value of organoids, and as the field has advanced, Kuo has continued to explore how they can be used to bring much greater precision to the treatment of disease.

His recent focus has been growing three-dimensional organoids that reproduce the cellular complexity of an entire healthy organ. (Other organoids may only reproduce the cellular lining.) "In our organoids, we don't want to only have simplistic models of tumor cells or the epithelial lining cells only in the normal organ. We want to build in the incredible diversity of cell interaction that's present *in vivo* in humans."

Much of his work has been devoted to using organoids to model cancer. He and his colleagues have succeeded in taking "healthy" colon, stomach, and pancreas organoids and making them "unhealthy" by adding cancerous mutations. These mutations then cause the organoids to replicate tumorlike behavior—metastasizing and invading—and to form tumors when implanted in mice.

According to Kuo, this ability to convert healthy tissues and organoids into cancer "represents a powerful system for discovering and proving the function of new cancer-causing mutations."

> Tumor cells often have hundreds if not thousands of mutations and other epigenetic alterations, but only a minority are critical "drivers" that cause cancer, versus the vast majority of irrelevant "passenger" mutations. With collaborators we utilize computational and systems biology principles to interrogate large tumor DNA sequencing data sets to identify candidate cancer driver genes. We then exploit the power of organoids for cancer gene discovery, systematically inserting mutations found in cancer cells to test if such mutations successfully convert the organoids to a cancerous phenotype. Accelerating the functional validation of cancer-causing mutation will allow therapies and diagnostics to be developed against these genes.

Kuo and his colleagues have succeeded in growing organoids that recapitulate the tumor cells but also the supporting cells of the tumor. These include the immune cells, which are extremely important for how tumors develop and the strategies to control tumors. Growing tumors in this more holistic way is seen as the next generation of organoids. One writer, summarizing a 2018 article in *Cell* coauthored by Kuo, labeled his work "Organoid 2.0" [43].

The breakthrough achieved by Kuo's lab has been to grow tumor organoids that preserve the tumor-infiltrating immune cells inside. They then apply FDA-approved immunotherapy agents, which target processes known as immune checkpoints (mechanisms by which tumor cells can repel the attacking immune cells). The tumor cells express certain proteins in the cell surface that then talk to other proteins on the attacking lymphocyte cell surface and repel the lymphocyte. The ability to manipulate the tumors so that lymphocytes will be able to attack them holds out the potential to predict which patients are going to respond to immunotherapy—a significant achievement, given that the response rate today is only about 25 percent. At a minimum, the ability to test the effectiveness of therapies, using tissue taken from individuals already afflicted with conditions such as cancer, should dramatically reduce the incidence of unnecessary treatments—and ensure the use of treatments that have a higher likelihood of success.

Kuo's lab is working with Stanford's Matt Porteus to grow organs out of cells taken from patients who have particular mutations and gene-correcting those organoids, with the goal of then putting them back into the patient. The poster child for this approach has been cystic fibrosis. It affects many different parts of the body—the lungs, the colon, and the pancreas, but also the nasal sinuses. Sinus tissue has the advantage of being very accessible—an ear, nose, and throat surgeon can easily extract it—and Kuo's lab has devised methods of using organoids to grow these sinus tissues from cystic fibrosis patients. From there, Porteus and his colleagues have been able to gene-correct them using CRISPR technology. The idea is to take this gene-corrected tissue from organoids and then reimplant it into the patient. Although this work is still in the research phase, it holds the potential for templating a process by which organoids are used to grow a patient's own tissue, which can then undergo gene correction of harmful mutations, followed by transplantation back into the patient.

Kuo is also exploring the use of organoids to create biobanks, which are biorepositories that store human samples for use in research. These are typically tissue samples taken from patients at the time of surgery that have been preserved on microscope slides for further study. Tissue in this state is "dead" in that it has been fixed and preserved. Kuo is pushing for the dead tissue samples to be replaced with live tissue, in the form of organoids. (The tissue is stored and frozen in liquid nitrogen as cryo vials and then can be thawed anytime someone wants to view it.) He says there are initiatives underway throughout the world to make cancer tissues as organoids, for the purpose of studying different types of cancer. "Every cancer is different," notes Kuo, "and every patient has different mutations. But a researcher may be able to find an organoid that has the genetic array of mutations that is similar to what he or she is interested in." These types of organoids can also be used to screen chemotherapy drugs on an array of cancers that have been converted to live organoids. Organoids could also be used to biobank tissues from diseases besides cancer, encompassing genetic or inflammatory conditions.

MAKING HEADWAY IN THE FIGHT AGAINST HIV-AIDS

I noted at the start of this chapter that the quest for medical cures is typically a very long—and very costly—process, with low odds of achieving a breakthrough. But there has been remarkably rapid progress in the effective treatment of one well-known condition: HIV-AIDS. Today there are medications available that make it possible for most people with AIDS to lead long and healthy lives. This progress has been "the biggest accomplishment in infectious diseases in the last 30 to 40 years," says Upinder Singh, a professor of medicine and of microbiology and immunology at Stanford.

It was only in 1981 that conditions resembling HIV-AIDS were first written about in the *New England Journal of Medicine* [44]. The following year, the U.S. government's Centers for Disease Control labeled the disease "acquired immuno-deficiency syndrome." At the time, the outlook was bleak, with no known treatments and diagnosis often leading to death. In the United States, the number of deaths steadily increased until 1995, reaching approximately 50,000 [45]. But since then, there has been a sharp reduction in HIV-related mortality rates. As of 2016, the age-adjusted HIV death rate was more than 80 percent lower than it had been in 1995 [46]. The fall in mortality rates has also been charted globally. The number of AIDS-related deaths has declined by more than 51 percent since peaking in 2004 [47].

The progress has been the product of a few different interrelated factors. For starters, the U.S. government took a leading role in researching the basic biology of the AIDS virus. This research was conducted at the National Institute of Allergy and Infectious Diseases as well as the National Cancer Institute, which was home to Robert Gallo, who in 1984 co-discovered the link between HIV and AIDS.

Pharmaceutical companies also played a critical role, making large investments in the development of antiretroviral drugs. Burroughs Wellcome (now part of GlaxoSmithKline) developed AZT, the first drug approved by the FDA to treat AIDS, in 1987. That pharmaceutical research continued for many years after, leading to the development of antiretroviral drugs that suppress HIV. Pharma companies and government researchers also collaborated in the search for treatments. "Everyone viewed this as a very important mission," recalls Dean Winslow, a professor of medicine at the Stanford Medical Center whose experience includes working in the pharmaceutical sector. "A lot of really good people, in the United States and Europe, put their egos aside and worked together to tackle this problem."

Amid all the research into HIV and AIDS, scientists also benefited from something entirely out of their control: some of the key elements of the disease could be understood and treated in ways that have proved more elusive for many other diseases. As Winslow points out,

> HIV is a lentivirus, and it produces immunosuppression largely through what's called a "cytopathic effect," meaning that it chews up its host cells in tissue culture in the lab, as well as in the lymph nodes of human beings.

So it's a bit more of a straightforward process by which HIV causes immune suppression in the host where it causes disease. Once the virus had been isolated, and once we had figured out how the virus assembles virus particles and replicates, then inhibitors could potentially be developed to interrupt its life cycle. And for researchers, developing those inhibitors was a much simpler problem to solve.

Public pressure also helped deliver progress. From the earliest days of HIV-AIDS, there was an energetic and vocal lobby pressing for government agencies and pharmaceutical companies to develop more advanced therapies. The activists clearly made a difference. "They played a very positive role," says Winslow, "in helping to ensure that AIDS was taken seriously and that the public and private sectors invested in it."

For all the progress, it's important to understand that there is still not a cure for HIV-AIDS. Anyone who is HIV-positive still needs to take the recommended medicine every day to counteract the disease. Although access to anti-retrovirals has expanded, particularly in Africa, the United Nations estimates that of the nearly 37 million people living with HIV in 2017, more than 15 million were not accessing antiretroviral therapy [48]. That's one reason why approximately 940,000 people throughout the world died from AIDS-related illnesses in 2017—a year when about 1.8 million people also became newly infected—demonstrating the clear need for heightened focus on both drug delivery and prevention. There is also research underway on a preventive HIV vaccine, which is focused on training an individual's immune system to recognize HIV and fight it, if ever exposed to the virus. Clinical trials are testing the vaccine, but it has not been approved by the FDA [49].

PERSISTENT THREATS TO TREATMENT OF INFECTIOUS DISEASES

HIV-AIDS is one of many infectious diseases found throughout the world. The discovery of antibiotics has significantly reduced the death rate from disease, but there are still huge gaps. Tuberculosis, for example, killed approximately 1.6 million people in 2017 [50]. And an emerging threat today is the spread of drug-resistant organisms and a rise in viral infections. Lucy Shapiro, whom I featured in chapter 3, has spoken with passion about this threat and the need for a remedy. The World Health Organization has also highlighted the threat: "New resistance mechanisms are emerging and spreading globally, threatening our ability to treat common infectious diseases, resulting in prolonged illness, disability, and death" [51]. A joint report published in 2016 by the UK government and Wellcome Trust noted that by 2050, 10 million lives per year would be at risk from drug-resistant infections—up from 700,000 in 2016—and most of the impact would be felt in low- and middle-income countries [52]. (Today, heart disease is responsible for more deaths annually—close to 10 million—than anything else [53].)

This phenomenon stems from several different factors. The expansion of cross-border travel means diseases can spread faster. Alterations to the environment, such as climate change, can also contribute. "Malaria is currently not prevalent in North America," points out Singh, "but the vector exists and as temperatures rise, infections can come back." There's also clear evidence that some medicines are becoming less effective in counteracting many infectious diseases. According to the WHO,

> Antimicrobial resistance occurs naturally over time, usually through genetic changes. However, the misuse and overuse of antimicrobials is accelerating this process. In many places, antibiotics are overused and misused in people and animals, and often given without professional oversight. Examples of misuse include when they are taken by people with viral infections like colds and flu, and when they are given as growth promoters in animals or used to prevent diseases in healthy animals [54].

Antimicrobial resistance could become one of the leading global public health challenges of the 21st century. Continued research and development by pharmaceutical companies will be critical, but the economics are challenging. As Singh points out,

> If a pharmaceutical company develops a new drug to treat high blood pressure or diabetes, there are always going to be a certain number of patients who have diabetes or high blood pressure, and they are going to take that medication daily for the rest of their life. With antibiotics, it costs the same to develop them as other drugs, but the patients are told, "Take for seven days and then stop." So the profit motive for pharma is minimal.

There are no easy answers to this challenge, but it's one that calls for more coordination from pharmaceutical companies, government officials, and academic medical centers.

HOW SURGERY IS BECOMING MORE EFFICIENT AND LESS INVASIVE

Although many recent advances in therapeutics have focused on the molecular and genetic components of disease, milestones in surgical therapies continue to be achieved. Everything is tailored to each patient, with a customized operation. Surgery can also be a center of innovation, as it often draws on many different disciplines, such as engineering and manufacturing.

Some of those important innovations have been launched at Stanford. In January 1968, Stanford's School of Medicine was home to the first adult heart transplant conducted in the United States. The procedure attracted global media coverage, and it also led the Santa Clara County coroner to threaten to bring murder charges against the surgeon, Norman Shumway. The coroner wisely did not pursue the matter, and many other surgery milestones have been achieved at Stanford. These include the world's first adult combined heart-lung transplant and the world's first surgical implantation of a ventricular assist device as a bridge to transplantation. Over the past decade, there have been multiple surgical innovations that advance precision and, in the process, improve patient outcomes.

One such innovation has been in the area of minimally invasive surgery. Although heart surgery typically involves opening the chest, Stanford has invented a variety of operations that involve small incisions on the side of the chest, with the heart accessed through the ribs. Patients see a range of benefits from this, including faster recovery, less pain, reduced risk of complications, minimal scarring, and shorter hospital stays.

Evelina Cavett, a Nevada resident, has always maintained a very active lifestyle during her 50 years as an educator, which has included teaching K–8 students, serving as a performing arts director at schools throughout the United States, and instructing ballroom dance for 35 years. But when she found herself experiencing high levels of fatigue and shortness of breath in 2017, she went to a doctor. He diagnosed her with what's known as *regurgitation*, which refers to the mitral valve not closing completely, causing blood to flow backward instead of forward through the valve. This can lead to heart failure. For decades, the standard treatment for mitral regurgitation was a median sternotomy, which involves making an incision along the sternum to get access to the heart—a highly invasive procedure that carries considerable risk, as well as a very long recovery for the patient.

But Cavett was referred to Joseph Woo, a cardiothoracic surgeon at Stanford, and in July 2018 he was able to conduct a minimally invasive mitral valve repair. This involves making a small, right-sided incision, which results in a direct view of the mitral valve that's superior to what's available in a median sternotomy.

For Cavett, the mitral valve repair was a two-hour procedure, and she was in intensive care for one day. But she had a much faster recovery than she expected, and within three months she had returned to teaching dance and other performing arts. She was so happy with how the procedure turned out that she told Woo she was going to use social media to spread the word about it. "People should know about this—not just in the United States, but worldwide."

Another heart surgery innovation has been a break with the decades-long practice of stopping the heart and stopping the lungs. Typically, patients are hooked up to a heart-lung machine, which was invented in the 1950s and hasn't changed much in the intervening years. It's basically one big tube taking blood out of a patient's body, a machine that adds oxygen to the blood, and one big tube returning it. The innovation at Stanford has been to operate on the heart without stopping it. Known as *beating heart surgery*—it is sometimes compared to changing the transmission in a car that has its engine running—it avoids some of the risks linked to conventional bypass surgery and being hooked up to the heart-lung machine, such as blood loss, stroke, and kidney failure.

A third innovation is called *natural repair*. It involves the use of as much of the heart's natural living tissues as possible to effect a repair, as opposed to replacing components inside the heart. Instead of removing a patient's diseased heart valve and replacing it with an artificial valve (typically made of animal parts, metal parts, or plastic), there has been a drive for surgeons to use patients' natural tissues to remodel, resculpt, cut, sew, and build new structures to make a repair. The use of living tissue will always be better than using something artificial, as the living tissue can heal, grow, and adapt.

Artificial heart pump devices have also benefited from innovation. Over the last 10 to 15 years, while the pumps have been getting smaller and easily fit inside the chest cavity, they still need to be powered through a driveline that comes out through the patient's skin. The next step is to power the device with *transcutaneous energy transmission*, which refers to charging by induction. Ideally, people with an artificial heart pump could have an induction coil inside their chest that's near the skin and that could be charged by an external device. Another innovation, which is in the works, will address the challenge posed by having artificial pumps in contact with blood. When anything other than the naturally smooth surface on the inside of human blood vessels touches blood, the blood detects a cut and immediately clots. To combat this, scientists and engineers have been trying to design bioengineered surfaces that can trick the blood vessels into thinking the machine is not a machine, and as of September 2018 this technology was part of early trials being conducted in Europe.

Another innovation being explored at Stanford involves coronary artery bypasses, which are the most common major operations performed in the United States—about 500,000 per year. Bypasses are designed to divert blood when there is a blockage in the patient's artery that is impeding blood flow. But despite the volume of bypasses performed, there are no specific guidelines on the optimal configuration. "Should I plug a vein into location A or location B? Should I change the angle? No one has any idea about what's best for each patient," says Joseph Woo, the Norman Shumway Professor and chair of the Department of Cardiothoracic Surgery at Stanford.

Woo is part of an interdisciplinary group, which includes physicians, engineers, and mathematicians, that is using imaging data to create a 3-D computational fluid dynamics model of each patient's disease and their native arteries, and drawing on that information to simulate what the blood flow should be. That information is then used in the operating room, with a flow probe determining the exact flow, which makes it possible to immediately corroborate what the calculations were. From this, different strategies for grafting can be developed, and optimal flow can be pinpointed. This work, which was in the pilot study phase in fall 2018, is an example of using engineering, science, and medicine together to precisely determine the best possible procedures for every patient.

Minimally invasive surgery is also utilized for other parts of the body. Mary Hawn, the Emile Holman Professor and chair of the Department of Surgery at Stanford, is one of the leaders in her field. She describes how surgical procedures have evolved:

> When I was a resident training in the '90s, we began to see the first major adoption of minimally invasive laparoscopic approaches for gastrointestinal surgery, known as laparoscopic cholecystectomy. This approach was a game changer for a procedure such as removing the gallbladder. Rather than making a big incision through the abdominal muscles, which meant the patient was in the hospital for five to seven days and couldn't work for six weeks, the surgery could be done through four small incisions, and the patient was discharged the same day in many instances. So it was amazing to do operations with minimal morbidity to patients, get them back to their lives much more quickly, and with better outcomes.

As Hawn and other surgeons became more experienced with minimally invasive surgery, they started extending laparoscopic surgery to other areas of the abdomen, including the appendix, the stomach, the esophagus, the colon, and the pancreas. Additionally, the philosophy of minimally invasive approaches extended to other disease processes. One such condition is called necrotizing pancreatitis, which involves an infection of the pancreas resulting in a buildup of dead tissue that needs to be removed. In the past, removing the tissue would have meant a big open operation, with the patient shuttled back and forth to the operating room multiple times. But with today's minimally invasive approaches, surgeons can use either a laparoscope to enter through the patient's abdominal wall or an endoscope to enter the necrotic cavity through the stomach. In the second case, there's no abdominal incision, which means less scar tissue, fewer issues with healing the surgical wounds, and less chance of developing a chronic fistula from the pancreas to the skin.

One of the breakthroughs in minimally invasive surgery has been the development of robotic tools. These procedures involve surgical instruments being manipulated by robotic arms that are moved by the surgeon. Operating around certain parts of the body, such as the pelvis, can be particularly challenging for surgeons. As Hawn explains,

> It's really hard to position yourself as a surgeon to access the pelvis in a way that is ergonomically friendly to the surgeon's body. If the surgery is being done laparoscopically, the surgeon often needs to reach over and lean across a body. This can lead to injuries for the surgeons. The robot also has instruments that articulate allowing better access to smaller cavities. That's why robotic surgery has been widely adopted by urologists, gynecologists, and colorectal surgeons in particular.

Hawn talks about how surgery has changed over the past two decades, with innovations in technology leading to innovations in surgical techniques. In the past, surgeons would do something called an *exploratory laparotomy*, which involved making an incision from the chest down to the lower abdomen, in order to explore the abdomen and figure out a path forward. Today, such procedures are uncommon.

> Going into an operation, we have a much broader understanding of the patient's anatomy and their pathology because we'll often have high-quality imaging—typically from a CT scan or MRI—beforehand. We can detect if a disease has spread and if there are other diseases that haven't already been identified. We can draw on all of this information to determine what the optimal operation is going to be. Then we can say, "All right, what is the best approach to this patient and to dealing with this disease or the pathology?"

Looking to the future, Hawn expects to see significant progress in image-guided surgery: "In minimally invasive surgery, we're already operating off of images, which means we're not looking directly at the tissue that we're operating on, but rather looking at an image on a screen. In the future, we're going to have ways to augment those images." She says that contrast agents will illuminate certain structures. Today, it's possible to light up the gallbladder and the bile duct by giving a contrast agent that's excreted into the bile that will fluoresce if the wavelength of the light is changed. Over time, says Hawn, "additional agents will be developed that will help make surgery more precise by defining each patient's individual anatomy more clearly."

Hawn is one of the leaders of a national initiative focused on predicting patient risk factors, with a special emphasis on those patients who are at higher risk for having poor postoperative outcomes. Using prediction models can help hospitals prepare to have resources available in situations where high-risk patients are undergoing high-risk surgeries. But these high-risk surgeries are conducted in an environment marked by lower overall risk associated with surgery, as well as expanded access. "We are doing procedures on patients that would have been considered too risky to do 20 years ago. That's one of the greatest legacies of minimally invasive surgery."

* * *

Cures, and the search to uncover new ones, have always been fundamental features of medicine—and they will continue to be. But as the examples above demonstrate, there is steady movement in the direction of remedies that are more precisely tailored to the needs of each patient. Whether immunotherapy that draws on the power of one's own cells to combat cancer, or the window for stroke treatment being determined by the size of one's stroke, there is less reliance on the one-size-fits-all treatments of the past.

This is an encouraging development, and it's going to continue to be enabled by those individuals and institutions that push the proverbial envelope in pursuit of what they believe to be a better way of treating diseases and other medical conditions. These innovators and disruptors often face resistance from those who are invested in the status quo (literally and figuratively), but their pioneering spirit is fundamental to continued medical progress.

ACHIEVING PRECISION HEALTH: THE OPPORTUNITIES—AND CHALLENGES—AHEAD

One hundred years ago, human health was in a parlous state. World War I had recently ended, but the armistice brought little to celebrate. Somewhere between 35 million and 40 million people—soldiers and civilians—had been killed, and as the war was winding down, the so-called Spanish flu epidemic was setting in [1]. With devastating efficiency, it would kill approximately 50 million people throughout the world in about 18 months [2]. *Before* these events, global life expectancy had been estimated at just 34 years [3]. By 1919, it was almost certainly lower.

But the end of that ruinous decade, and the start of a new one, marked a radical new era of health and medicine. Investments in research started to pay dividends. A vaccine for tuberculosis was first administered to a human in 1921. Insulin was also discovered in 1921—changing diabetes from a near-certain death sentence to a manageable condition. Penicillin's discovery came a few years later, providing new ammunition to fight bacterial infections and saving millions of lives in the decades that followed. In the 1920s, several important vitamins were discovered (A, B, C, D, E, K). The decade also saw the first use of the iron lung, which enabled people with polio, whose respiratory functions were often impaired, to breathe easier.

Just as we look back at 1919 as an inflection point, I hope that 100 years from now someone will look back at 2019 and recognize its significance—a moment when there was renewed focus on the extraordinary potential enabled by the convergence of digital health technology, big data, artificial intelligence, genomics, metabolomics, proteomics, and cell-free DNA detection. Together, these things—and others like them—have dramatically expanded our knowledge about the determinants of health and disease. That makes it possible to completely transform our approach to the study of health and the delivery of health care. The Precision Health vision I've laid out in this book can be at the center of this new approach.

Discovering Precision Health: Predict, Prevent, and Cure to Advance Health and Well-Being, First Edition. Lloyd Minor and Matthew Rees.
© 2020 John Wiley & Sons Ltd. Published 2020 by John Wiley & Sons Ltd.

Fundamental to today's transformation is a focus on something that links us to the efforts of a century ago. One of the cornerstones of Precision Health is trying to prevent numerous diseases before they strike. We are distinguished from our early-20th-century predecessors by the ability to draw on new knowledge and new technology to predict the likelihood of disease, which can lead to early and well-targeted interventions. Similarly, that new knowledge and new technology gives us the ability to be precise in our approaches to health and medical care—tailoring them to individual variations so that doctors can recommend therapies that are based on a comprehensive understanding of individual patients (and other patients like them).

The innovations and disruptions I featured in chapter 3, coupled with the discovery-based, fundamental research I described in chapter 4, hold the keys to many of the transformative changes in health and health care delivery that we will see in the future. We are likely to see even more changes as companies like Amazon, Apple, and Google focus on consumer health. Amazon, for example, has teamed up with JPMorgan and Berkshire Hathaway on a venture that's focused on reducing health care costs. In a CNBC interview, the CEO of JPMorgan, Jamie Dimon, spoke to how the venture will proceed:

> We think together we have the right people, a long-term view, we're not profit-seeking, and that we can do what we're doing a lot better. We don't expect progress in the immediate future—like a year or two—but if we come up with some great stuff, we're going to share it with everybody....
>
> We're going to give it our best shot and be very patient. I'll remind people that Jeff Bezos, when he started Amazon, he might have had visions about the "everything store," but he started with books. And he spent 10 years getting books right. So we may spend a bunch of time getting one piece of it right, and testing various things to see what works [4].

I am encouraged by this approach and the long-term focus in particular. Because health insurers and health care providers are running their day-to-day businesses and having to meet quarterly earnings expectations, it's very difficult for them to take the long view. By contrast, these three companies can take the time they need, and because they're not coming from the health care sector, they can put forward the kind of unorthodox ideas that may lead to comprehensive changes.

As for Apple, its partnership with Stanford on the atrial fibrillation study is indicative of the company's growing interest in health. In 2018, the company announced that consumers could aggregate their EHR data on their iPhones. Apple CEO Tim Cook laid out his vision for the company's legacy during a January 2019 interview with CNBC:

> If you zoom out into the future, and you look back, and you ask the question, "What was Apple's greatest contribution to mankind?" it will be about health. ...
> We are democratizing it. We are taking what has been with the institutions and empowering the individual to manage their health [5].

Google has also prioritized work on health. It is sponsoring a major study of human health, which I describe below, and it started a research and development company called Calico, which is dedicated to expanding understanding of the biology that controls life-span. Google has hired several leading health care executives, such as David Feinberg, who had served as CEO of the Pennsylvania-based Geisinger Health System, and Toby Cosgrove, who had been CEO of the Cleveland Clinic. Jeff Dean, a senior Google executive, describes how the company views its health care work.

> Google's origins are in taking information in the world and then organizing it for people so that it's useful. It's pretty clear that health care is a specific domain where there's lots of information available in distributed form, and there are lots of complexities in the ecosystem. But being able to organize that information can make a real difference in patient care. It can lead to people living longer and getting better decisions, and it can lead to doctors feeling more confident in the decisions they make. So this is a real significant effort for us that plays to our natural strengths.

These companies bring a deep understanding of something that's often lacking in health care: the customer experience. That can translate to increased utilization of digital health tools. "If consumers are not afraid of the technology, they will want to access it," says Sue Siegel, an entrepreneur and former chief innovation officer at GE and CEO of GE Ventures. "That alone is going to improve the health of those consumers. And if the process can be educational, consumers will develop a better understanding of how to prevent illness and how to stay healthy."

It's too early to tell if Amazon, Apple, and Google will achieve their objectives, but given their success—and disruptive impact—in other sectors, I am glad to see each of them moving into health care. Even so, progress in health is far from preordained. As I detailed in different chapters, health care innovation is difficult (and often extremely expensive)—whether it's new drugs, new devices, or new tools, like IBM's Watson, which has struggled to deliver the health information insights that its leaders touted [6]. Regulation factors into the slow pace of progress; so does the extraordinarily complex structure of the U.S. health care system.

There are many other challenges ahead. It's distressing to see the many different medical and technological advances I've described in this book coincide with a global trend of only modest progress in reducing the incidence of noncommunicable diseases, such as cancer, cardiovascular disease, and diabetes [7]. It's estimated that in 2016, 71 percent of all deaths, throughout the world, stemmed from such diseases [8]. Direct or indirect exposure to just one product—tobacco—kills more than seven million people each year. That's more than 19,000 every day [9].

Similarly, the United States and other advanced economies are home to many health-related challenges, with significant health disparities based on differences in income and education. The United States in particular has poor outcomes on broad measures of health despite high levels of spending on medical care.

We should see gradual improvements in health as new medicines and new technologies—many of which I've described in the preceding chapters—become available. But in the United States and other advanced economies, the biggest gains are likely to come from addressing the social, environmental, and behavioral factors that play such a major role in determining individual health. As I mentioned in chapter 6, the dramatic decline in smoking rates over the past 50 years reminds us that life-threatening behaviors can change. More recently, there has been a significant decline in mortality rates from heart disease in the United States—falling 28 percent from 2003 to 2015 [10].

But there are still significant challenges ahead—with several troubling indicators. In 2017, for example, there were 70,000 deaths from drug overdoses—a record number, and more than quadruple the number in 1999. Drug abuse was far from the only condition ailing the United States. As one journalist noted, "In the nation's 10 leading causes of death, only the cancer death rate fell in 2017. Meanwhile, there were increases in seven others—suicide, stroke, diabetes, Alzheimer's, flu/pneumonia, chronic lower respiratory diseases and unintentional injuries" [11]. Even with the decline in cigarette smoking, it is still the leading cause of preventable death—responsible for approximately 480,000 deaths in the United States each year [12].

The spread of claims that are not grounded in science poses a very different kind of challenge. Emblematic of this trend is the turn away from child vaccinations. The World Health Organization named voluntary resistance to vaccines one of the top 10 global health threats for 2019 [13]. In California's Marin County, which has one of the best-educated populations of any county in the country, nearly one in five children under the age of 36 months has not been fully vaccinated, according to a 2015 Kaiser Permanente study. U.S. government data show that since 2001 there has been a quadrupling of the percentage of children who have not been vaccinated. This is largely because of fears about side effects—fears that are not supported by science. Reduced vaccination rates heighten the risk of people becoming infected with measles—a potential threat that was realized in early 2019, leading officials in Clark County, Washington, to declare a public health emergency [14].

Overcoming these challenges, and others like them, will take time and will require specifically tailored solutions. As we strive to meet them, we can't lose sight of a longer-term goal: deepening our understanding of human biology and focusing on translating what we learn into new therapies. Fundamental research has been—and always will be—our most constant and reliable source of discovery and progress. That research is being conducted throughout the world, and it's one of the many reasons I remain very optimistic about the future. I expect two research initiatives in particular to yield valuable insights and help advance the Precision Health vision.

One of those initiatives, the Project Baseline Health Study, is the most ambitious study of human health ever conducted. Its goal is to enroll up to approximately 10,000 individuals, beginning at sites in the San Francisco Bay Area, North

Carolina, and Los Angeles. The study will recruit a broad range of participants across the entire health spectrum. It will include those who are healthy as well as an enriched population with an elevated risk of cardiovascular disease, lung cancer, and breast/ovarian cancers. The project, which is being underwritten by Verily, is an academic-industry partnership including Stanford Medicine and the Duke School of Medicine. It will be measuring just about everything imaginable, including saliva, stool, the microbiome, cardiac imaging, and the genome. The subjects will also use wearable devices for continuous monitoring, and there will be sensors in their residence to monitor sleep patterns. They will be tracked longitudinally, and, for the first time, there will be enough baseline data so that when individuals experience a health condition, it will be possible to look back and identify what might have predicted that condition. All the participants have given their consent to have their data analyzed, and the researchers have engaged heavily with local individuals and institutions to create a community of participants, to enhance the research experience for them. The ultimate goal is to make the Project Baseline Health Study data available to the public.

The other initiative is called All of Us. It is loosely modeled on the Framingham Study (as is Project Baseline), which I mentioned in the introduction, with the chief difference being that it draws from people throughout the country, with more diversity in terms of the people participating, the health conditions being followed, and the data captured. Launched in May 2018, and sponsored by the National Institutes of Health, the effort calls for recruiting approximately one million people to participate in the study, by 2023, with 70 to 75 percent of those enrolled to be representatives of groups who have been historically underrepresented in biomedical research, and 50 percent to be ethnic and racial minorities. Enrollees will agree to share their health data over many years, and that de-identified data will be made available publicly, to help drive research into different diseases and to explore possible linkages between the environments in which people live and different health outcomes. (Some researchers, approved by All of Us, will be able to see individual health data.) Given its size, and the profiles of those being enrolled, All of Us has the potential to help unlock valuable new knowledge and advance the Precision Health objectives of predicting, preventing, and curing disease—precisely.

* * *

I began this book by describing a scenario in which you face a high risk of pancreatic cancer—one of the deadliest forms of cancer, given the difficulty of early detection. But through a program of close surveillance and monitoring, complemented by close coordination with your physician and targeted therapies, a tiny pancreatic tumor is destroyed at an early stage of development. Given the developments I've described through this book, I hope you can understand even better how predicting, preventing, and curing conditions such as pancreatic cancer is not a pie-in-the-sky goal—it is truly within our grasp.

I expect there to be steady progress in our powers of predicting, preventing, and curing disease—precisely. But that progress depends on continuing to nurture the innovative and disruptive spirit—in places like research universities and academic medical centers, pharmaceutical companies, and the digital health sector. That spirit is what gives rise to breakthroughs such as Stan Cohen and Herb Boyer unlocking the ability to clone genes or, more recently, Karl Deisseroth developing the discipline of optogenetics.

Achieving the full potential of Precision Health will also require much more focus on the social, environmental, and behavioral determinants of health. As described in chapter 2, these determinants have far more impact on health than our investments and areas of focus have reflected in the past. They are also among the most difficult areas to address. But as discussed in this book, meaningful progress is underway across the landscape of health and health care. Improving air quality reduces the incidence of asthma in children. Digital health tools are enabling better outcomes for people living with conditions such as diabetes. New technologies are expanding our understanding of the mechanisms of psychiatric conditions—such as depression—and providing insights on effective treatments.

While developments like these are a critical piece of the future health care puzzle, maximizing the opportunities ahead will also depend on steady infusions of fresh thinking about science, health, and the practice of medicine. That thinking will enable discovery-focused, fundamental research to continue unraveling the mysteries of the human body and help lay the foundation for more effective ways of predicting and preventing disease. Just as important will be refining how we approach the social determinants of health. Finally, those who are on the front lines of health—doctors, nurses, and other health care professionals—will need to continually adapt to evolving patient desires, while also continuing to play critical roles in treating disease, and helping their patients understand how to get healthy and stay healthy.

One of the central themes of this book has been that digital tools are destined to make deeper inroads into the health care system. A technology-focused columnist for the *Wall Street Journal,* Andy Kessler, has written, "Doctors don't scale, so the real future of medicine is digital diagnosis. The best doctor sees one patient at a time, but a clever piece of code can be used by countless people" [15]. This is true, up to a point. Artificial intelligence, for example, will help democratize access to knowledge, as certain diagnoses will not be entirely dependent on experts who may be in short supply in certain parts of the world. But a study of ClickWell, which I mentioned in chapter 6, found that although young people are open to receiving care virtually, they still want their first interaction to be with a human health care professional [16]. I don't see that dynamic changing anytime soon.

I'm hopeful that the vision for Precision Health I've spelled out in this book can be a catalyst for that new thinking and help spur the long-term changes that lead to better health and wellness, and accelerated human progress, throughout the world.

NOTES

INTRODUCTION

1. https://www.cancer.net/cancer-types/pancreatic-cancer/stages
2. http://pancreatic.org/pancreatic-cancer/pancreatic-cancer-facts/
3. https://www.cancer.org/content/dam/cancer-org/research/cancer-facts-and-statistics/annual-cancer-facts-and-figures/2017/cancer-facts-and-figures-2017.pdf
4. "Reports and Papers Presented at the Meetings of the American Public Health Association," 1873. Accessed online March 2, 2018: https://tinyurl.com/yc5ukpde
5. https://www.framinghamheartstudy.org/fhs-about/history/epidemiological-background/
6. https://www.framinghamheartstudy.org/fhs-risk-functions/
7. "How Tech Can Turn Doctors Into Clerical Workers," *New York Times*, May 16, 2018. https://www.nytimes.com/interactive/2018/05/16/magazine/health-issue-what-we-lose-with-data-driven-medicine.html
8. http://med.stanford.edu/news/all-news/2018/02/5-questions-sam-gambhir-on-progress-in-precision-health.html
9. Ibid.
10. http://stanmed.stanford.edu/2016winter/target-health.html
11. http://med.stanford.edu/news/all-news/2018/02/5-questions-sam-gambhir-on-progress-in-precision-health.html
12. "Defeating the ZIP Code Health Paradigm: Data, Technology, and Collaboration are Key," Health Affairs blog, August 6, 2015. https://www.healthaffairs.org/do/10.1377/hblog20150806.049730/full/
13. https://www.healthsystemtracker.org/chart-collection/u-s-life-expectancy-compare-countries/
14. https://www.healthsystemtracker.org/chart-collection/infant-mortality-u-s-compare-countries/#item-infant-mortality-higher-u-s-comparable-countries
15. "Sound- and/or pressure-induced vertigo due to bone dehiscence of the superior semicircular canal," *Archives of Otolaryngology—Head & Neck Surgery*, March 1998. https://jamanetwork.com/journals/jamaotolaryngology/fullarticle/219008
16. Thomas Goetz, *The Decision Tree: Taking Control of Your Health in the New Era of Personalized Medicine* (New York: Rodale Books, 2010).
17. https://obamawhitehouse.archives.gov/photos-and-video/video/2015/01/30/president-obama-speaks-precision-medicine-initiative

18. "A New Initiative on Precision Medicine," *New England Journal of Medicine*, February 26, 2015. https://www.nejm.org/doi/full/10.1056/NEJMp1500523

19. Disclosure of relationships that leaders of academic institutions and medical centers have with industry is important in ensuring the integrity of the mission of these institutions. As of May 2019, I am a member of advisory boards for the following companies for which I receive compensation for my activities: Ancestry, Mammoth Biosciences, Mission Bio, and Sensyne Health. I am also a compensated advisor to General Atlantic, a private equity firm. I am a member of the advisory board of Thrive Global, for which I receive no compensation. As a part of my role as Dean of Medicine at Stanford, I am on an advisory board focused on exploring collaborations between Novartis and academic institutions in the area of digital health. I receive no compensation from Novartis in this role. I own common stock in Apple and in Alphabet. This stock was purchased before any significant digital health collaborations between the Stanford School of Medicine and these companies, and I have not bought or sold stock in these companies since that time.

CHAPTER 1

1. https://www.youtube.com/watch?v=ssw0QanLS74

2. https://www.cdc.gov/nchs/data/nvsr/nvsr66/nvsr66_04.pdf (Table 19)

3. https://www.cia.gov/library/publications/the-world-factbook/rankorder/2102rank.html

4. https://data.worldbank.org/indicator/SP.DYN.LE00.IN?year_low_desc=true

5. "Inequalities in Life Expectancy Among US Counties, 1980 to 2014: Temporal Trends and Key Drivers," *JAMA Internal Medicine,* July 2017. https://jamanetwork.com/journals/jamainternalmedicine/fullarticle/2626194

6. "The Association Between Income and Life Expectancy in the United States, 2001–2014," *Journal of the American Medical Association*, April 26, 2016. https://jamanetwork.com/journals/jama/article-abstract/2513561

7. Ibid.

8. "Wealth Inequality in the United States since 1913: Evidence from Capitalized Income Tax Data," *Quarterly Journal of Economics*, May 2016, 519–578. https://doi.org/10.1093/qje/qjw004

9. "Socioeconomic Differences in the Epidemiologic Transition from Heart Disease to Cancer as the Leading Cause of Death in the United States, 2003 to 2015: An Observational Study," *Annals of Internal Medicine*, December 18, 2018. https://annals.org/aim/article-abstract/2715460/socioeconomic-differences-epidemiologic-transition-from-heart-disease-cancer-leading-cause

10. "U.S. Health in International Perspective: Shorter Lives, Poorer Health," National Academies Press; 2013. www.ncbi.nlm.nih.gov/books/NBK115854/

11. "US Burden of Disease Collaborators. The State of US Health, 1990–2010 Burden of Diseases, Injuries, and Risk Factors," *Journal of the American Medical Association,* August 14, 2013. https://jamanetwork.com/journals/jama/fullarticle/1710486

12. https://jamanetwork.com/data/Journals/JAMA/936922/joi180029t1.png

13. Ibid.

14. "Prevalence of obesity among adults and youth: United States, 2015–2016," National Center for Health Statistics. 2017. https://www.cdc.gov/nchs/products/databriefs/db288.htm

15. "World-wide trends in body mass index, underweight, overweight, and obesity from 1975–2016: a pooled analysis of 2416 population-based measurement studies in 128.9 million children, adolescents, and adults," *The Lancet*, December 16, 2017.

16. "Health Effects of Overweight and Obesity in 195 Countries Over 25 Years," *New England Journal of Medicine*, July 6, 2017. http://www.nejm.org/doi/full/10.1056/NEJMoa1614362

17. "U.S. Health Care Quality Ratings Among Lowest Since '12," Gallup, November 30, 2017.

18. "Americans Still Hold Dim View of U.S. Healthcare System," Gallup, December 11, 2017.
19. "The fax of life: Why American medicine still runs on fax machines," Vox, January 12, 2018. https://www.vox.com/health-care/2017/10/30/16228054/american-medical-system-fax-machines-why
20. "How Tech Can Turn Doctors Into Clerical Workers," *New York Times Magazine*, May 16, 2018. https://www.nytimes.com/interactive/2018/05/16/magazine/health-issue-what-we-lose-with-data-driven-medicine.html
21. "Physician Burnout in the Electronic Health Record Era: Are We Ignoring the Real Cause?" *Annals of Internal Medicine*, May 8, 2018. https://annals.org/aim/article-abstract/2680726/physician-burnout-electronic-health-record-era-we-ignoring-real-cause
22. "The Future of Electronic Health Records," Stanford Medicine, September 2018. http://med.stanford.edu/content/dam/sm/ehr/documents/SM-EHR-White-Papers_v12.pdf
23. "Death by a Thousand Clicks: Where Electronic Health Records Went Wrong," *Fortune*, March 18, 2019. http://fortune.com/longform/medical-records/
24. https://www.cms.gov/research-statistics-data-and-systems/statistics-trends-and-reports/nationalhealthexpenddata/nhe-fact-sheet.html
25. http://stats.oecd.org/Index.aspx?DataSetCode=SHA
26. "How does health spending in the U.S. compare to other countries?" Kaiser Family Foundation, December 7, 2018. https://www.healthsystemtracker.org/chart-collection/health-spending-u-s-compare-countries/#item-average-wealthy-countries-spend-half-much-per-person-health-u-s-spends
27. Elisabeth Rosenthal, *An American Sickness: How Healthcare Became Big Business and How You Can Take It Back* (Penguin, 2017), p. 2.
28. "Remarks on Value-Based Transformation to the Federation of American Hospitals," March 5, 2018. https://www.hhs.gov/about/leadership/secretary/speeches/2018-speeches/remarks-on-value-based-transformation-to-the-federation-of-american-hospitals.html?new
29. "Medical errors may stem more from physician burnout than unsafe health care settings," Stanford Medicine, July 8, 2018. https://med.stanford.edu/news/all-news/2018/07/medical-errors-may-stem-more-from-physician-burnout.html
30. "Physician Well-Being: The Reciprocity of Practice Efficiency, Culture of Wellness, and Personal Resilience," *NEJM Catalyst*, August 7, 2017. https://catalyst.nejm.org/physician-well-being-efficiency-wellness-resilience/
31. "Research Shows Shortage of More than 100,000 Doctors by 2030," Association of American Medical Colleges, March 14, 2017. https://www.aamc.org/news-insights/research-shows-shortage-more-100000-doctors-2030
32. http://wellmd.stanford.edu/content/dam/sm/wellmd/documents/2017-ACPH-Hamidi.pdf
33. "Symptoms of burnout common among medical residents; UW taking steps to help," *UW News*, March 4, 2002. http://www.washington.edu/news/2002/03/04/symptoms-of-burnout-common-among-medical-residents-uw-taking-steps-to-help/
34. "Intervention to promote physician well-being, job satisfaction, and professionalism: a randomized clinical trial." *JAMA Internal Medicine*, April 17, 2014. https://www.ncbi.nlm.nih.gov/pubmed/24515493
"A randomized controlled trial evaluating the effect of COMPASS (Colleagues Meeting to Promote and Sustain Satisfaction) small group sessions on physician well-being, meaning, and job satisfaction," *Journal of General Internal Medicine*, April 2015.
35. "Physician and Nurse Well-Being: Seven Things Hospital Boards Should Know," *Journal of Healthcare Management*, November/December 2018. https://www.ncbi.nlm.nih.gov/pubmed/30418362
36. "Making the Case for the Chief Wellness Officer in America's Health Systems: A Call to Action," Health Affairs blog, October 26, 2018. https://www.healthaffairs.org/do/10.1377/hblog20181025.308059/full/

CHAPTER 2

1. "The Case for More Active Policy Attention to Health Promotion," Health Affairs, March/April 2002. https://www.healthaffairs.org/doi/10.1377/hlthaff.21.2.78
   American Journal of Preventive Medicine, February 2017, pp. 129–135. https://www.ajpmonline.org/article/S0749-3797(15)00514-0/fulltext
   Commission on Social Determinants of Health, The World Health Organization, 2008. https://www.who.int/social_determinants/thecommission/finalreport/en/
   "The Key Role of Epigenetics in Human Disease Prevention and Mitigation," *New England Journal of Medicine*, April 5, 2018. https://www.nejm.org/doi/full/10.1056/NEJMra1402513
2. "Prevalence of Obesity Among Adults, by Household Income and Education—United States, 2011–14," Centers for Disease Control and Prevention, December 22, 2017. https://www.cdc.gov/mmwr/volumes/66/wr/pdfs/mm6650a1-H.pdf
3. "Cigarette Smoking and Tobacco Use Among People of Low Socioeconomic Status," Centers for Disease Control and Prevention. https://www.cdc.gov/tobacco/disparities/low-ses/index.htm
4. Robert M. Kaplan and Arnold Milstein, "Contributions of Healthcare to Longevity: A Review of Four Estimation Methods," *Annals of Family Medicine*, May/June 2019. http://www.annfammed.org/content/17/3/267.full
5. "Bad genes don't mean you are doomed to heart disease and early death," *Washington Post*, February 27, 2018. https://www.washingtonpost.com/national/health-science/bad-genes-dont-mean-you-are-doomed-to-heart-disease-and-early-death/2018/02/23/ddf19a78-0b73-11e8-8890-372e2047c935_story.html?
6. "Genes can push you toward obesity, but there are things you can do to prevent that," *Washington Post*, August 13, 2017. https://www.washingtonpost.com/national/health-science/genes-can-push-you-toward-obesity-but-there-are-things-you-can-do-to-prevent-that/2017/08/11/5bb7a80e-77ad-11e7-8f39-eeb7d3a2d304_story.html?
7. "Friends and Family May Play a Role in Obesity," National Institutes of Health, August 13, 2007. https://www.nih.gov/news-events/nih-research-matters/friends-family-may-play-role-obesity
8. "Obesity Is 'Socially Contagious,' Study Finds," UCSD News Center, July 25, 2007. https://ucsdnews.ucsd.edu/archive/newsrel/soc/07-07ObesityIK-.asp
9. "Physical Activity Attenuates the Influence of *FTO* Variants on Obesity Risk: A Meta-Analysis of 218,166 Adults and 19,268 Children," *PLOS Medicine*, November 1, 2011. https://journals.plos.org/plosmedicine/article?id=10.1371/journal.pmed.1001116
10. "Well now: What humans need to flourish," Stanford Medicine, Summer 2016. https://stanmed.stanford.edu/2016summer/well-now.html
11. "The thrifty phenotype hypothesis: Type 2 diabetes, *British Medical Bulletin*, November 2001. https://academic.oup.com/bmb/article/60/1/5/322752
12. "Association of Improved Air Quality with Lung Development in Children," *New England Journal of Medicine*, March 5, 2015. https://www.nejm.org/doi/full/10.1056/NEJMoa1414123
13. "FEAST: Empowering community residents to use technology to assess and advocate for healthy food environments," *Journal of Urban Health*, 2017.
    Buman MP, Winter SJ, Baker C, Hekler EB, Otten JJ, King AC, "Neighborhood Eating and Activity Advocacy Teams (NEAAT): engaging older adults in policy activities to improve food and physical environments." *Transl Behav Med* 2012, 2(2):249–253.
14. "A qualitative study of shopper experiences at an urban farmers' market using the Stanford Healthy Neighborhood Discovery Tool," *Public Health Nutrition*, April 2015. https://www.ncbi.nlm.nih.gov/pubmed/24956064
15. "Harnessing Technology and Citizen Science to Support Neighborhoods That Promote Active Living in Mexico," *Journal of Urban Health*, December 2016. https://www.ncbi.nlm.nih.gov/pubmed/27752825

16. "Maximizing the promise of citizen science to advance health and prevent disease," *Preventive Medicine*, February 2019. https://www.ncbi.nlm.nih.gov/pubmed/30593793

17. "The Stanford Healthy Neighborhood Discovery Tool: a computerized tool to assess active living environments," *American Journal of Preventive Medicine*, April 2013. https://www.ncbi.nlm.nih.gov/pubmed/23498112

18. "Well now," Stanford Medicine, Summer 2016.

19. "Smart phones could be game-changing tool for cardiovascular research," Stanford Medicine News Center, December 14, 2016. https://med.stanford.edu/news/all-news/2016/12/smartphones-could-be-game-changing-tool-for-cardiovascular-research.html

20. "Arianna Huffington Thought 'Huff Post' Would Be Her Last Chapter. Was She Ever Wrong." *Entrepreneur,* October 26, 2018. https://www.entrepreneur.com/article/322204

21. "How to make healthy life changes from tiny habits," WRVO, August 13, 2016. https://www.wrvo.org/post/how-make-healthy-life-changes-tiny-habits

CHAPTER 3

1. "2018 Year End Funding Report: Is digital health in a bubble?" Rock Health. https://rockhealth.com/reports/2018-year-end-funding-report-is-digital-health-in-a-bubble/

2. "Internet Trends 2017—Code Conference," May 31, 2017. https://www.kleinerperkins.com/perspectives/internet-trends-report-2017

3. "6 Reasons Why Digital Health Startups Will Fail (Obamacare Repeal Won't Be One of Them)," Medtech Boston, January 9, 2017. https://medtechboston.medstro.com/blog/2017/01/09/6-reasons-why-digital-health-startups-will-fail-obamacare-repeal-wont-be-one-of-them/

4. Ibid.

5. "The secret weapon of World War II," *Baltimore Sun,* January 11, 1993. http://articles.baltimoresun.com/1993-01-11/news/1993011049_1_fuse-proximity-smart-weapons

6. Ibid.

7. "The Cell's Integrated Circuit: A profile of Lucy Shapiro," *The Scientist,* August 1, 2018. https://www.the-scientist.com/profile/the-cells-integrated-circuit--a-profile-of-lucy-shapiro-64496

8. Ibid.

9. "More can benefit from stroke treatment," *Stanford Medicine Newsletter*, Summer 2018. https://med.stanford.edu/communitynews/2018summer/more-can-benefit-from-stroke-treatment.html

10. "Prompt clot-grabbing treatment produces better stroke outcomes," American Heart Association, January 25, 2018. http://newsroom.heart.org/news/prompt-clot-grabbing-treatment-produces-better-stroke-outcomes

11. "Thrombectomy for Stroke at 6 to 16 Hours with Selection by Perfusion Imaging," *New England Journal of Medicine*, February 22, 2018. https://www.nejm.org/doi/full/10.1056/NEJMoa1713973

12. "Stanford-led clinical trials shows broader benefits of acute stroke therapy," Stanford Medicine News Center, January 24, 2018. https://med.stanford.edu/news/all-news/2018/01/clinical-trial-shows-broader-benefits-of-acute-stroke-therapy.html

13. "More can benefit from stroke treatment," *Stanford Medicine Newsletter*, Summer 2018.

14. Ibid.

15. "Greg Albers: Changing the face of the stroke stopwatch," *The Lancet,* January 5, 2017. https://www.thelancet.com/journals/laneur/article/PIIS1474-4422(16)30386-6/fulltext

16. "Purification and characterization of mouse hematopoietic stems cells," *Science*, July 1, 1988. http://science.sciencemag.org/content/241/4861/58

17. "Long-Term Outcome of Patients with Metastatic Breast Cancer Treated with High-Dose Chemotherapy and Transplantation of Purified Autologous Hematopoietic Stem Cells," *Biology of Blood and Marrow Transplantation*, January 2012. https://www.bbmt.org/article/S1083-8791(11)00299-0/fulltext

18. "Survival of stage IV breast cancer patients improves with stem cell treatment, study finds," Stanford Medicine News Center, July 22, 2011. https://med.stanford.edu/news/all-news/2011/07/survival-of-stage-iv-breast-cancer-patients-improves-with-stem-cell-treatment-study-finds.html

19. "Anti-CD47 cancer therapy safe, shows promise in small clinical trial," Stanford Medicine News Center, October 31, 2018. https://med.stanford.edu/news/all-news/2018/10/anti-cd47-cancer-therapy-safe-shows-promise-in-small-trial.html

20. Ibid.

21. "Efficient transplantation via antibody-based clearance of hematopoietic stem cell niches," *Science*, November 23, 2007. https://www.ncbi.nlm.nih.gov/pubmed/18033883; "Hematopoietic stem cell transplantation in immunocompetent hosts without radiation or chemotherapy," *Science Translational Medicine*, August 10, 2016. https://www.ncbi.nlm.nih.gov/pubmed/27510901

22. "How One Thing Led to Another," *Annual Review of Immunology*, May 2016. https://www.annualreviews.org/doi/10.1146/annurev-immunol-032414-112003

23. Mark M. Davis, "A Prescription for Human Immunology," *Immunity*, December 19, 2008.

24. "1 in 3 adults don't get enough sleep," Centers for Disease Control and Prevention," February 18, 2016. https://www.cdc.gov/media/releases/2016/p0215-enough-sleep.html

25. "A harrowing journey through disordered sleep," *Nature*, February 27, 2018. https://www.nature.com/articles/d41586-018-02510-3

26. "Artificial Intelligence May Unlock the Mysteries of Sleep Testing," Thrive Global, December 10, 2018. https://thriveglobal.com/stories/this-device-may-be-key-to-finding-out-why-you-arent-sleeping/

27. "Neural network analysis of sleep stages enables efficient diagnosis of narcolepsy," *Nature*, December 6, 2018. https://www.nature.com/articles/s41467-018-07229-3

28. "A harrowing journey through disordered sleep," *Nature*, February 27, 2018.

29. "Prevalence and Severity of Food Allergies Among US Adults," JAMA Network Open, January 4, 2019. https://jamanetwork.com/journals/jamanetworkopen/fullarticle/2720064?mod=article_inline

30. "The Public Health Impact of Child-Reported Food Allergies in the United States," *Pediatrics*, December 2018. http://pediatrics.aappublications.org/content/142/6/e20181235?mod=article_inline

31. "Trends in Allergic Conditions Among Children: United States, 1997–2011," National Center for Health Statistics, May 2013. https://www.cdc.gov/nchs/products/databriefs/db121.htm

32. https://www.nimh.nih.gov/health/statistics/mental-illness.shtml

33. https://med.stanford.edu/psychiatry/special-initiatives/precisionpsychiatry/pmhw.html

34. "To Diagnose Mental Illness, Read the Brain," *Scientific American*, June 25, 2016. https://www.scientificamerican.com/article/to-diagnose-mental-illness-read-the-brain/

35. "Initial Severity and Antidepressant Benefits: A Meta-Analysis of Data Submitted to the Food and Drug Administration," *PLOS Medicine*, February 2008. https://www.ncbi.nlm.nih.gov/pmc/articles/PMC2253608/

36. https://es-la.facebook.com/worldeconomicforum/videos/10153794471101479/

37. https://www.dailymotion.com/video/x31jyrp

38. "To Diagnose Mental Illness, Read the Brain," *Scientific American*, June 25, 2016.

39. https://es-la.facebook.com/worldeconomicforum/videos/10153794471101479/

40. "Data & Statistics on Autism Spectrum Disorder," Centers for Disease Control and Prevention. https://www.cdc.gov/ncbddd/autism/data.html

41. "Randomized, Controlled Trial of an Intervention for Toddlers with Autism: The Early Start Denver Mode," *Pediatrics*, January 2010. http://pediatrics.aappublications.org/content/125/1/e17.short

42. "The urgent need to shorten autism's diagnostic odyssey," Spectrum, July 15, 2014. https://www.spectrumnews.org/opinion/viewpoint/the-urgent-need-to-shorten-autisms-diagnostic-odyssey/

43. "Cognoa's AI platform for autism diagnosis gets first FDA stamp," *TechCrunch*, February 21, 2018. https://techcrunch.com/2018/02/21/cognoas-ai-platform-for-autism-diagnosis-gets-first-fda-stamp/

44. "Screening in toddlers and preschoolers at risk for autism spectrum disorder: Evaluating a novel mobile-health screening tool," *Autism Research*, July 2018. https://www.ncbi.nlm.nih.gov/pubmed/29734507 See also, "Machine learning approach for early detection of autism by

combining questionnaire and home video screening," *Journal of the American Medical Informatics Association*, August 2018. https://doi.org/10.1093/jamia/ocy039

45. "Exploratory study examining the at-home feasibility of a wearable tool for social-affective learning in children with autism," *npj Digital Medicine*, August 2, 2018. https://www.nature.com/articles/s41746-018-0035-3

46. "Innovation in the pharmaceutical industry: New estimates of R&D costs," *Journal of Health Economics*, May 2016. https://www.sciencedirect.com/science/article/abs/pii/S0167629616000291?via%3Dihub

47. "Her one-in-a-million baby," Stanford Children's Health. https://www.stanfordchildrens.org/en/service/fertility-and-reproductive-health/one-in-a-million-baby

48. "Meet Rhiju Das," Biomedical Beat Blog—National Institute of General Medical Sciences, July 9, 2014. https://biobeat.nigms.nih.gov/2014/07/meet-rhiju-das/

49. Rhiju Das, Benjamin Keep, Peter Washington, and Ingmar H. Riedel-Kruse, "Scientific discovery games for biomedical research," *Annual Review of Biomedical Data Science*, 2019.

50. Ibid.

51. "Principles for Predicting RNA Secondary Structure Design Difficulty," *Journal of Molecular Biology*, February 27, 2016. https://doi.org/10.1016/j.jmb.2015.11.013

52. "Power to the people: Does Eterna signal the arrival of a new wave of crowd-sourced projects?" *BMC Biochemistry*, October 23, 2013. https://www.ncbi.nlm.nih.gov/pmc/articles/PMC3854504/

53. "Diagnosing suspected arrhythmias: An interview with Uday Kumar of iRhythm," Stanford Byers Center for Biodesign. https://biodesign.stanford.edu/our-impact/technologies/irhythm.html

54. https://tedmed.com/talks/show?id=292997

55. Ibid.

56. http://10newtons.com/whatwedo/datascience/

57. "Sensor Technology in Assessments of Clinical Skill," *New England Journal of Medicine*, February 19, 2015. https://www.nejm.org/doi/full/10.1056/NEJMc1414210

58. http://10newtons.com/new-technology-seeks-to-teach-proper-self-breast-exam-techniques/

59. https://tedmed.com/talks/show?id=292997

60. https://vimeo.com/76445878

61. "Getting real: Medical residents experience global health needs firsthand," *Stanford Medicine*, Winter 2019. http://stanmed.stanford.edu/2019winter/residents-global-health-needs-firsthand.html

62. "Interventions to Improve Adherence to Self-Administered Medications for Chronic Diseases in the United States: A Systematic Review," *Annals of Internal Medicine*, December 4, 2012. http://annals.org/aim/fullarticle/1357338/interventions-improve-adherence-self-administered-medications-chronic-diseases-united-states

63. https://faq.impossiblefoods.com/hc/en-us/articles/360018936694-What-is-Impossible-Foods-mission-

64. https://impossiblefoods.com/mission/2019impact/

65. "Our Meatless Future: How the $90B Global Meat Market Gets Disrupted," CB Insights, January 16, 2019. https://www.cbinsights.com/research/future-of-meat-industrial-farming/?

66. "Why Most Published Research Findings Are False," *PLOS Medicine*, August 30, 2005. https://doi.org/10.1371/journal.pmed.0020124

67. "Primary Prevention of Cardiovascular Disease with a Mediterranean Diet," *New England Journal of Medicine*, April 4, 2013. https://www.nejm.org/doi/full/10.1056/NEJMoa1200303

68. "Retraction and Republication: Primary Prevention of Cardiovascular Disease with a Mediterranean Diet," *New England Journal of Medicine*, June 21, 2018. https://www.nejm.org/doi/full/10.1056/NEJMc1806491

69. "Science mapping analysis characterizes 235 biases in biomedical research" *Journal of Clinical Epidemiology*, November 2010. https://www.researchgate.net/publication/43182837_Science_mapping_analysis_characterizes_235_biases_in_biomedical_research

70. "Reproducible Research Practices and Transparency across the Biomedical Literature," *PLOS Biology*, January 4, 2016. http://journals.plos.org/plosbiology/article?id=10.1371/journal.pbio.1002333

71. "Reproducible research practices, transparency, and open access data in the biomedical literature, 2015–2017," *PLOS Biology*, November 20, 2018. https://journals.plos.org/plosbiology/article?id=10.1371/journal.pbio.2006930

72. https://www.sec.gov/litigation/complaints/2018/comp-pr2018-41-theranos-holmes.pdf

73. "Stealth Research: Is Biomedical Innovation Happening Outside the Peer-Reviewed Literature?" February 17, 2015. https://jamanetwork.com/journals/jama/article-abstract/2110977

74. http://www.demog.berkeley.edu/~andrew/1918/figure2.html

75. https://www.cdc.gov/nchs/data/databriefs/db293.pdf

CHAPTER 4

1. "Science: The Endless Frontier," A Report to the President by Vannevar Bush, Director of the Office of Scientific Research and Development, July 1945. https://www.nsf.gov/about/history/vbush1945.htm

2. Donald E. Stokes, *Pasteur's Quadrant: Basic Science and Technological Innovation* (Brookings Institution Press, 1997), pp. 73–74.

3. https://parkinsonsdisease.net/basics/statistics/

4. https://www.pbs.org/newshour/health/the-real-story-behind-the-worlds-first-antibiotic

5. "Francisco Mojica, the scientist who discovered CRISPR and DNA editing," ABC.net.au, June 14, 2018. https://www.abc.net.au/news/2018-06-15/francisco-mojica-scientist-who-discovered-crispr-dna-editing/9864070

6. Ibid.

7. Horace Freeland Judson, *The Eighth Day of Creation: The Makers of the Revolution in Biology* (Simon & Schuster, 1979) p. 326.

8. As quoted in Errol C. Friedberg, *A Biography of Paul Berg: The Recombinant DNA Controversy Revisited* (World Scientific Publishing, 2014), pp. 71–72.

9. Friedberg, *A Biography of Paul Berg*, p. 73.

10. Ibid.

11. Siddhartha Mukherjee, *The Gene: An Intimate History* (Scribner, 2017), p. 234.

12. Sally Smith Hughes, *Genentech: The Beginnings of Biotech* (University of Chicago Press, 2011), p. 10

13. Hughes, *Genentech*, pp. 10–11.

14. Hughes, *Genentech*, p. 11.

15. "DNA cloning: A personal view after 40 years," *PNAS*, September 24, 2013. https://www.pnas.org/content/110/39/15521

16. Stanley N. Cohen, M.D., "Science, Biotechnology, and Recombinant DNA: A Personal History," an oral history conducted by Sally Smith Hughes in 1995, Regional Oral History Office, The Bancroft Library, University of California, Berkeley, 2009.

17. https://www.nobelprize.org/prizes/medicine/2006/press-release/

18. "Potent and specific genetic interference by double-stranded RNA in *Caenorhabditis elegans*," *Nature*, February 19, 1998. https://www.nature.com/articles/35888

19. http://news.bbc.co.uk/2/hi/health/5398844.stm

20. https://www.nobelprize.org/prizes/chemistry/2012/kobilka/biographical/

21. "Stanford scientist Brian Kobilka wins Nobel Prize for Chemistry," Stanford News, October 10, 2012. https://news.stanford.edu/news/2012/october/nobel-prize-kobilka-101012.html

22. https://www.nobelprize.org/prizes/chemistry/2013/levitt/facts/

23. http://med.stanford.edu/news/all-news/2013/10/the-science-behind-michael-levitts-nobel-prize.html

24. https://www.nobelprize.org/prizes/medicine/2013/sudhof/biographical/
25. "Lighting the Brain: Karl Deisseroth and the optogenetics breakthrough," *The New Yorker*, May 11, 2015. https://www.newyorker.com/magazine/2015/05/18/lighting-the-brain
26. https://news.stanford.edu/features/2014/optogenetics/
27. "A Look Inside the Brain," *Scientific American*, October 2016. http://clarityresourcecenter.org/pdfs/Deisseroth_SciAm2016.pdf
28. The acronym is based on the following construction: "*c*lear *l*ipid-exchanged *a*crylamidehybridized *r*igid *i*maging/immunostaining/in situ hybridization-compatible *t*issue-hydrogel."
29. "Turning back time with emerging rejuvenation strategies," *Nature Cell Biology*, January 2, 2019. https://www.nature.com/articles/s41556-018-0206-0
30. https://web.stanford.edu/group/brunet/research%20interests.html
31. https://www.ted.com/talks/tony_wyss_coray_how_young_blood_might_help_reverse_aging_yes_really?language=en
32. "Redefining differentiation: Reshaping our ends," *Nature Cell Biology*, May 30, 2012. https://www.nature.com/articles/ncb2506?draft=collection
33. Ibid.
34. "Profile of Helen M. Blau," *Proceedings of the National Academy of Sciences*, October 31, 2017. https://www.pnas.org/content/114/44/11561 OF I L
35. "Plasticity of the differentiated state," *Science*, November 15, 1985. https://www.ncbi.nlm.nih.gov/pubmed/2414846
36. "Nuclear reprogramming to a pluripotent state by three approaches," *Nature*, June 9, 2010. https://www.nature.com/articles/nature09229
37. "Differentiation requires continuous regulation," *Journal of Cell Biology*, March 1991. https://www.ncbi.nlm.nih.gov/pubmed/1999456
38. https://med.stanford.edu/news/all-news/2010/12/new-mouse-model-for-duchenne-muscular-dystrophy-implicates-stem-cells-researchers-say.html
39. "Re'evolutionary' regenerative medicine," *Journal of the American Medical Association*, January 5, 2011. https://jamanetwork.com/journals/jama/article-abstract/644485
40. "Identification and specification of the mouse skeletal stem cell," *Cell*, January 15, 2015. https://doi.org/10.1016/j.cell.2014.12.002
41. https://med.stanford.edu/news/all-news/2015/01/researchers-isolate-stem-cell-that-gives-rise-to-bones-cartilage.html
42. "Identification of the human skeletal stem cell," *Cell*, September 20, 2018.
43. https://med.stanford.edu/news/all-news/2018/10/skeletal-stem-cells-regress-when-tasked-with-extensive-regeneration.html
44. "Human Skeletal Stem Cell Found," *The Scientist*, September 20, 2018. https://www.the-scientist.com/news-opinion/human-skeletal-stem-cell-found-64830
45. https://med.stanford.edu/news/all-news/2018/09/study-identifies-stem-cell-that-gives-rise-to-new-bone-cartilage.html
46. https://med.stanford.edu/news/all-news/2018/10/skeletal-stem-cells-regress-when-tasked-with-extensive-regeneration.html
47. "Genetics, FACS, Immunology and Redox: A Tale of Two Lives Intertwined," *Annual Reviews of Immunology*, December 16, 2003. https://www.annualreviews.org/doi/full/10.1146/annurev.immunol.22.012703.104727
48. "Leonard Herzenberg, geneticist who developed key cell-sorting technology, dies," Stanford Medicine News Centers, October 31, 2013. http://med.stanford.edu/news/all-news/2013/10/leonard-herzenberg-geneticist-who-developed-key-cell-sorting-technology-dies.html
49. https://www.nytimes.com/2013/11/11/us/leonard-herzenberg-immunologist-who-revolutionized-research-dies-at-81.html
50. http://med.stanford.edu/news/all-news/2013/10/leonard-herzenberg-geneticist-who-developed-key-cell-sorting-technology-dies.html
51. http://archive.sciencewatch.com/inter/aut/2008/08-apr/08aprNolan/

52. "Single-cell mass cytometry of differential immune and drug responses across a human hematopoietic continuum," F1000 Prime, May 6, 2011. https://f1000.com/prime/10641956?key=qllgw6hpwr306f5#

53. https://med.stanford.edu/news/all-news/2018/05/slac-stanford-open-facility-for-cryogenic-electron-microscopy.html

54. "Visualizing virus assembly intermediates inside marine cyanobacteria," *Nature*, October 9, 2013. https://www.nature.com/articles/nature12604

55. https://www.nobelprize.org/prizes/chemistry/2017/press-release/

56. "Refinement and Analysis of the Mature Zika Virus Cryo-Em Structure at 3.1 Å Resolution," *Cell*, June 26, 2018. https://www.cell.com/structure/fulltext/S0969-2126(18)30170-9

57. "Cryo-EM stuctures of tau filaments from Alzheimer's disease," *Nature*, July 5, 2017. https://www.nature.com/articles/nature23002

CHAPTER 5

1. https://www.canaryfoundation.org/about-canary/founders-story/

2. https://www.canaryfoundation.org/about-canary/

3. https://www.ncbi.nlm.nih.gov/books/NBK338586/

4. "New center sets out to stop disease before it starts," Stanford Medicine News Center, May 16, 2018. https://med.stanford.edu/news/all-news/2018/05/new-center-sets-out-to-stop-disease-before-it-starts.html

5. "QnAs with Stephen Quake," *Proceedings of the National Academy of Sciences*, August 2, 2016. https://www.pnas.org/content/113/31/8557

6. "Noninvasive diagnosis of fetal aneuploidy by shotgun sequencing DNA from maternal blood," *Proceedings of the National Academy of Sciences,* October 21, 2008. https://www.pnas.org/content/105/42/16266

7. "Cell-free DNA Analysis for Noninvasive Examination of Trisomy," *New England Journal of Medicine*, April 23, 2015. https://www.nejm.org/doi/full/10.1056/NEJMoa1407349

8. https://www.washingtonpost.com/national/health-science/a-safe-prenatal-genetic-test-is-gaining-popularity-with-young-moms-to-be-and-their-doctors/2019/01/04/746516a2-f4f2-11e8-bc79-68604ed88993_story.html?utm_term=.fbb1d97567b6

9. "Disruptive Technology: Dr. Diana Bianchi Talks Prenatal DNA Testing," *The NICHD Connection*, June 2019. https://science.nichd.nih.gov/confluence/display/newsletter/2017/09/07/Disruptive+Technology%3A+Dr.+Diana+Bianchi+Talks+Prenatal+DNA+Testing

10. "What are common treatments for Down syndrome?" National Institute of Child Health and Human Development. https://www.nichd.nih.gov/health/topics/down/conditioninfo/treatments#f2

11. https://www.cancer.org/cancer/breast-cancer/screening-tests-and-early-detection/mammograms/limitations-of-mammograms.html

12. "Ultrasound Molecular Imaging with BR55 in Patients with Breast and Ovarian Lesions: First-in-Human Results," *Journal of Clinical Oncology*, March 14, 2017. http://ascopubs.org/doi/abs/10.1200/JCO.2016.70.8594

13. http://med.stanford.edu/news/all-news/2017/04/ultrasound-and-microbubbles-flag-malignant-cancer-in-humans.html

14. "Cost-effectiveness of Screening for Breast Cancer with Magnetic Resonance Imaging in BRCA1/2 Mutation Carriers," *JAMA*, May 24, 2006. https://jamanetwork.com/journals/jama/fullarticle/202909

15. "American Cancer Society guidelines for breast screening with MRI as an adjunct to mammography." *CA: A Cancer Journal for Clinicians*, March–April 2007. https://www.ncbi.nlm.nih.gov/pubmed/17392385

16. "Effect of screening and adjuvant therapy on mortality from breast cancer," *New England Journal of Medicine*, October 27, 2005.

17. "Association of Screening and Treatment with Breast Cancer Mortality by Molecular Subtype in US Women, 2000–2012," *Journal of the American Medical Association*, January 9, 2018. https://jamanetwork.com/journals/jama/fullarticle/2668347

18. https://www.statnews.com/feature/retro-report/the-code/

19. https://www.genome.gov/12011238/an-overview-of-the-human-genome-project/

20. https://stanmed.stanford.edu/2017winter/could-genetic-mosaicism-have-caused-a-deadly-heart-arrhythmia-long-qt-syndrome.html

21. https://med.stanford.edu/news/all-news/2018/06/study-solves-mystery-of-genetic-test-results-for-patient-with-heart-condition.html.

22. https://newsroom.heart.org/news/gene-editing-technology-may-improve-accuracy-of-predicting-individuals-heart-disease-risk

23. "A Geneticist's Research Turns Personal," *New York Times*, June 2, 2012. https://www.nytimes.com/2012/06/03/business/geneticists-research-finds-his-own-diabetes.html

24. http://med.stanford.edu/news/all-news/2012/03/revolution-in-personalized-medicine-first-ever-integrative-omics-profile-lets-scientist-discover-track-his-diabetes-onset.html

25. "Personal Omics Profiling Reveals Dynamic Molecular and Medical Phenotypes," *Cell*, March 16, 2012. https://www.cell.com/cell/abstract/S0092-8674(12)00166-3

26. "NIH-Wide Strategic Plan: Fiscal Years 2016–2010," National Institutes of Health. https://www.nih.gov/sites/default/files/about-nih/strategic-plan-fy2016-2020-508.pdf, p. 20

27. *To Err Is Human: Building a Safer Health System* (Institute of Medicine, 2000). https://www.nap.edu/catalog/9728/to-err-is-human-building-a-safer-health-system

28. "Study Suggests Medical Errors Now Third Leading Cause of Death in the U.S.," Johns Hopkins Medicine, May 3, 2016. https://www.hopkinsmedicine.org/news/media/releases/study_suggests_medical_errors_now_third_leading_cause_of_death_in_the_us

29. "Your Sweat Will See You Now," *New York Times*, January 18, 2019. https://www.nytimes.com/2019/01/18/health/wearable-tech-sweat.html?

30. https://www.nejm.org/doi/full/10.1056/NEJMoa1901183?

31. "Predicting patient 'cost blooms' in Denmark: a longitudinal population-based study," *British Medical Journal*, January 11, 2017. https://bmjopen.bmj.com/content/7/1/e011580.info

32. "Bedside Computer Vision—Moving Artificial Intelligence from Driver Assistance to Patient Safety," *New England Journal of Medicine*, April 5, 2018. https://www.nejm.org/doi/10.1056/NEJMp1716891

33. "Identifying facial phenotypes of genetic disorders using deep learning," *Nature Medicine*, January 7, 2019. https://www.nature.com/articles/s41591-018-0279-0

34. "Scalable and accurate deep learning with electronic health records," *npj Digital Medicine*, May 8, 2018. https://www.nature.com/articles/s41746-018-0029-1

35. Ibid.

36. "Dermatologist-level classification of skin cancer with deep neural networks," *Nature*, January 25, 2017. https://www.nature.com/articles/nature21056

37. https://news.stanford.edu/2017/01/25/artificial-intelligence-used-identify-skin-cancer/

38. "Deep learning for chest radiograph diagnosis: A retrospective comparison of the CheXNeXt algorithm to practicing radiologists," *PLOS Medicine*, November 20, 2018. https://journals.plos.org/plosmedicine/article?id=10.1371/journal.pmed.1002686

39. "Deep-learning-assisted diagnosis for knee magnetic resonance imaging: Development and retrospective validation of MRNet," *PLOS Medicine*, November 27, 2018. https://journals.plos.org/plosmedicine/article?id=10.1371/journal.pmed.1002699

40. Bernard Lown, *The Lost Art of Healing: Practicing Compassion in Medicine* (Random House, 1999), pp. 9–10.

CHAPTER 6

1. "Association Between Dietary Factors and Mortality From Heart Disease, Stroke, and Type 2 Diabetes in the United States," *Journal of the American Medical Association*, March 7, 2017. https://jamanetwork.com/journals/jama/article-abstract/2608221

2. https://www.statista.com/chart/13945/the-words-that-make-groceries-less-appealing/

3. "Save the World, Prevent Obesity: Piggybacking on Existing Social and Ideological Movements," *Obesity*, February 2010.

4. http://www.who.int/dg/speeches/2013/health_promotion_20130610/en/

5. Thomas N. Robinson, "Stealth Interventions for Obesity," in Kelly Brownell and B. Timothy Walsh (eds.), *Eating Disorders and Obesity* (Guilford Press, 2018) p. 610.

6. "A Randomized Controlled Trial of Culturally Tailored Dance and Reducing Screen Time to Prevent Weight Gain in Low-Income African American Girls," *Archives of Pediatric Adolescent Medicine*, November 1, 2010. https://jamanetwork.com/journals/jamapediatrics/fullarticle/383967

7. Robinson, "Save the World, Prevent Obesity."

8. "Effects of a College Course About Food and Society on Students' Eating Behaviors," *American Journal of Preventive Medicine*, May 2010. https://www.ncbi.nlm.nih.gov/pubmed/20227847

9. "Association Between Indulgent Descriptions and Vegetable Consumption: Twisted Carrots and Dynamite Beets," *JAMA Internal Medicine*, August 2017. https://jamanetwork.com/journals/jamainternalmedicine/article-abstract/2630753

10. Rachel Herz, *Why You Eat What You Eat: The Science Behind Our Relationship with Food* (Norton, 2018), p. 143.

11. Richard H. Thaler and Cass R. Sunstein, *Nudge: Improving Decisions About Health, Wealth, and Happiness* (Penguin, 2009), p. 6.

12. Justin Sonnenburg and Erica Sonnenburg, *The Good Gut: Taking Control of Your Weight, Your Mood, and Your Long-Term Health* (Penguin, 2016), p. 2.

13. *The Good Gut*, p. 5.

14. https://www.youtube.com/watch?v=1XJtNYxMF9U

15. https://www.nih.gov/news-events/news-releases/nih-launches-human-microbiome-project

16. *The Good Gut*, pp. 27–28.

17. https://www.genome.gov/27549144/

18. "The human gut microbiome in early-onset type 1 diabetes from the TEDDY study," *Nature*, October 24, 2018. https://www.nature.com/articles/s41586-018-0620-2

19. "Duodenal Infusion of Donor Feces for Recurrent *Clostridium Difficile*," *New England Journal of Medicine*, January 31, 2013. https://www.nejm.org/doi/full/10.1056/NEJMoa1205037

20. A study published in the *New England Journal of Medicine* in 2019 revealed that a patient had died following a fecal transplant, but the group performing the fecal transplant failed to screen for a pathogen that should have disqualified the donor sample.

21. http://med.stanford.edu/prematurity.html

22. "Temporal and spatial variation of the human microbiota during pregnancy," *Proceedings of the National Academy of Sciences*, August 17, 2015. https://www.pnas.org/content/112/35/11060.short

23. https://www.cmqcc.org/resources-tool-kits/toolkits

24. https://letsgethealthy.ca.gov/goals/healthy-beginnings/reducing-infant-mortality/

25. https://fred.stlouisfed.org/series/SPDYNIMRTINUSA

26. https://www.cdc.gov/nchs/data/databriefs/db316.pdf

27. https://www.cmqcc.org/who-we-are

28. https://www.cmqcc.org/research/ca-pamr-maternal-mortality-review

29. "A shocking number of U.S. women still die from childbirth. California is doing something about that," *Washington Post*, November 4, 2018. https://www.washingtonpost.com/national/health-science/a-shocking-number-of-us-women-still-die-from-childbirth-california-is-doing-something-about-that/2018/11/02/11042036-d7af-11e8-a10f-b51546b10756_story.html?utm_term=.f6b2a9fa545b

30. "Can Early Childhood Interventions Improve Health and Well-Being?" Robert Wood Johnson Foundation, March 1, 2016. https://www.rwjf.org/en/library/research/2016/03/can-early-childhood-interventions-improve-life-outcomes-.html

31. "Live Video Diet and Exercise Intervention in Overweight and Obese Youth: Adherence and Cardiovascular Health," *Journal of Pediatrics*, September 2015. https://www.jpeds.com/article/S0022-3476(15)00598-3/abstract
32. Patient correspondence with Seda Tierney.
33. "Finding missing cases of familial hypercholesterolemia in health systems using machine learning," *npj Digital Medicine*, April 11, 2019. https://www.nature.com/articles/s41746-019-0101-5
34. "How do health expenditures vary across the population?" Kaiser Family Foundation, January 16, 2019. https://www.healthsystemtracker.org/chart-collection/health-expenditures-vary-across-population/#item-discussion-health-spending-often-focus-averages-spending-varies-considerably-across-population_2015
35. https://www.livongo.com/news/livongo-demonstrates-cost-savings-for-employers/
36. "Use of a Connected Glucose Meter and Certified Diabetes Educator Coaching to Decrease the Likelihood of Abnormal Blood Glucose Excursions: The Livongo for Diabetes Program," *Journal of Medical Internet Research*, July 2017. https://www.jmir.org/2017/7/e234/
37. https://www.omadahealth.com/press/press-release-omada-health-achieves-full-cdc-approval
38. https://www.cnbc.com/2017/04/12/nearly-every-american-spent-money-at-wal-mart-last-year.html
39. "Humanwide: A Comprehensive Data Base for Precision Health in Primary Care," *Annals of Family Medicine*, May/June 2019. http://www.annfammed.org/content/17/3/273.full

CHAPTER 7

1. https://www.neuro.duke.edu/research/faculty-labs/lo-lab
2. "The quest for the cure: The science and stories behind the next generation of medicines," *Journal of Clinical Investigation*, November 1, 2011. https://www.jci.org/articles/view/59328
3. Siddhartha Mukherjee, *The Emperor of All Maladies: A Biography of Cancer* (Scribner, 2010), pp. 39–41.
4. Ibid., p. 44.
5. Ibid., p. 45.
6. Clifton Leaf, *The Truth in Small Doses* (Simon & Schuster, 2013), p. 178.
7. This description provided the title for Mukherjee's book.
8. https://www.npr.org/sections/health-shots/2015/12/28/459218765/cutting-edge-cancer-treatment-has-its-roots-in-19th-century-medicine
9. Mukherjee, *The Emperor of All Maladies*, p. 161.
10. http://med.stanford.edu/news/all-news/2010/04/5-questions-jacobs-on-her-new-biography-of-cancer-fighter-henry-kaplan.html
11. Ibid.
12. https://stanmed.stanford.edu/2017fall/car-t-immunotherapy-targets-elusive-cancer-cells-in-children.html
13. https://www.cancer.net/blog/2018-01/car-t-cell-immunotherapy-2018-advance-year
14. https://www.cartercenter.org/news/pr/carter-center-statement-120615.html
15. https://www.fda.gov/newsevents/newsroom/pressannouncements/ucm574058.htm
16. "T cells expressing CD19 chimeric antigen receptors for acute lymphoblastic leukaemia in children and young adults: a phase 1 dose-escalation trial," *The Lancet,* October 12, 2014. https://www.thelancet.com/journals/lancet/article/PIIS0140-6736(14)61403-3/fulltext
17. Each parent of an SMA patient has one copy of chromosome 5 that contains SMN1, but the gene is missing from their other chromosome 5; each child with SMA inherits the bad chromosome 5 from each parent and thus has no copies of SMN1.
18. "New Stanford drug saves child with deadly genetic disease," *Mercury News*, August 25, 2017. https://www.mercurynews.com/2017/08/24/child-is-worlds-first-patient-to-receive-new-stanford-drug-for-deadly-genetic-disease/

19. https://www.fda.gov/newsevents/newsroom/pressannouncements/ucm534611.htm

20. http://prahs.com/blog/2017/05/09/the-latest-in-als-research-challenges-and-progress/

21. "Therapeutic reduction of ataxin-2 extends lifespan and reduces pathology in TDP-43 mice," *Nature*, April 12, 2017. https://www.nature.com/articles/nature22038

22. "CRISPR–Cas9 screens in human cells and primary neurons identify modifiers of *C9ORF72* dipeptide-repeat-protein toxicity," *Nature Genetics*, March 5, 2018. https://www.nature.com/articles/s41588-018-0070-7

23. https://www.clinicalleader.com/doc/on-rare-disease-day-are-we-making-progress-for-patients-in-need-0001

24. https://stanmed.stanford.edu/2018winter/CRISPR-for-gene-editing-is-revolutionary-but-it-comes-with-risks.html

25. Ibid.

26. David Baltimore, Paul Berg, Michael Botchan, Dana Carroll, R. Alta Charo, George Church, Jacob E. Corn, George Q. Daley, Jennifer A. Doudna, Marsha Fenner, Henry T. Greely, Martin Jinek, G. Steven Martin, Edward Penhoet, Jennifer Puck, Samuel H. Sternberg, Jonathan S. Weissman, Keith R. Yamamot, "A Prudent Path Forward for Genomic Engineering and Germline Gene Modification," *Science,* April 3, 2015. https://science.sciencemag.org/content/348/6230/36. summary

27. Rasmus O. Bak, Natalia Gomez-Ospina, and Matthew H. Porteus, "Gene Editing on Center Stage," *Trends in Genetics*, June 13, 2018. https://doi.org/10.1016/j.tig.2018.05.004

28. https://www.ncbi.nlm.nih.gov/pmc/articles/PMC3560868/

29. "Adopt a moratorium on heritable genome editing," *Nature*, March 13, 2019. https://www.nature.com/articles/d41586-019-00726-5

30. "Scientists for Moratorium to Block Gene-Edited Babies," *Wall Street Journal*, March 13, 2019. https://www.wsj.com/articles/scientists-call-for-moratorium-to-block-gene-edited-babies-11552500001?mod=hp_lead_pos9

31. https://www.youtube.com/watch?v=zO7fgp0Hxjg

32. http://scopeblog.stanford.edu/2015/07/08/life-with-epidermolysis-bullosa-pain-is-my-reality-pain-is-my-normal/

33. https://med.stanford.edu/news/all-news/2014/11/blistering-skin-disease-may-be-treatable-with-therapeutic-reprog.html

34. "Assembling human brain organoids," *Science*, January 11, 2019. https://science.sciencemag.org/content/363/6423/126.summary

35. https://vimeo.com/295847090

36. http://stanmed.stanford.edu/2018winter/lab-grown-brain-balls-could-aid-understanding-of-neurological-diseases.html

37. https://vimeo.com/295847090

38. https://www.sciencedirect.com/science/article/pii/S0735109716010263?via%3Dihub

39. https://www.stemcell.com/pluripotent-profiles-joseph-wu

40. "Human induced pluripotent stem cell-derived cardiomyocytes recapitulate the predilection of breast cancer patients to doxorubicin-induced cardiotoxicity," *Nature Medicine*, April 18, 2016. https://www.ncbi.nlm.nih.gov/pubmed/27089514

41. https://www.stemcell.com/pluripotent-profiles-joseph-wu

42. "Sustained in vitro intestinal epithelial culture within a Wnt-dependent stem cell niche," *Nature Medicine*, April 27, 2009. https://www.nature.com/articles/nm.1951

43. "Organoid 2.0," Nature Reviews Cancer, January 22, 2019. https://www.nature.com/articles/s41568-019-0108-x

44. "*Pneumocystis carinii* Pneumonia and Mucosal Candidiasis in Previously Healthy Homosexual Men—Evidence of a New Acquired Cellular Immunodeficiency," *New England Journal of Medicine*, December 10, 1981. https://www.nejm.org/doi/full/10.1056/NEJM198112103052401

45. https://www.cdc.gov/mmwr/preview/mmwrhtml/00046531.htm

46. https://www.kff.org/hivaids/fact-sheet/the-hivaids-epidemic-in-the-united-states-the-basics/

47. http://www.unaids.org/en/resources/fact-sheet
48. http://www.unaids.org/en/resources/fact-sheet
49. https://aidsinfo.nih.gov/understanding-hiv-aids/fact-sheets/19/96/what-is-a-preventive-hiv-vaccine-
50. https://www.tballiance.org/why-new-tb-drugs/global-pandemic
51. http://www.who.int/en/news-room/fact-sheets/detail/antimicrobial-resistance
52. https://amr-review.org/sites/default/files/160525_Final%20paper_with%20cover.pdf
53. https://www.who.int/news-room/fact-sheets/detail/the-top-10-causes-of-death
54. http://www.who.int/en/news-room/fact-sheets/detail/antimicrobial-resistance

CONCLUSION

1. The epidemic did not start in Spain and had no specific connection to the country. But because Spain was independent in World War I, Spanish media were able to report on it freely—other countries faced wartime censorship—and thus many came to associate the country with the epidemic.
2. https://www.cdc.gov/features/1918-flu-pandemic/index.html
3. "Estimates of Regional and Global Life Expectancy, 1800–2001," *Issue Population and Development Review*. Population and Development Review, September 2005. https://onlinelibrary.wiley.com/doi/pdf/10.1111/j.1728-4457.2005.00083.x
4. https://www.cnbc.com/2018/07/30/jamie-dimon-says-health-care-initiative-with-buffett-and-bezos-may-sta.html
5. https://www.cnbc.com/2019/01/08/apple-ceo-tim-cook-and-cnbcs-jim-cramer-talk-china-qualcomm.html
6. "IBM Has a Watson Dilemma," *Wall Street Journal*, August 11, 2018. https://www.wsj.com/articles/ibm-bet-billions-that-watson-could-improve-cancer-treatment-it-hasnt-worked-1533961147?mod=djemalertNEWS
7. https://www.thelancet.com/journals/lancet/article/PIIS0140-6736(18)31992-5/fulltext
8. Ibid.
9. https://www.who.int/news-room/fact-sheets/detail/tobacco
10. "Socioeconomic Differences in the Epidemiologic Transition From Heart Disease to Cancer as the Leading Cause of Death in the United States, 2003 to 2015: An Observational Study," *Annals of Internal Medicine*, December 18, 2018. https://annals.org/aim/article-abstract/2715460/socioeconomic-differences-epidemiologic-transition-from-heart-disease-cancer-leading-cause
11. https://www.statnews.com/2018/11/29/u-s-life-expectancy-declines-again-in-sobering-wake-up-call/
12. https://www.cdc.gov/tobacco/data_statistics/fact_sheets/fast_facts/index.htm
13. https://www.who.int/emergencies/ten-threats-to-global-health-in-2019
14. https://www.king5.com/article/news/nearly-all-children-with-measles-in-washington-state-are-unvaccinated/281-ccbb10a3-0281-4b75-ac97-1a53e0209bca
15. "It's Time to Fire Your Doctor," *Wall Street Journal*, February 10, 2019. https://www.wsj.com/articles/its-time-to-fire-your-doctor-11549829009
16. "New Delivery Model for Rising-Risk Patients: The Forgotten Lot?" *Telemedicine and e-Health*, April 2017.

INDEX

academia, and industry, 43–45, 57, 89, 150
acyladenylates, 115
Affordable Care Act (Obamacare), 18
African Americans, 17, 220
aging, 128, 130–133
air quality, 38
Albers, Greg, 52–55
Alizadeh, Ash, 154
allergies, 59, 62–64, 182
Allison, James, 44, 211
All of Us initiative, 12, 241
Altman, Russ, 164–166
Alzheimer's disease, 18, 123, 128, 132–133,
    143, 146, 216, 240
Amazon, 19, 101, 187, 189, 198, 238–239
amniocentesis, 48, 152
amyotrophic lateral sclerosis (ALS), 215–216
Anacor, 50
anchoring fibrils, 222
antibiotics
    discovery, 50–51, 114, 231, 237
    resistance, 51, 183, 185, 232
antidepressants, 66–67, 69, 165
antimicrobials, 49–51, 231–232
antisense oligonucleotide (ASO), 214–216
Apple, 21, 40, 46, 106, 167, 189, 238–239
Apple Watch, 167–168
artificial heart pump, 234
artificial intelligence (AI), 6, 7, 21, 45, 74, 75,
    167–173, 226, 237, 242
atrial fibrillation, 67, 162–163, 167–168, 175, 238
Ashkin, Arthur, 126, 127
Ashley, Euan, 5, 160–161
autism, 73–78, 182, 225
autologous stem cell transplant, 220–221
Avey, Linda, 108
aviation, 148
Azar, Alex, 25

Baltimore, David, 135
Barry, Michele, 99–101
Bassik, Michael, 216
behavioral factors, and health, 7, 13, 26, 33–41,
    179–180, 240
Behr, Barry, 80–82
"bench to bedside" time, 7
Benkovic, Steve, 50
Berg, Paul, 115–116, 119–120, 144
Bertozzi, Carolyn, 208–209
BEST Touch, 96
Bezdek, Trevor, 101–102
Bezos, Jeff, 154, 238
Bianchi, Diana, 152
biobanks, 229
biomarkers, 39, 72, 73, 149–155
biomedical sciences, 6, 15–16, 111–112,
    138–142
biotechnology, 16, 116–118
biotypes, and depression, 66–67
Blau, Helen, 133–137
Block, Steven, 127
blood tests, 151–156
Bohman, Bryan, 26
Bohr, Niels, 112–113
Boyer, Herbert, 117–118, 242
Bradley, Elizabeth, 22
brain, 224–226
    circuits, 65, 67, 69, 70, 128
    development, 127–130, 225–226
    neuron communication, 122–123
    optogenetics, 123–126, 242
    three-dimensional, 225
BRCA1 and BRCA2 genes, 158
breast cancer, 10, 56, 82–84, 155, 157–159,
    165, 175, 227
Brown, Michael, 122
Brown, Pat, 102–104

Discovering Precision Health: Predict, Prevent, and Cure to Advance Health and Well-Being,
First Edition. Lloyd Minor and Matthew Rees.
© 2020 John Wiley & Sons Ltd. Published 2020 by John Wiley & Sons Ltd.